THE GREAT SHUTDOWN

Praise for *The Great Shutdown*

The Great Shutdown is a detailed account of what the country has been through during the two years of the COVID-19 pandemic. It is also an excellent account of the ad hoc decisions and bungling of official responses at each stage, the effect of this on ordinary people trapped without work and money far from home and the crisis hitting sundry businesses. This has been a seminal event that will live in people's memories for decades, and therefore is a story that needs to be told. Jyoti Mukul has told the story with an admirable mastery of detail and a reporter's eye for the telling anecdote.

—**T.N. Ninan**, columnist and former editor, *Business Standard*

We are still struggling to wrap our minds around the phenomenon of COVID-19, caught as we are between individual tragedies and national and global crises. We are inundated with information and stand bewildered. *The Great Shutdown* is an excellent collation of organized information and analyses, needed to unpack most of our confusions. A must-read for every concerned citizen.

—**Aruna Roy**, Ramon Magsaysay Award winner and founder,
Mazdoor Kisan Shakti Sangathan (MKSS)

THE GREAT SHUTDOWN

A Story of Two Indian Summers

JYOTI MUKUL

HarperCollins *Publishers* India

First published in India by HarperCollins *Publishers* 2022
Building No. 10, Tower A, 4th Floor, DLF Cyber City, Phase II
Gurugram, Haryana – 122002
www.harpercollins.co.in

2 4 6 8 10 9 7 5 3 1

P-ISBN: 978-93-5489-280-6
E-ISBN: 978-93-5489-287-5

Typeset in 11.5/15.2 Adobe Garamond Pro at
Manipal Technologies Limited, Manipal

Printed and bound at
Thomson Press (India) Ltd

FSC MIX Paper FSC® C010615

This book is produced from independently certified FSC® paper
to ensure responsible forest management.

To Erick Massey's mother

CONTENTS

PART V: THE SECOND WAVE

PART VI: THE ALTERNATIVES

INTRODUCTION

WHEN CONFINEMENT IS INVOLUNTARY, it can work as a push factor for needing to move even more. The COVID-19 pandemic, its pain in the death and in the disease itself, has the force to overshadow the moment when life came to a standstill in India and millions decided to take to the road because of economic distress. Loss of life due to the disease, however, will be just another number unless it comes with a chronicle of why it happened, how it happened near us and whether those happenings had anything to do with how India lived through those days, months and years. Conscious of the fact that many authors, globally and in India, would be able to chronicle COVID-19 from a medical lens, and others would be able to comment on the 2020 Indian lockdown and the migrant crisis from the expert perspectives of an activist or a labour specialist, it was necessary to take up a subject that was not only different but more importantly, chronicling something that was mundane and yet, was at the heart of both the contagion as well as the migrant crisis. The snapping of transport links needed a work to itself. It was the single most important factor which differentiated the national lockdown of 2020 from the localized lockdowns that India witnessed in 2021. If 2020 was harsh because of the ineptitude of the Union and state governments in handling a pandemic, it was also because governance failed each day to anticipate the next crisis. Rightfully, the 2020 lockdown was compared to the 2016 demonetization of currency notes, not just by commentators but also by a politically aware Ekdashi Kumar of Bihar, who just withdrew all his cash from an ATM machine when the lockdown started in Bengaluru because he did not want to run out of cash and add to his woes.

The book was conceived the moment the Union Ministry of Home Affairs (MHA) decided that the Indian Railways would no longer carry passengers and that airlines would be grounded. The almost 68,000 km-long railway network is the only means of travel for people who work outside their home states and cannot afford air travel. Long-distance buses have also become an option in the past decade but these are arduous journeys, usually undertaken only if a confirmed railway ticket is not available because of travel at short notice, or if it is cheaper to travel by road than by train. Besides the Indian Railways, other long- and short-distance travel links were also snapped in 2020 within the span of a few days, some before and some after the railway shutdown. The decisions taken by the states and the Union governments for other modes of travel to prevent a contagion needed to be chronicled. Mentioning all decisions of each state, however, would have yielded similar results. The approach, therefore, was to capture the Union government's lockdown directives on all activities which were not permitted, broadly, and on transport sector, specifically. Some state government decisions prior to the national lockdown have been included to give an idea of the build-up to a complete shutdown.

Though the tales and travails of individuals caught in the lockdown are important, the focus of the book is not the 'reverse migration'[1] of the labour force, or what some people call the going away of the 'guest workers' (India is the only country which calls its own people migrants, even if all they are doing is moving from one state to another). The book instead goes into how the sudden cessation of transport operations for a billion-plus people created not just uncertainty of movement, but also the emotional crisis of being separated from family back home at a time when an unknown disease could have claimed their lives. It was, however, neither possible nor appropriate to take the people out of the story. Besides, restricting the narrative to just government notifications, decisions and Prime Minister Narendra Modi's addresses to the nation ran the same risk as journalistic reports: it could easily be termed 'one side of the story,' apart from becoming banal.

It was, therefore, important to analyse the government's decisions minutely, and also record the voices of those severely impacted: some already heard but many gone unheard. Conversations with such people have been conducted largely over phone calls, though their pain, as well as the stubborn belief of some that there was nothing called COVID in India was palpable even through the airwaves. 'I do not believe there is anything like corona. We stayed back with 400 people in one place last year (2020) and nothing happened to anyone. Then, I came home and later went back to Bengaluru. We have only heard about corona; we have not seen it happen,' said Jitendra Yadav of Ballia district in May 2021 (chapter 11), even after he learnt of people dying in scores after contracting fever in neighbouring villages during the second wave (chapter 11).

Some authentic first-hand accounts from published news and feature reports have also been interwoven with the government directives to give a sense of the unprecedented situation in 2020. This also breaks the mundane tone of government directives, which sometimes begin with a DO number or phrases like inter alia, and can put off even an avid reader. DO is short for demi-official, and indicates a personalized letter to an officer on a specific aspect of a decision already taken or proposed to be taken, while inter alia is Latin for something as simple as 'among other things.'

The 2020 lockdown in India was undoubtedly among the most stringent in the democratic world, and even perhaps brutal. There were many cases of policemen fatally hitting people for violations both during the stricter 2020 lockdown and during the more relaxed localized lockdowns of 2021. Thirty-two-year-old Lal Swami in West Bengal's Howrah went out to buy milk on 25 March 2020, the first day of the national lockdown. Policemen on duty there were dispersing people in the market to prevent crowding and, as is common in India, the baton-wielding constables used force inconsiderately. One of them struck Swami, already suffering from heart ailments. He suffered a cardiac arrest and later died.[2] In May 2021, Faisal, in the Bangarmau Kotwali area of Unnao district of Uttar Pradesh, ran into an argument with the police when he was selling vegetables on a cart in a wholesale market. 'The police thrashed him and took him to the station, where he was found dead. The police then left him at the hospital,' Faisal's brother was quoted as saying in an ANI report dated 22 May 2021.[3] Faisal was just seventeen.

Lockdowns in more evolved democracies were debated and protested against openly. For instance, Governor Tony Evers of Wisconsin state of the United States issued Executive Order 72, declaring a health emergency on 12 March 2020. A day later, the state's Supreme Court struck down a 'stay at home' order, numbered 28, issued by Andrea Palm, secretary-designee of the Department of Health Services (DHS). 'This case is about the assertion of power by one unelected official, Andrea Palm, and her order to all people within Wisconsin to remain in their homes, not to travel and to close all businesses that she declares are not "essential" in Emergency Order 28,' the court said.[4] Order 28 said the transgressor could face imprisonment for thirty days, a $250 fine or both. But the court observed that she broke the law when issuing Emergency Order 28 since emergency rule procedures were not followed, and that she exceeded her authority by ordering everyone to stay home, closing all 'non-essential' businesses, prohibiting private gatherings of any number of people who were not part of a single household and forbidding all 'non-essential' travel.

The Wisconsin case was filed by the Republican legislature of the state, which was politically opposed to restrictions. Seven days after the Wisconsin Supreme Court order, a group of seventeen petitioners, including salon owners, a pastor, a protest organizer and a candidate for Congress, petitioned a federal court on 20 May 2020, saying the local orders infringed their First Amendment rights.[5] Federal Judge William Griesbach, however, rejected the petitions on 21 July, saying, 'Leaving aside the now invalidated (state-wide stay-at-home order), each plaintiff is subject to different orders implemented by different individuals on behalf of different governmental entities in different parts of the State in which presumably different rates of infection, population density, and other pertinent conditions exist.'[6]

Though restrictions were eventually put in place in Wisconsin and other American states, there were open protests and deliberate violations of lockdown rules across the US and Europe. The approach of the police and of those implementing lockdowns in the US and even in Europe was not to force, but to convince. There was, nonetheless, no merit in such protests in these countries. They should, in fact, be seen as the obverse of a stringent lockdown that was being imposed in other countries.

The US federal government under Donald Trump, on its part, was reluctant to impose a nationwide lockdown but unlike India in 2020, the states were the key players in taking COVID-19 prevention measures in the US. While one reason is the nature of American democracy, which gives states more freedom, it also had a lot to do with the invoking of the Disaster Management Act, 2005, by the Narendra Modi government. This legislation gives more powers to the Union government than to state governments in India. Many states had invoked the Epidemic Diseases Act, 1897 while imposing restrictions, but the Disaster Management Act can override it. The only leeway which the Centre gave to the states under the Disaster Management Act in the 2020 national lockdown was that they could impose any rule stricter than the Union government's directives.

Even before India started 'unlocking' in June 2020, various state governments and the Indian Railways had been facilitating the travel of those stranded in the cities, initially through buses and then via trains. This facilitation was forced by the huge public pressure arising out of the humanitarian crisis of migrant workers stranded in the cities, especially when they started walking or using cycles and carts to reach their villages hundreds of kilometres away. But controversies arose over who was paying for the train travel and also over the deaths reported on these special trains. Nonetheless, this movement of people by train helped in easing the angst among migrant labourers, many of whom had lost their jobs in the cities. There was, however, a fear of the contagion spreading in rural areas, but deaths and disease did not spread as widely in 2020 as in 2021, when bodies were found floating in the waters, or buried on the banks of the holiest of Hindu rivers, the Ganga, in Bihar and Uttar Pradesh. An *Indian Express* analysis of government data published on 8 May 2021 showed that 243 districts covered by the Backward Region Grant Fund (BRGF) had more than 3.92 million infected with COVID-19 as of 5 May. This was more than four times the 950,000 infections at the peak of the first wave on 16 September 2020.[7] Though the number of infections in these districts as a percentage of total infections in the country remained almost the same, at 18.6 per cent, '... the contribution of deaths from these districts had risen significantly. By 16 September last year, deaths in these districts accounted for 11.5 per cent of the national death toll of 83,198. On May 5 (2021), however, this contribution had increased to 16 per cent,' said the analysis.

The cessation of long-distance travel might not have contained the spread of infection during the second COVID-19 wave in India. Travel, however, can spread infection, which is why Mahatma Gandhi had called the railways a 'gigantic evil' and the reason for the spread of the plague in British India. Socially ahead of his times, Mohandas Karamchand Gandhi is often criticized for his harsh words on the rail network. 'Is it any wonder that plague has become endemic in India? Any other result is impossible where passengers always leave some dirt where they go and take more on leaving ... The existence of the awful war cannot be allowed to stand in the way of removal of this gigantic evil. War can be no warrant for tolerating dirt and overcrowding,' he wrote in a letter to the editor of *Leader*, an English-language daily published from Allahabad and founded by Madan Mohan Malviya in 1909.[8]

Railway services had been running in India for sixty-four years when Gandhi wrote the letter from Ranchi on 25 September 1917. 'One could understand an entire stoppage of passenger traffic in a crisis (war) like this, but never a continuation or accentuation of insanitation and conditions that must undermine health and morality,' he wrote in the letter 'Third Class Travelling on Indian Railways.' Gandhi, however, was lamenting the unhygienic conditions on trains, the 'packing of passengers like sardines' and even refreshments being 'previously sampled by millions of flies.' He was also comparing the lot of lower class travel with the luxury of first-class travel on trains. The fact that he sent a copy of the letter on 31 October 1917 to the secretary, Department of Commerce and Industries, in Delhi, making suggestions for improvements in railway services, shows that much has been made of his criticism of the railways. Perhaps, considering the plight of scores of migrant labourers in 2020, Gandhi would have never wanted the rail network to shut down during COVID-19.

Just a few months after Gandhi wrote the letter, the first signs of a virulent form of influenza appeared in India in June of 1918. 'In the city of Bombay towards the end of that month, many employees of offices, banks and so forth, were incapacitated by fever. The disease began to spread over India and before long the mortality, at first low, began to rise in an alarming degree,' says L.F. Rushbrook Williams, officer on special duty in the Home Department, Government of India, in a report for years 1917 and 1918, prepared for presentation to the British Parliament under Section 26 of the Government of India Act.[9] He admits India suffered more severely than any other country in the world; and 'influenza was responsible in British India alone for a death roll of approximately five million. Detailed information with regard to the incidence of the disease in the Indian States is not available, but it is unlikely that the influenza mortality therein fell short of one million.' Williams here was trying to give desegregated data for death in the British-ruled Indian territory as well as the princely states. 'Within the space of four or five months, influenza was thus responsible for the death of 2 per cent of the total population of British India. In some places, the Central Provinces, for example, two months of influenza caused twice as many deaths as 22 years of plague,' he says. The number of deaths, however, were grossly underreported. John M. Barry in *The Great Influenza* says it is likely that close to 20 million died in the Indian subcontinent, and quite possibly the deal toll exceeded that number. 'Throughout the Indian sub-continent there was only death. Trains left one station with the living. They arrived with the dead and dying, the corpses removed as the trains pulled into station. British troops, Caucasians, in India suffered a case mortality rate of 9.61 per cent.

For Indian troops, 21.69 per cent of those who caught influenza died,' says Barry.[10]

The British did not close the railway system despite the influenza, also called the Spanish flu. In fact, running trains was a necessity because of the movement of men and material due to the First World War. More passengers, in fact, moved by train in 1918-19, the period when the influenza infected Indians, than in the previous year. 'The increase in the passenger traffic compared with 1917-18 was chiefly due to the larger movement of pilgrims and marriage parties and also of troops, especially drafts and labour parties, and men on war furloughs and under demobilization,' says Rushbrook Williams in the 1919 annual report.[11]

Stopping air or rail travel would not have made much of a difference during the second wave of COVID-19 in 2021, though many people did fall ill after travel. One reason was that India had already started vaccinating its population from 16 January 2021. The drive began with medical workers and then moved on to frontline workers on 1 February. By 1 March, the government had allowed the administration of either of the two approved vaccines, Covishield and Covaxin, to senior citizens above sixty years of age and those above forty-five years suffering from comorbidities. Whatever the shortcomings of India's vaccine programme, it gave people a sense of comfort in that the severity of infections would be low. However, even fully vaccinated people were contracting infection and dying.

The other reason that shutting down of transport would not have helped much during the second wave was the superspreader events of assembly elections and the Mahakumbh. There was no social distancing being followed in election rallies and the religious gathering in Haridwar. Elections were held in multiple states between 2 March 2021 and 4 May 2021. It was only on 22 April 2021 that Prime Minister Modi decided to cancel his election rallies. 'Tomorrow, will be chairing high-level meetings to review the prevailing COVID-19 situation. Due to that, I would not be going to West Bengal,' he announced in a tweet that day.[12]

Besides, even local lockdowns, first called 'curfews', were able to control infections only marginally since the disease had spread rapidly within housing complexes all across the country. The infection was officially declared airborne and could travel from one house to another, even if the people in those houses did not interact.

On 30 April 2021, the World Health Organization (WHO) acknowledged for the first time that COVID-19 was airborne. 'Evidence suggests that the virus spreads mainly between people, who are in close contact with each other, typically within 1 metre (short-range). A person can be infected when aerosols or droplets containing the virus are inhaled or come directly into contact with the eyes, nose, or mouth. The virus can also spread in poorly ventilated and/or crowded indoor settings, where people tend to spend longer periods of time. This is because aerosols remain suspended in the air or travel farther than 1 metre (long-range),' it said in a Q&A section on its website in April 2021.[13] This was in contrast to what it said on 29 March 2020. 'According to current evidence, COVID-19 virus is primarily transmitted between people through respiratory droplets and contact routes. In an analysis of 75,465 COVID-19 cases in China, airborne transmission was not reported,' it had said in the 29 March 2020 scientific brief on modes of transmission of the disease. It further said droplet transmission occurs when a person is in close contact (within 1 metre) with someone who has respiratory symptoms (coughing or sneezing) and is, therefore, at risk of having his/her mucosae (mouth and nose) or conjunctiva (eyes) exposed to potentially infective respiratory droplets. Transmission, it said, may also occur through fomites in the immediate environment around the infected person. Therefore, transmission of the COVID-19 virus can occur by direct contact with infected people and indirect contact with surfaces in the immediate environment or with objects used on the infected person (for example, stethoscope or thermometer). 'Airborne transmission is different from droplet transmission as it refers to the presence of microbes within droplet nuclei, which are generally considered to be particles <5 micrometre or microns (μm) in diameter, can remain in the air for long periods of time and be transmitted to others over distances greater than 1 m,' it had emphatically claimed in March 2020.[14]

One of the challenges of writing on contemporary subjects is that the situation keeps changing. This was especially true in the case of COVID-19 and the human and economic crises it induced. Governments changed their strategies within days, and India moved in less than a year from the strictest lockdown of 2020 to a relaxed spring of 2021. Getting information from the government on simple things, like data or details of discussions that went into a particular decision, through the Right To Information (RTI) Act was a herculean task. The Department of Economic Affairs, for instance, in its reply dated 31 March 2021, said it had no information on the Stringency Index, which chief economic advisor K.V. Subramanian had mentioned in Volume 1 of his Economic Survey 2020–21 in January 2021 while justifying the national lockdown. An appeal was filed but despite the legal requirement of an answer within thirty to forty-five days with reasons for the delay, a reply to the first appeal in the Union Ministry of Finance came after seventy-five days. It only said, 'CPIO to obtain information from Economic Division and provide the information or transfer under 6(3).'

The practice of transferring RTIs is actually shifting of responsibility. A total of eight RTIs were filed. The breaking of these applications into different questions to be addressed by different divisions within the same ministry, transfer of the RTIs and appeals against unsatisfactory answers led to a situation where the total number of applications ballooned more than seven times to sixty-two, of which twelve remained unanswered even after seven months till December 2021. When the Department of Personnel and Training was asked how many Union government employees got COVID-19, and how many of them died due to it, it did not have any clue. The application was first transferred to the Union Ministry of Labour and Employment, then to the MoHFW. This shirking of the responsibility to provide information went on to such an extent that myriad departments under the Ministry of Labour and Employment across the country, from Surat in Gujarat to Jowai in Meghalaya, replied with information on how many Union government employees they had even, if they had to just say 'nil'. This showed that the Indian government had no clue about the health of its own employees, even though it was at the helm of the fight against the pandemic.

Another instance of making information-seeking tough was when data was sought from the National Highways Authority of India (NHAI) and the Indian Railways. Both these bodies did not seem to have consolidated numbers of simple things like monthly toll collections from the national highways and money spent on providing refreshments to Shramik Special passengers. RTIs filed seeking this information were also sent all around the country, with each Project Information Unit of the NHAI sending its own information, all in varied formats. Meanwhile, in a classic case of the right hand not knowing what the left is doing, Ajay Mishra, chief general manager in the NHAI and its first appellate authority, in a reply on 29 June 2021 to an appeal filed on 9 April 2021, said, 'It is important to note that only such information can be supplied under the Act that is available and existing and is held by the public authority. The PIO [public information officer] is not supposed to create information that is not a part of the record of the public authority.' This implied that the NHAI did not have any data on how much total toll was being collected every month from the country's national highways. Without such data, how could the government analyse a trend in traffic volumes during and after the lockdown, or gauge any recovery in the economy?

Railway departments, like the Firozpur division and the Indian Railway Catering and Tourism Corporation, also sent their own replies. The responses not only showed a woeful lack of data-keeping at the level of administrative ministry despite the Modi government's Digital India push, but also a deliberate attempt to exasperate applicants till they gave up. Except for two applications filed with the MoHFW and with the Delhi Metro Rail Corporation, the remaining were transferred or came up with replies that were unsatisfactory.

The primary source of information on government decisions, however, were websites, both of the Union and the states, which mostly provided information on COVID-19 regulations. Beyond these, officials, both serving and retired, were not willing to talk, citing confidentiality reasons, though everything about the lockdowns was of public interest. Two police officers in Haryana and Karnataka, who had done a lot of work on the ground during the lockdown, however, gave useful insights into the migrant labourer crisis.

When the first draft of this manuscript was almost finalized in April 2021, the second wave overwhelmed everything. The anxiety was so pervasive that writing felt meaningless. After regaining the have-to-tell-the-story spirit of a reporter, a separate section on the second wave was added to capture the tale of India's woeful medical infrastructure. There was an important link between the two waves beyond the contagion itself. While lack of transport created a humanitarian crisis and impacted businesses between March and June 2020, the same transport network across all modes became all-important and was requisitioned for dealing with oxygen, medicine and ventilator shortages during the second wave. This link helped in keeping the book's focus on transport challenges.

The sections of the book chronicle the COVID-19 regulations implemented at various times. They deal with events prior to the national lockdown and during the lockdown, the humanitarian challenges that came up, the unlocking, the second wave, and the alternatives that were available and could have been made available to keep travel going.

PART I

THE PRELUDE

1

FROM CLOSING TO BEING SHUTTERED OUT

IT WAS 10 JANUARY 2020 and COVID-19 cases had already been reported in China. The World Health Organization (WHO), however, in its advice that day did not recommend any specific measure for travellers,[1] though it acknowledged for the first time that on 31 December 2019 'a cluster of pneumonia of unknown etiology' was reported in Wuhan city, Hubei province, China. The Chinese authorities had officially announced this to the media on 9 January. What WHO did flag was the usual precautionary measures for which there were well-established international conventions. It quoted its World Health Regulations (WHR) of 2005 where Article 23 specifically mentions 'health measures on arrival and departure' of persons from areas that have been infected.

This first travel advice from WHO for COVID-19 was similar to those of diseases relating to the family of corona viruses that range from the common cold to the Middle East Respiratory Syndrome (MERS) and the severe acute respiratory syndrome

(SARS). Its previous corona-related advice was for MERS-CoV, on 16 September 2018, where it said almost the same thing as that in the 10 January 2020 advice on the novel coronavirus disease.[2] A reading of the September 2018 advice clearly indicates WHO did not itself believe in entry screening. Passengers might travel during the incubation period of virus, and hence might be asymptomatic, while in other cases, symptoms such as fever, coughing and diarrhoea could be due to other infectious diseases or even due to factors such as consuming hot beverages or menstrual period in women. Besides, it said fever measurement could be inaccurate due to inadequate calibration of thermal scanners. Passengers could also conceal their fever by taking antipyretic drugs before travel, or conceal accurate reporting of travel history and exposure to risk factors. Passengers with MERS-CoV infection might not show typical symptoms during screening procedures and, therefore, the infection could be missed. 'Entry screening at destination, including temperature checks and/or health questionnaires, is unlikely to detect passengers with MERS-CoV infection … it is generally considered that entry screening offers little benefit while requiring considerable resources. WHO does not recommend entry screening at points of entry for MERS, nor does it recommend the application of any travel or trade restrictions,' said the 16 September 2018 advisory for MERS-CoV.

The 10 January advice on travel, too, categorically stated: 'It is generally considered that entry screening offers little benefit, while requiring considerable resources. In case of symptoms suggestive to respiratory illness before, during or after travel, the travellers are encouraged to seek medical attention and share travel history with their healthcare provider. WHO advises against the application of any travel or trade restrictions on China based on the information currently available on this event.' It is, therefore, perplexing why

WHO later advised screening even though it had earlier maintained that it was of no use. The screening clearly was meant only as a way of keeping travel going since it consistently did not advise against travel.

These screening advices were based on International Health Regulations (IHR) (2005),[3] which provide 'an overarching legal framework that defines countries' rights and obligations in handling public health events and emergencies that have the potential to cross borders.' These regulations are an instrument of international law and are legally binding on 196 countries, including the 194 WHO member states. While IHR grew out of the response to deadly epidemics of Europe, it put in place only safeguards 'to protect the rights of travellers and other persons in relation to the treatment of personal data, informed consent and non-discrimination in the application of health measures under the regulations.'

Under IHR, countries are to ensure that routine measures, trained staff, appropriate space and stockpile of adequate equipment is in place at departure points for assessing and managing travellers detected ill before travel, on board conveyances (such as planes and ships) and at entry points; procedures and means are in place for communicating information on ill travellers between conveyances and points of entry, as well as between points of entry and national health authorities; safe transportation of symptomatic travellers to hospitals or designated facilities for clinical assessment and treatment is available; and a functional public health emergency contingency plan is in place at entry points to respond to public health events.

Article 2 of IHR states that the purpose and scope of the regulations are 'to prevent, protect against, control and provide a public health response to the international spread of disease in ways that are commensurate with and restricted to public health risks, and which avoid unnecessary interference with international traffic and trade.' This means that the regulations are designed to *prevent* any stoppage of movement.

India took its first step in preventing COVID-19 on 17 January when it announced a basic health screening at airports.[4] This was a week after the WHO advisory came and just three days after China had put similar screening measures in place. According to the 21 January 2020 situation report of WHO, China had had thirty-five infrared thermometers installed at airports, railway stations, long-distance bus stations and ferry terminals since 14 January 2020. For a country the size of China, with some 1.4 billion people, thirty-five is certainly a small number, even if the reported cases of COVID-19 were a few hundred.

Till 17 January, in fact, there were no advisories for international travellers from the Indian government. Considering that screening was put in place only at three airports first and in line with the 10 January advice of WHO, only for passengers travelling from China, it is clear that the anticipated risk was not high at that time. The MoHFW announced that travellers from China would be screened with thermal scanners at Delhi, Mumbai and Kolkata airports. On the same day, a separate advisory was issued for travellers coming from China,[5] requiring them to self-declare and report any subsequent symptoms to government helpline numbers. The first case of COVID-19, which till then was called novel coronavirus, was reported in India thirteen days later, on 30 January 2020.[6] This was a student studying medicine in Wuhan, who returned to Kerala on 24 January 2020.

India extended health screening to those coming from Hong Kong on 21 January[7] and to a total of eight airports, including Chennai, Bengaluru, Hyderabad and Cochin, apart from the three airports in Delhi, Mumbai and Kolkata that were notified earlier. Subsequently, other countries were added to the list, with Singapore and Thailand included on 5 February, Nepal, Indonesia, Vietnam and Malaysia on 23 February, and Italy and Iran on 2 March. The Directorate General of Civil Aviation (DGCA) included Macau in the list the very next day as an afterthought.

Before screening of all international passengers was announced on 4 March, passengers from twelve countries were already being screened. At a media briefing, Union Health Minister Harsh Vardhan announced universal screening of all international travellers and said that a total of twenty-eight persons had officially tested positive for the virus, of which one person was from Delhi, six were his relatives in Agra, sixteen were Italian travellers to India and their Indian driver, one in Telangana, and three early cases in Kerala.[8] At that time, a total of 589,000 people had been screened at various airports across the country and over 1,00,000 at borders with Nepal; around 27,000 were under community surveillance.

Health screening and keeping track of persons who had travelled back from affected regions and countries was the initial response of countries for containing the spread of the virus, but soon it was realized that the infection could spread through asymptomatic persons as well. In fact, WHO travel advisories throughout 2019 and 2018 related to diseases like yellow fever, Zika and Ebola were steadfast on how infections spread through asymptomatic carriers too.

An updated WHO travel advisory related to COVID-19 coincidently came on 24 January 2020, the day India reported its first COVID-19 case.[9] It continued to advise against 'the application of any restrictions of international traffic based on the information currently available on this event.' The advisory, in fact, maintained that measures to limit the risk of exportation or importation of the disease should be implemented, 'without unnecessary restrictions of international traffic.'

By April, when most countries had already shut down travel especially for international passengers, WHO listed some measures for suppressing community transmission.[10] Among those, it said, authorities must immediately adopt and adapt population-level distancing measures and movement restrictions in addition to other public health and health-system measures to reduce exposure and suppress transmission, in countries and sub-national regions in which community transmission had become established or which were at risk of entering the phase. This, it said, should include measures 'to reduce the risk of importation or reintroduction of the virus from high-transmission areas, such as limits on national and international travel, enhanced screening and quarantine.'

The WHO, however, modified its stance on quarantine in May 2021. 'Evidence for the usefulness of quarantine to prevent transmission of SARS-CoV-2 is of low to very low certainty at best and based on a limited number of modelling studies and a few observational series available at the time of closure of the literature search on 13 November 2020,' it said. WHO made this new observation in 'Evidence Review—Public Health Measures in the Aviation Sector in the Context of COVID-19: Quarantine and Isolation on 21 May 2021.'[11] In October 2020, the WHO Guideline Development Group (GDG) for International Travel and Health (ITH) met to evaluate the evidence. Though ITH GDG said isolation of symptomatic and/or travellers who tested positive remains 'an integral, WHO-endorsed response strategy' to the pandemic, public health interventions such as quarantine for travellers might have the greatest impact in countries with low COVID-19 incidence and many international arrivals. WHO said in the review, 'In countries at the tipping point of exponential growth. The undesirable effects may exceed the benefits in countries that already have a high incidence and/or exponential growth.'

The review said that the quarantine of travellers should be feasible from the perspective of border management and cost, and be accompanied by clear communication. The modelling studies it considered demonstrated that, on balance, 'quarantine of sufficient duration, with high compliance, implemented in such a way as to mitigate any unintended harm to equity and human rights, is likely to slightly or even largely reduce or prevent further community transmission from arriving travellers. Quarantine, therefore, could be both an effective and an appropriate intervention, depending on each country's circumstances; however, robust, high certainty evidence to support this conclusion is lacking.' The 2019 version of WHO-INTEGRATE evidence-to-decision framework, which combines global health norms and values of WHO and the United Nations system, was used to contextualize data on effectiveness, to facilitate decision-making.

The framework has six criteria: balance of health benefits and harms, human rights and sociocultural acceptability, health equity, equality and non-discrimination, societal implications, financial and economic considerations and feasibility, and health system considerations. Based on this framework and limited modelling studies, the 21 May 2021 review noted that combining quarantine of travellers with virological testing, particularly when repeated during the quarantine period, might improve the effectiveness and reduce the duration of quarantine. WHO, however, has always been in favour of allowing free flow of travel and commercial interests of travel industry appeared to be piggy riding on the human rights and equity angles to this inference by its ITH GDG since quarantine requirements mandated by governments for international and even domestic travel do dissuade people from undertaking even essential travel.

WHO has, in fact, been widely criticized for its late responses to COVID-19-related incidences and even some erroneous observations. Its first travel advisory relating to COVID-19 came eleven days before its first situation report on 21 January 2020, which meant its official assessment of the disease came after its suggestions on travel. The situation report put the number of confirmed COVID-19 cases at 282.[12] Four Chinese regions were reported to be impacted, and the majority, 258 cases, were from the Hubei province, which includes Wuhan. Cases in Japan, in the Republic of Korea and in Thailand were reported to have been 'exported' from Wuhan. The 10 January advice of WHO on international trade and travel maintained that the cause of the pneumonia seemed to be a novel coronavirus but the transmission potential and modes of transmission remained unclear. 'Therefore, it would be prudent to reduce the general risk of acute respiratory infections while travelling in or from affected areas (currently Wuhan city) by avoiding close contact with people suffering from acute respiratory infections; frequent hand-washing, especially after direct contact with ill people or their environment; avoiding close contact with live or dead farm or wild animals; travellers with symptoms of acute respiratory infection practicing cough etiquette (maintain distance, cover coughs and sneezes with disposable tissues or clothing, and wash hands).'

Later, its 24 January advisory had two parts: 'exit screening in countries or areas with ongoing transmission of the novel coronavirus 2019-nCoV (currently People's Republic of China)' and 'entry screening in countries/areas without transmission of the novel coronavirus.'[13] It continued to cast doubts on screening but admitted that during the current outbreak, the majority of exported cases were detected through entry screening. 'The risk of importation of the disease may be reduced if temperature screening at entry is associated with early detection of symptomatic passengers and their referral for medical follow up,' it said.

On 5 February, Indians were advised 'to refrain from travelling to China.'[14] While the Union government started taking measured steps that did not anticipate a huge level of infection, voluntary restrictions or stopping of travel by companies occurred even before the government responded. According to PricewaterhouseCoopers, businesses spend more than $300 billion each year on corporate travel, approximately 20 per cent of which is on airfare.[15] For airlines, corporate travellers represent 12 per cent of passengers and generate as much as 75 per cent of profit on certain routes. Even before 4 March, when screening of all international travellers started, companies like Tata Consultancy Service, Wipro, HCL Technologies and Infosys restricted travel by their employees to certain geographies.[16]

Ernst & Young (EY) concluded a survey in September 2020 that captured the views of executives from travel-intensive sectors across India, explored how their businesses were impacted by COVID-19, how the pandemic has affected their corporate travel policy and the steps these businesses are taking to evolve. The bulk of respondents (92 per cent) reported that their businesses had been adversely impacted by the pandemic at the time of taking the survey. While an almost identical percentage of respondents expect recovery in their businesses by the end of 2022, a combination of employee health concerns, reduced business activity and limited flight options led to corporate travel restrictions in most respondent companies. 'Despite having expectations that business travel will get resumed next year (2021) most respondents are of the opinion that corporate travel policies will be revised to limit strategically important business development and revenue enhancement activities. This, the majority believe, will be a result of the proven effectiveness of video conferencing tools. Others hold that reduced business activity and budget limitations will also impact corporate travel,' said EY in the survey summary.

It took a full forty-eight days, from 17 January to 4 March, for India to extend universal health screening to all persons travelling from any other country at all its airports, but it was not the first time such screening was being done in the country. Eleven years earlier, on 29 April 2009, the DGCA had issued a circular asking airlines to get a form filled by passengers and crew arriving from swine flu-affected countries, which included Mexico, the United States and Canada. The form was designed by Airport Health Organization (APHO) and had just three straight questions on fever, cough and whether the person had been in the proximity of a person with flu. The questions were to be answered if the person had visited or transited any of the three countries in the previous ten days.

Clearly, the Union government's restrictions came in a graded manner, which could also be termed as late and full of execution loopholes, showing its lack of preparedness to deal with the COVID-19 pandemic. Stricter and more effective screening and even stopping of all international travel in early March could have been termed as an overreaction at that point of time but potentially could have stopped the spread of infection in the initial phase. The point at which the curbs on international travel should have been implemented would now appear to be February, though this can only be said with the benefit of hindsight.

Health screening was followed by suspension of visas. As with screening, visas were also suspended in a graded way. E-visas issued to Chinese passport holders or persons of other nationalities residing in China were first suspended on 3 February.[17] Within two days, the DGCA issued another circular, on 5 February, suspending all visas issued to Chinese passport holders and foreign nationals travelling from China. Even after twenty-five days, the government did not appear to be sure how exactly it wanted to move on visa restriction, so while on 28 February, it suspended visa on arrival facilities for nationals of Japan and South Korea, it allowed persons from these countries holding e-visa or regular visa to come in provided they had not visited China after 15 January. On 3 March, regular and e-visas issued to nationals of Italy, Iran, South Korea and Japan, who had not yet entered India, were suspended. Even visas issued to other foreign nationals who had travelled to these countries or to China on or after 1 February and who had not yet entered India stood suspended.

A day later, health screening for all international passengers was announced. On 5 March, the DGCA announced that beginning 10 March, anyone travelling from Italy and the Republic of Korea needed a COVID-19 negative test certificate. From 11 March, regular and e-visas issued to nationals of France, Germany and Spain were also suspended. The next day, on 12 March, however, a new circular announced the suspension of all visas issued to nationals of other countries except to those issued to diplomats, employees of the United Nations and international organizations, and project visas. This change in position certainly had to do with the WHO declaring COVID-19 a pandemic on 11 March.[18] 'Pandemic is not a word to use lightly or carelessly. It is a word that, if misused, can cause unreasonable fear, or unjustified acceptance that the fight is over, leading to unnecessary suffering and death,' said WHO in its media briefing. 'Describing the situation as a pandemic does not change WHO assessment of the threat posed by this virus. It doesn't change what WHO is doing, and it doesn't change what countries should do,' it said.

While acknowledging that some countries implemented entry screening for air travellers, United Nations' International Civil Aviation Organization (ICAO) also said in its 18 March 2020 letter to member states, 'Evidence, however, has shown that entry screening may miss infected cases and States are reminded not to rely on entry screening as a stand-alone measure. Screening measures should be part of a multilayer strategy.'[19] It asked countries to strike 'a fine balance between protecting public health, respecting human rights and minimizing economic and social disruption.' The emphasis was on undisrupted movement of cargo across the countries.

The situation across the world, however, did keep changing, with governments, including the Indian government, taking decisions according to what they were dealing with at that point. 'We have never before seen a pandemic sparked by a coronavirus. This is the first pandemic caused by a coronavirus. And we have never before seen a pandemic that can be controlled, at the same time.' These words of WHO were clearly too optimistic, considering what the world witnessed in the subsequent months.

India's suspension of visas was to initially come into effect from 13 March 2020 to 15 April 2020. Visa-free travel facility for OCI card holders was also suspended for that period. This suspension of permission to travel was valid for all modes of travel—by air, sea and land—but it did not affect the visas of those already in India. The 12 March DGCA circular[20] also made a fourteen-day quarantine mandatory for incoming travellers, including Indians, from seven countries: China, Italy, Iran, the Republic of Korea, France, Spain and Germany.

People travel overseas for both work and leisure. A vast population of students also move countries, so while India was reviewing measures on how to deal with international travellers almost on a daily basis, there was a most vulnerable section among foreign travellers, students, who found themselves stranded when hostels and universities abroad shut down, even as the window to travel back home to India shrunk to a small one.

Twenty-three-year-old Mihir Tak boarded a flight back home to India from New York on 13 March 2020. 'I believe I booked the second last seat available on the flight,' she says.[21] This was a day after a COVID-19 case was detected a few blocks away from her workplace in New York. India had not shut itself at that point. A student enrolled in a business and merchandising course at Indiana University, she says, 'I was in New York and there was a COVID-19 case detected on 12 March 2020 two blocks away from my workplace, so everything was shutting down. My management was in talks to start work from home and even schools and colleges were looking to shut down. Alarmed by the scarcity of resources such as sanitizers, wipes, staple food items [beans, rice, pasta, grains and even sugar] in my nearest supermarket, I decided to come back to India. My parents pushed me to get out of the city as early as the next day.'

When she departed from the John F. Kennedy airport, she was surprised to find that there were no protocols being followed, even though the virus was spreading in the city. 'They were only allowing Indian nationals to get on the flight, though. I remember, a girl was flying to India to see her extended family but was an American passport holder. She was detained from flying,' she says.

Upon landing at the Mumbai airport, the flight attendants separated people into groups for temperature checks and the officials at the airport took down all the details of their final destinations. 'I was contacted a few hours later over a call and was given instructions about home quarantining,' says Mihir. Once at home in Rajasthan's Udaipur, she faced what proved to be a badge of suspicion for people who had travelled from abroad. A sticker outside her house cautioned neighbours to stay away from a possible source of infection.

In an additional advisory issued on 10 March, the MoHFW for the first time laid isolation guidelines for overseas travellers.[22]

'All passengers having travel history to China, Hong Kong, the Republic of Korea, Japan, Italy, Thailand, Singapore, Iran, Malaysia, France, Spain and Germany are advised to undergo self-imposed quarantine for a period of 14 days from the date of their arrival. If such passengers are working in some organizations/institutions, their respective employers are advised to facilitate work from home during this period,' it said. These rules were soon extended to more countries and then to all overseas travellers. Working on data from the immigration department, local authorities affixed stickers outside the homes of returnees, asking everyone to not interact with the person. These stickers also ensured that neighbours kept a vigil on the person asked to remain in isolation.

'Within two days [of returning to Udaipur], a team of government workers came home to check my temperature and marked my house as a quarantine area, making everyone in my locality aware of it. After fifteen days, I got a phone call to inquire if I had any symptoms and to check if I needed to be quarantined for a longer period,' says Mihir. Fortunately, it turned out well for Mihir, who thinks returning home was 'a great decision because New York then became the epicentre of the virus and I felt I was much safer at home. If I am being completely honest, I thought I would rather catch the virus at home [where I have people to take care of me] than alone in my apartment in New York.'

At the Delhi airport, Videh Kumar Jaipuriar, chief executive officer, Delhi International Airport Ltd (DIAL), saw a mother crying because her daughter, who had come on an Air India flight from San Francisco, was inside the airport but she could not speak to her. 'The Central Industrial Security Force (CISF) was not allowing her to come to the visitor area. Finally, I took the details. She calmed down and a senior CISF officer sat with her. There were thousands of persons inside, but they found her and made her talk through a CISF personnel's phone,' he says.[23] As things became difficult, many more started heading back home. Aishwarya Airy was at the Northwestern University's Medill School of Journalism. She took an Air India flight from Washington DC on 20 March 2020. Some five days earlier, the school had informed that their programme was going to go remote. 'That's when it first hit me that this is something serious, and with the way things were going, both in the US and in India, I decided that the best thing for me to do would be to come back home. At that moment, no other international student in my programme was going back, so it was definitely a risk because there was a good chance that I wouldn't be able to come back for my last quarter.'[24] She weighed the pros and cons and decided she rather be with her family in India. 'Once I decided I wanted to go back, the next thing to do was to find a flight. My aim was to get a direct flight and I guess I was lucky because I found an Air India direct flight for 20 March.' Leaving was not as simple since she was staying in a shared apartment with two other flatmates and the lease was up in May. 'With the way things were going, I had a feeling I wouldn't be back by the time our lease ended, so I decided to pack up my things and move them into storage. So it was a really chaotic few hours, but I am glad I was able to get everything done before I left because I didn't get back until July.'

The fare for this flight, which was probably one of the last ones from the US before the shutdown, was much higher than for regular flights—it was even costlier than a regular return journey. At the departing airport, Dulles, her experience was similar to that of Mihir Tak. 'There was no protocol as such being followed. There were still no mandatory mask requirements. It was just like any regular flight at that point.'

Upon landing, it was absolute chaos at the airport. 'It took me almost twelve hours after deboarding to exit the airport. The ground staff was just as confused. There were passengers from flights that came much before ours waiting to get their temperature check clearances. They said a three-step check was in place. We were all made to wait at the gates (the area right after getting off the plane, with travelators and vending machines).' They were called in flight-wise for temperature checks and then allowed to go forward. 'At that moment, it felt so much riskier to be at the airport. There was obviously no social distancing. People were literally sticking to each other at one point. It felt like 7 p.m. at Rajiv Chowk Metro station on a weekday,' says Aishwarya.[25] After letting them leave in batches from the waiting area, they took our passports because there had to be another check at the exit gate, and formed groups of 10. Another wait started to get to the medical makeshift facility at the exit gates. There were older people, families with little children—everyone was stuck in what seemed like an endless, complex affair. Passengers were losing their cool and getting into fights with airport staff because a process that takes 40–60 minutes was taking eight hours and they did not know how much longer it would be.

Aishwarya narrated her experience in a series of tweets. 'The airport staff was trying their best, but trying to manage hundreds of anxious passengers is not easy. So, it was just chaotic for everyone. Around 10.30–11 p.m., we made it to the gates. We were now waiting for our turn to go into the makeshift facility and be examined one last time before leaving the airport. Then the airport staff came with food and water packages and distributed some refreshments. When I made it to the final level of this ordeal, it was rather underwhelming,' she wrote. The doctors asked passengers if they had travelled to certain places in the past few days, about any symptoms, and gave a number to call if they developed symptoms later. 'They then put a quarantine stamp [on hand] and told me to quarantine at home. They took down my address and phone number as well. After this, I was free to go. It was rather confusing for me because the only medical check that had happened in those twelve hours was a temperature check right at the beginning and this conversation with a doctor at the end,' she says.

There was limited knowledge about the disease at that time. 'The government was also learning and coming with new notification every day. We had a huge rush of people coming back because they were being evacuated and suddenly there was a new process which was being put in place. There was a huge mess at the airport because airport is usually only about people coming in and coming out,' says Jaipuriar of DIAL.

Jaipuriar says the airport had never handled the extra processes in the past. The Central government had put in place processes which health officials had to follow. There was another process put in place by the immigration for which a form was to be submitted. The Delhi government put up its own processes. It were three government agencies doing similar kind of processes causing huge grief to people. 'There were cases where people had to wait for 10-12 hours,' he says. 'There were counters for food and water but they (passengers) did not want to leave the queue (for medical screening). We tied up with flight catering and started distributing food,' he says.

DIAL started monitoring flight-wise to see how much time completing of processes was taking and found that thirteen-and-a-half hours was going into these things. A triage facility was created at the airport (for medical screening), where it was decided where an incoming passenger should go based on where the person was coming from. 'We got the information from the Delhi government that nobody will be allowed to go till they go through this triage facility, whether they are asymptomatic or symptomatic or risk or high-risk country. It was decided at the triage whether a person would go through institutional or home quarantine. First two days there was a problem because of the number of doctors appointed by the Delhi government were not enough,' says Jaipuriar.

Seven doctors a shift were posted in the triage area and the processing time was 10–15 minutes for every passenger. This led to situation wherein it took about seven to nine hours to clear passengers from a single flight, says Jaipuriar. The number of doctors was later increased to nineteen.

The processes and management of anxious people were not the only challenges DIAL had to deal with. There was Edgard Ziebat, for instance, who landed in India on 17 March 2020 from Hanoi by a VietJet flight VJ-971. 'He was a German national and had to go to Istanbul via Riyad. While he reached here, the onward flights were cancelled. He did not have a visa for India and was in no-man's land,' says Jaipuriar. He was medically examined at the airport. 'We had no other option but to keep him in the international transfer area since he could not go out because he did not have Indian visa. We got in touch with the Ministry of External Affairs (MEA) and the German embassy and requested them to get him evacuated and or put him up in the embassy but when embassy officials came and met him four to five days later, he refused to go back to Germany because he had a legal case there.'

The Indian government, early May, also tried to fly Ziebat on an evacuation flight to Ankara but Turkish authorities refused since the flight was only for their citizens or permanent card holders.[26] DIAL gave him food, water and toiletries while hosting him for 55 days in the international transfer area. He finally took a KLM evacuation flight to Amsterdam on 12 May 2020, says Jaipuriar.

India stopped all international flights on 22 March 2020. In a 19 March circular, the DGCA said flights for India would not take off beginning 0001 hours GMT (0.50 a.m. IST), 22 March 2020 onwards.[27] While a 20-hour travel was permissible, disembarkation beyond 2001 hours GMT (1.30 a.m. IST on 23 March 2020). The circular was to remain in force till 0001 hours GMT on 29 March 2020. Just four days later, however, on 26 March, another circular was issued which extended the suspension of flights to 14 April.[28] Another extension till 3 May was announced on 14 April[29] and subsequently, it was extended till 17 May,[30] then 31 May,[31] and then till 30 June.[32] On 26 June, a new circular[33] extended the suspension of international flights till 15 July but added that competent authorities could allow scheduled flights on select routes on a case-to-case basis. This was extended via the October 27 circular[34] till 30 November, in a 26 November circular[35] till 31 December, and then till 30 June 2021.[36] Later in December 2021, India decided to reopen regular international flights but had to take back the decision following the spread of Omicron variant of COVID-19. It decided to continue the ban on scheduled international flights till 30 January 2022.

Stopping of domestic and international flights did not mean that the airports were shut. 'The airports were closed for passengers but there were cargo and evacuation flights which were in service. I got a call from the Air Traffic Control [ATC] at the Delhi airport whether they can operate in one shift since flight operations were limited and they had some cases of [COVID-19] infection,' says Jaipuriar. ATC normally works 24×7. The request, however, could only be accepted by the director-general of civil aviation, so Jaipuriar called the DGCA and asked if there could only be one shift because there were only three to four evacuation flights and about ten to fourteen cargo flights coming in. 'The problem is ATC not only supports flights coming to Delhi but also planes crossing the city's air space so it is not possible for an airport like Delhi to stop ATC,' he says. Shops inside the airport had to be shut down from 23 March 2020 but none of the shops at the Delhi airport had shutters. 'The only way was to cover them with cyclophilin sheets but security was important. We gave 24 hours to shops to put some cover or remove their merchandise and shut shop. Some of them wanted to keep one guard so those many numbers we allowed,' says Jaipuriar.

Crucial to the cancellation of all travel and visas was the issue of how and when the journey could be resumed. While this was uncertain, especially since the government kept extending the travel ban, a large segment wanted their fare refunded. A circular issued by DGCA, the same day India suspended all visas, asked airlines to support passengers by waiving of cancellation and reschedule charges but added a caveat of 'any other option,' which meant that passengers were not reimbursed the travel money but given a credit for future travel. This credit shell was supported by DGCA and meant that traveller money was blocked. Later, the matter went to the courts and on 1 October 2020, the Supreme Court ruled that if tickets were booked before the lockdown period that started 25 March, then credit could be given, but if the ticket was booked after that, then all airlines had to issue refunds. Subsequently, the DGCA issued a notification on 7 October 2020, enforcing the Supreme Court order on refunds.[37]

The decisions taken by the Indian government from January to March 2020 were similar to those its neighbour Pakistan took. Pakistan also started screening passengers from China at four airports.[38] Due to Pakistan's geographical proximity to Iran, which was one of the earliest countries to see an increase in COVID-19 cases, it was especially vulnerable. In fact, the early cases of COVID-19 in Pakistan were of people who travelled to Iran.[39] It also shares land borders with China. From 13 March 2020 onwards, it closed its land borders and limited international flights to Karachi, Lahore and Islamabad airports. Though it planned to resume normal operations at all airports from 21 March 2020 after making COVID-19 testing mandatory, the plan changed. In a statement, the Pakistani civil aviation ministry said, '(The) government of Pakistan has decided to suspend operation of all international passenger, chartered and private flights to Pakistan, effective from 21 March till 4 April.' At that time, the number of confirmed COVID-19 cases was 645, with 4,046 suspected cases across Pakistan.[40]

Both India and Pakistan extended the suspension of international as well as domestic air services several times. This is in contrast to what was happening in the United States, where stopping flights altogether was unthinkable.[41] Yet, the curbs on international travel in the US started much earlier. A presidential proclamation on 'suspension of entry of immigrants and non-immigrants of persons who pose a risk of transmitting 2019 Novel Coronavirus' came on 31 January 2020.[42] Following the proclamation, from 5 p.m. on 2 February 2020, the US government allowed the return of US citizens or lawful permanent residents who had travelled to mainland China within the previous fourteen days only through eleven approved airports, where a screening mechanism was put in place. Foreign nationals who had travelled to mainland China within the last fourteen days, however, were denied permission to travel to the US.[43] There were similar restrictions on travellers from Iran and the Schengen area. But even before these, on 29 January 2020, American Airlines announced the suspension of services from Los Angeles airport to Shanghai Pudong Airport (PVG) and Beijing Capital International Airport (PEK) from 9 February to 27 March 2020 because of 'significant decline in demand for travel to and from China.'[44]

Though there were subsequent cuts in flight schedule, most of them were due to a lack of demand. American Airlines on 18 May, for instance, announced it will cut capacity in summer 2020 to address record low customer demand, including suspending 70 per cent of domestic and 80 per cent of international capacity for June versus the same period the previous year. The airline also said it would delay the start of some international services that were to begin in May and June.[45]

When the second COVID-19 wave swept India in early 2021, the United States, like many other countries, decided to impose a travel ban on India. On 30 April 2021, American president Joseph R. Biden Jr said, 'I have determined that it is in the interests of the US to take action to restrict and suspend the entry into the US, as nonimmigrants, of noncitizens of the US ("noncitizens") who were physically present within the Republic of India during the 14 day period preceding their entry or attempted entry into the US.'[46] The country's Centers for Disease Control and Prevention (CDC), within the Department of Health and Human Services, along with the Department of Homeland Security, had concluded that India was experiencing widespread, ongoing person-to-person transmission of COVID-19. 'The magnitude and scope of the COVID-19 pandemic in the Republic of India is surging; the Republic of India accounts for over one-third of new global cases, and the number of new cases in the Republic of India is accelerating at a rapid rate. There have been more than 300,000 average new daily cases in the Republic of India over the past week,' said the White House proclamation.

A variant strain of the virus, known as B.1.617, was also circulating in the Republic of India, along with other variant strains, including B.1.1.7, first detected in the United Kingdom, and B.1.351, first detected in the Republic of South Africa, said the proclamation. According to CDC, these variants had 'characteristics of concern which may make them more easily transmitted and have the potential for reduced protection afforded by some vaccines.' Two days earlier, the US embassy in New Delhi said its citizens should leave if they wished. 'Access to all types of medical care is becoming severely limited in India due to the surge in COVID-19 cases. US citizens, who wish to depart India should take advantage of available commercial transportation options, now. Direct flights between India and the United States are offered daily, with additional flight options available to US citizens via transfers in Paris and Frankfurt.'[47] Hospitals were reporting shortages of supplies, oxygen and beds for both COVID-19 and non-COVID-19 related patients. US citizens were reporting being denied admittance to hospitals in some cities due to a lack of space, it said.

While Canada banned direct flights from India and Pakistan on 22 April 2021, it insisted that RT-PCR (reverse transcription polymerase chain reaction) test be done in third country for people coming from India. 'During that period, passengers who travel to Canada from India via an indirect route will need to obtain a pre-departure negative COVID-19 molecular test result from a third country before continuing their journey to Canada,' said the Canadian government.[48] This, however, was tough since some countries did not allow entry or transit for passengers from India or for passengers who had previously tested positive for COVID-19.

Britain, too, banned entry from India from 23 April 2021 onwards, except British and Irish citizens, by putting the country on the 'red' list.[49] The UK rated countries red, amber or green depending on COVID-19 related risks and rules they needed to follow to enter England. Neighbouring Sri Lanka, Bangladesh and Nepal were all on the red list.

The journey for students from India to some countries, including China, the United States, Canada, Germany and Australia, was not easy either, despite the Indian government allowing them priority vaccination. Australia, which had strict COVID-19 related restrictions throughout, was one of the toughest destinations. Even as later as September 2021, Union External Affairs Minister S. Jaishankar had to raise the issue with his Australian counterpart Marise Payne, during the first India-Australia 2+2 dialogue of defence and foreign ministers in New Delhi.[50] To this, Payne said

Australia would follow a four-phase pathway for progression out of COVID-19 restrictions. Reopening began after enough Australians were vaccinated, with students returning in phases three and four. Later, on 1 October 2021, Australian Prime Minister Scott Morrison announced that fully vaccinated Australian citizens and permanent residents would be eligible for international travel without seeking a travel exemption from November 2021. There were over thirty countries that imposed flight restrictions on India from April to June 2021, in contrast to what happened in 2020, when India shut its borders with other countries in order to contain the virus. The situation had reversed for Indians.

2

AT SEA WITH THE PANDEMIC

'REQUEST TO [THE] INDIA government total 160 Indian crew rescue from ship [Japan].' There was no storm on the high seas when Binay Kumar Sarkar of Siliguri, a chef de partie, said this desperate line in a video message he uploaded on his Facebook account aboard *Diamond Princess.* He had other Indian crew members standing next to him in the kitchen of the cruise ship that became the only other place outside of Wuhan, China, to have a high concentration of COVID-19 cases in the initial phase. It was 7 February 2020, and according to Sarkar, the cruise ship had 137 COVID-19 positive cases. So he sought help from the Indian government for rescue.

Diamond Princess was not to be just 'a treasure trove of exceptional delights waiting to be discovered,' where tourists could dine on 'freshly prepared sashimi in Kai Sushi, watch street performers in the dazzling Atrium, or take in a lavish production show in our state-of-the-art theater. And for a unique treat, visit the Izumi Japanese Bath, the largest of its kind at sea.'[1] From being a princess of the sea, it had become an abandoned child docked at Japan with its occupants waiting to deboard and be treated, prompting Sarkar to send the desperate video message.[2]

Bearing cruise number M003, the ship was anchored at the Yokohama port since 3 February 2020 after it had cut short its tour by a day. This was also two days after the Hong Kong government notified that one of the passengers who had deboarded at Kai Tak Cruise Terminal in Hong Kong on 25 January had tested positive for COVID-19.

There were 2,666 passengers on board, of which 1,281 were Japanese, and 1,045 crew members from a total of fifty-six countries.[3] The ship had started from the Yokohama port on 20 January 2020 and during its sixteen-day voyage touched shores of Hong Kong, Chan May Port and Cai Lan in Vietnam, Keelung in Taiwan and Naha in Japan. It was to return to Yokohama on 4 February. This meant a journey of four countries and six cities. But on 1 February 2020, the Hong Kong government announced that pneumonia due to COVID-19 was confirmed in an eighty-year-old passenger on the *Diamond Princess*. He had disembarked on 25 January.

Hong Kong's Centre for Health Protection (CHP) under the Department of Health (DH) reported this 'one additional case of novel coronavirus' infection on 1 February: 'The patient is an 80-year-old man who lives in Luk Kwai House, Kwai Chung Estate, New Territories with good past health. He presented with cough since 19 January and started having fever since 30 January. He sought medical attention at the Accident and Emergency Department at Caritas Medical Centre on 30 January and was admitted for isolation and management.'[4] The bulletin also said the patient went to the Mainland (China) for a few hours through Lo Wu border control point on 10 January. Subsequently, he took a flight from Hong Kong to Tokyo (Japan) on 17 January and boarded a cruise at Yokohama on 20 January. He deboarded *Diamond Princess* when it arrived at Kai Tak Cruise Terminal in Hong Kong on 25 January.

On 4 February, Princess Cruises, the cruise liner that ran *Diamond Princess* and is part of the New York Stock Exchange-listed Carnival Corporation, issued a statement cancelling the next voyage of the vessel 'to help facilitate the health screening and records review process.'[5] *Diamond Princess* was due to depart Yokohama (4 February 2020) for another eight-day round-trip cruise. 'However, the decision was made to cancel the cruise because of the time needed for the authorities to complete their comprehensive review. All guests will receive a full refund. Each guest will also receive a one hundred percent future cruise credit,' it said.

Companies like to be diplomatic with governments, especially if they are foreign governments in whom they have a business interest, so despite a humanitarian crisis on their hands and the Japanese government's changing stance on quarantine, the statement also politely thanked the Japan Ministry of Health for their 'thorough review of the health status of guests and crew aboard *Diamond Princess.*'

By the next day, on 5 February, there were ten confirmed cases on *Diamond Princess*. This made the Japanese government set a fourteen-day health observation period but infection spread on board. On 16 February, there were at least two confirmed cases of Indians being infected and by 23 February, when passengers began disembarking, the number of confirmed cases rose to 691.[6] Infection had also been confirmed in five quarantined officers and healthcare workers on 21 February. There were two deaths on 20 February and another on 23 February.

The United States, Canada, Australia and Hong Kong started coordinating with the Japanese government and the cruise management for repatriation of their citizens, both guests and crew, on board. Jan Swartz, Princess Cruises' president, was in Japan on 19 February to coordinate response operations and prepare for the disembarkation of guests.

In response to a question in the Rajya Sabha on 19 March, Minister of State for External Affairs V. Muraleedharan said there were a total of 138 Indian nationals, including 132 crew members, on board the *Diamond Princess*. 'Of these, 119 Indian nationals were brought back to India on a special Air India flight on 27 February 2020. Upon their return, these were quarantined in an Indian Army facility at Manesar, Haryana,' he said.[7] Sixteen Indian nationals on board the cruise had tested positive for COVID-19. They were treated in onshore medical facilities in Japan. All of them were discharged after the completion of their treatment and as per available information, have returned to India. Three Indian nationals chose to stay back and were quarantined at an onshore facility in Japan.

The interesting fact, however, remains that the Santa Clarita, California based Princess Cruises announced withdrawal of all its cruise trips more than two months later, on 12 March 2020.[8] This it called a 'proactive response to the unpredictable circumstances evolving from the global spread of COVID-19.' And, 'in an abundance of caution,' it announced that it will voluntarily pause global operations of its eighteen cruise ships for two months (sixty days), impacting voyages departing 12 March to 10 May.

Diamond Princess was not to be alone. There were other ships landing in deep waters, too. Even as the crisis was unfolding at Yokohama, Japanese Prime Minister Shinzo Abe on 6 February announced the country would refuse entry to foreigners on the cruise ship *MS Westerdam*, scheduled to dock in Okinawa on 8 February. *Westerdam* was on a fourteen-day Taiwan and Japan cruise that departed Hong Kong on 1 February. There were 1,455 guests and 802 crew on board, of which 687 guests were continuing on the 1 February sailing, from the previous voyage.[9] The ship had been scheduled to call at Ishigaki Island, Naha, Okinawa, Nagasaki and

Fukuoka (Hakata), before its scheduled turn in Yokohama on 15 February, where the next cruise was scheduled to embark.

The ship was refused entry under the Immigration Control Law, Article 5.1 (14), entitled 'Persons with a reason to be deemed likely to harm Japan's interests and public interest.' This clause, which has been applied only once since 1945, was cited as the reason for the response after a Japanese National Security Council meeting that positioned COVID-19 as a national security issue.[10]

At 1 p.m. on 7 February, Holland America Line, the company that runs *Westerdam* cruise, issued a statement that also reflected its helplessness because of the apathy of governments that wanted to keep any suspicious case of COVID-19 off their shores: '*Westerdam* is currently sailing on a southwesterly course off the coast of Taiwan to best position the ship to access potential port locations where we can disembark our guests. We are evaluating several options and working with different governments for a swift resolution.'[11] Japan was not the only one to refuse docking of the vessel. On 10 February, Holland America announced *Westerdam* was sailing for Laem Chabang, Bangkok, Thailand, where the current cruise that departed 1 February would end on Thursday, 13 February. 'Guests will be disembarking in Laem Chabang and transfer to Bangkok for their forward travel home,' it said. But that was not to be as Thailand's Public Health Minister Anutin Charnvirakul announced the country would not allow the cruise ship from Japan to let passengers disembark at the Laem Chabang port.[12]

According to a BBC report, besides Thailand, Taiwan, Guam, the Philippines and Japan, a total of five nations had turned away the ship.[13] Finally, it was Cambodia which allowed *Westerdam* to anchor. On 12 February, it agreed to let the *MS Westerdam* dock and allow passengers to disembark. Cambodian Prime Minister Hun Sen told the media, 'The real disease is fear, not the virus.' While the WHO Director-General Tedros Adhanom also praised Cambodia and the 'international solidarity'[14] in situations where cruise ships are denied entry 'without an evidence-based risk assessment,' it did nothing to issue an advisory for such cruises stranded in the middle of nowhere.

Malaysia's Deputy Prime Minister Dr Wan Azizah Wan Ismail announced on 15 February at a press conference that a *Westerdam* guest who disembarked the ship to fly home was reported positive for Covid-19. The guest departed *Westerdam* on 14 February and later reported feeling ill at the Kuala Lumpur, Malaysia airport. The guest's travelling companion, however, tested negative for COVID-19.[15] But on 21 February, Ismail again announced that the guest tested earlier was a 'false positive.' The Cambodian government, in fact, cleared all persons on board the *Westerdam* as having tested negative for COVID-19. It took ten days from the docking of the ship at Cambodia to get all passengers tested and disembark.

Late in June 2020, WHO did laud Cambodia as 'A Small Country with Big Heart' in a featured article.[16] It said, 'One important lesson learned is that leadership and solidarity can be as crucial as the technical elements of public health responses. An effectively coordinated response goes well beyond the scope of the health sector and must include a whole-of-government approach, steered by the country's leaders. Cambodia's response to the *MS Westerdam* crisis demonstrates that a country with fewer resources can contribute to global health security. It can take a humanitarian approach in a public health crisis and deliver a measured, coordinated response despite the uncertainty and complex challenges.' There was, however, no mention of countries that did not allow *Westerdam* to dock and what should have been the approach of countries in such a crisis.

The long days and weeks of sea travel means quarantine is possible on board itself though the duration depends on the distance between the last port of call and the final destination. The reason cruise ships were looked at with suspicion is because they, more than cargo carriers, could potentially be the single biggest superspreader for any country due to the thousands they sail in a restricted and closed environment, which leads to intermixing of people for fun and food. While there was a humanitarian crisis on board cruise ships, countries tightened the regulations around shipping vessels to prevent any influx of infection coming from people and material via the sea route.

What happened to subsequent cruises was obvious as the world shut both its doors and its shores. *Diamond Princess*, however, was set to resume operations. On 3 December 2020, its operator, Princess Cruises, announced that upon approval to return to service in 2021, its global fleet will feature 'the MedallionClass Experience,' offering a number of new features that leverage touchless technologies and significantly enhance and personalize the guest experience, as well as support new health protocols. 'The line of smart ships is expanding as ship transformation has continued during the pause. *Coral Princess*, *Diamond Princess*, *Emerald Princess*, *Grand Princess*, *Island Princess*, *Majestic Princess* and *Sapphire Princess* will return as MedallionClass ships along with the new Enchanted Princess.'[17] A MedallionClass cruise offers safer stay like an OceanMedallion, a quarter-sized wearable device that enables touch-free boarding to locate family and friends anywhere on the ship, as well as services delivered to the passengers.

Diamond Princess, however, would not sail for two years. It was scheduled to begin new journeys only in 2022, with a series of cruises in Southeast Asia, the Malaysian Peninsula and Japan. Part of the reason for this long intermission was restrictions across various countries due to the deadlier 2021 waves in Asia.

Westerdam, too, had its itinerary chalked out though it was not sailing the geography where it was left ashore. According to Holland

America website, *Westerdam* sailed for twenty-four days, from Barcelona, Spain, on 20 April 2021, to Piraeus (Athens), Greece, on 14 May 2021.[18] But not all cruise ships were setting sail again. Many were landing up for scrapping because the business was not good. *MV Karnika* and *Ocean Dream* were among those that reached Alang in Gujarat for an end of their lifecycle scrapping.[19]

The source of COVID-19 infection was supposed to be not just men but also material, especially in the initial months when every packaged handled was viewed with suspicion. Nevertheless, while regulations and restrictions from the governments came in for sea travel along with air travel itself, there was not much thought given to the handling of material at ports. The first advisory in India from the Directorate General of Shipping (DGS) came on 28 January 2020. It merely said: 'All Indian seafarers are advised to comply with WHO recommendation and MoHFW advisory ... Also, all Indian ships are required to exercise due caution while calling at ports of the regions where such infection is reported.'[20]

On 4 February 2020, the DGS issued a second advisory which merely added a few more guidelines to be followed by seafarers, including those spelt out by the International Maritime Organisation. An exhaustive list of what is to be followed came from Director-General of Shipping Amitabh Kumar on 16 March. Apart from seafarers, it laid down the protocol to be followed by recruiters and marine training institutes.[21] Seafarers were to avoid availing shore leave in infected regions and consider the risks involved before going ashore in other regions. 'Availing shore leave during the pandemic may need to be avoided and used only in exigencies with necessary precautions. Seafarers, who have travelled abroad to infected regions, are advised to self-quarantine immediately on arrival in India for at least a period of 14 days,' it said.

The norms subsequently issued by the DGS included the time taken for sailing in the number of days required for quarantine since a ship will be at sea for those many days. The Jawaharlal Nehru Port Trust (JNPT) in Navi Mumbai, the country's largest container handler, had on its hand the case of *The Moon*, which came from Iran and had Turkish and Indian crew.[22] It was put under quarantine for fourteen days, with precautions being undertaken since some of the crew members had deboarded at Iran, which was at that time recording the second-highest number of COVID-19 cases after China.

In the seventh month of the calendar or of the pandemic hitting the world, the maritime world became conscious of the anxiety of seafarers since many of them were not able to end their contracts and return home to be with their families. A maritime meet organized virtually by the United Kingdom and attended by a total of fifteen countries recognized that at least 200,000 seafarers required immediate repatriation, with many serving on extended crew contracts overdue to return home. 'In addition, a similar number of seafarers urgently need to join their ships in order to allow the world's internationally trading vessels to continue to operate safely,' observed a joint statement by these nations on crew changes.[23]

Yet, even in December 2020, Indian crew in at least two cargo ships were stuck on board in China. Clearly, nine months into the pandemic, the world had not learnt how to deal with humans that were stuck in the middle of nowhere. On *MV Anastasia*, a forty-seven-year-old tried to commit suicide because of his longing for his family after he heard they were down with COVID-19 back in India.[24] When he attempted suicide, the ship was stuck in the Chinese waters for over 140 days with sixteen Indian crew members since it could not offload the cargo it was carrying from Australia. Owned by MSC Crewing Services Private Ltd, Mumbai, the ship was on anchorage near Caofeidian port in China since 20 September 2020. Its parent company, MSC Mediterranean Shipping Company, headquartered in Geneva, said that though it supported COVID-19 health and sanitation requirements wherever it operates, 'the impact of restrictions on crew changes has taken its toll on hundreds of thousands of seafarers globally, throughout the pandemic crisis.'[25]

While China cited the pandemic and the fear of contagion, the crew believed it had a political reason of a trade war between China and Australia. MSC believed that 'those in control in similar situations should work to prioritise the well-being of seafarers and their families above commercial interests, as human suffering and lives are at stake.' It maintained that dozens of ships were stuck off the coast of China in late 2020 amid a trade dispute, which created uncertainty over whether cargo merchants could deliver coal to buyers in China. 'MSC understands that the company which initially chartered *Anastasia* from MSC had sub-chartered the vessel to a third party and that the commercial parties involved in the selling and buying of the cargo onboard were caught in the ensuing political uncertainty around the trade issue,' said the statement.

MSC, which maintained the vessel and organized its crew, said it had exhausted all possible options for crew change, including efforts at a diplomatic level between Indian and Chinese authorities, and so it was left with no other option but to advise the master of *Anastasia* to make 'a short hop to Japan on 4 February (2021) after already grave concerns for the safety and well-being of the seafarers intensified.' The crew, later in February, was back in India.

There was also the case of *MV Jag Anand* that was stuck since 13 June 2020 with twenty-three Indian sailors. Owned by the Mumbai-based Great Eastern Shipping Company, it was anchored near the Jingtang port, the People's Republic of China. The MEA, in a reply to a question in the Lok Sabha on 3 February 2021, said the two ships could not offload their cargo and carry out crew rotation due to the strict regulations introduced by China in view of the COVID-19 pandemic. The Indian government took up the issue of early crew change with the Chinese authorities both at the provincial level and with the Chinese ministry of foreign affairs. The Indian ambassador in Beijing also took up the matter with the vice foreign minister of People's Republic of China. The Chinese side conveyed the shipping company/agent can apply for crew rotation from a different port. The ship carried out crew change in Chiba, Japan on 18 January 2021. All the twenty-three crew members who were on board *MV Jag Anand* later arrived in India.[26]

Though the origin of COVID-19 is traced to China and countries put restrictions on Chinese nationals and others coming from there, tables turned very quickly. China itself followed rigorous rules for seafarers of other countries, leading to distress among mariners. When the second wave sent India to the top of global COVID-19 headlines, one Indian joined the crew of *MT Sonangol Rangel* on 31 March 2021. MT is short for 'motor tanker' vessels that carry liquid cargo. It was scheduled for dry docking in the Xinya Shipyard in the Zhoushan region of China. 'Just 48 hours before the arrival, however, it was refused entry because one Indian crew had joined the vessel on 31 March. The earlier rule was that no crew change within the last 30 days of arrival at the shipyard. As our ship was arriving at the shipyard on 5 May, we were complying with regulations, but overnight after the second wave the rule was changed to no crew change within the last 90 days and we were left high and dry,' says master of the Bahama-flagged vessel Rahul Srivastava. The 2011 vintage ship belongs to Stena Sonangol Suezmax Pool, a joint venture between Stena Bulk and Sonangol, the Angolan government-owned energy company. There was a last moment scramble to find a new shipyard, since the vessel was already off-hire from charterers and was scheduled for dry docking for a five-yearly repair planned well in advance. 'The manning company has no option but to stop crew change to comply with these regulations but no one has thought what the crew will do. What about the crew who have already finished the majority of their contracts?'

MT Sonangol Rangel sails across the world and before docking at China, it had finished a delivery of crude oil. The oil was loaded at Novorossiysk in Russia and travelled through the Suez Canal in Egypt to unload at Ulsan in Korea. After discharging in Korea, the vessel was taken out of service for the five-yearly repairs. 'I have sixteen crew out of twenty-three who have finished their contract. With present restrictions, crew change does not look possible for the next few months,' says Srivastava, whose four-month contract ended in May 2021 but who was still on board in June. He was commanding eleven Indian and thirteen Filipino crew. 'Some of the Filipinos have finished nine months on board and looks like they might end up doing eleven to twelve months. This is exactly what happened last year [2020]. Restrictions from the [Chinese] port do not allow crew change. No shore leaves,' he says.

Besides China, several other countries, including Singapore, Canada, the UK and the United Arab Emirates, put restrictions on Indian crew due to the second wave. This made the DGS issue a circular asking Indian seafarers not to sign off from vessels for one month. 'The second wave of COVID-19 pandemic in India has led to re-imposition of movement restrictions to and from India by several countries. The spread of coronavirus and the cross-border movement restrictions imposed by these countries has made repatriation of seafarers unsafe and difficult once they sign off at foreign ports,' said the circular. Stating that getting replacement seafarers was also difficult, it 'strongly' advised Indians to desist from signing off from the vessel, 'except in case of extreme emergency/ medical exigencies for a period of one month or till the situation improves.' It asked Indian seafarers whose tenure exceeded eleven months to put in a repatriation request through a portal with the DGS for 'advice'.

A year earlier, when India was closing its shores, the DGS on 24 March 2020 clarified the government orders that were being used to deny requests of sign off for Indian seafarers at Indian ports.[27] There was no restriction of sign on/sign off of Indian seafarers in ports in India, it said. Indian seafarers, though, were advised to 'exercise utmost caution in respect of sign off in foreign ports due to the international and domestic travel restrictions imposed by various international and national authorities.' It also said the MHA order of 23 March 2020, which stopped immigration of passenger traffic at 107 check posts, including all seaports, was 'applicable only for passengers and not crew.'

On 17 December, the DGS removed the quarantine restrictions that had been put in place on 20 March 2020, for ships before they berth. By then, much of the lockdown restrictions had been eased, though airline and railway operations were yet to resume normal operations. 'Representations have been received from stakeholders to review the DGS Order 04 of 2020 to remove the mandatory quarantine period of 14 days so that the vessels are not required to wait for their berthing turn,' said the new order.[28]

Beginning March 2020 and until December 2020, it had been a whirlpool of a ride for tourists and crew locked inside quarantined vessels and for cargo that logged in at ports but had restrictions on their movement. The crew, however, yearned to be with their families even during the second wave.

Binay Kumar Sarkar, a continental chef who became a mascot of the troubled crew that countries initially did not bother to take note, is grateful.[29] His distress video changed the course for him and his colleagues on board *Diamond Princess*. 'I thought, social media has a lot of power and I wanted to give a message to India and families of crew members so that we can be brought back at the earliest and we could stay in India for the quarantine period.' He was scared, and the situation was getting out of hand. The crew felt that the infection might come through the ventilation system. The precautions that could have been taken there would not be as adequate as what can be done while quarantining on land. Nevertheless, the code of conduct of his job did not allow him to use social media. 'I could have lost job but my contract was completing [on 12 February 2020] and I was not alone. My colleagues were with me. I wanted to be at home at the earliest,' he says. Later, the Indian government responded to his request. External Affairs Minister Jaishankar spoke to him while he was still on the ship. 'We were brought back and kept in a nice place in Manesar for seventeen days.' Married for two years then in February, Sarkar says he is very close to his family, including his brother, and they all were anxious.

'We did not know whether we will live or die. We felt like it was a war,' he says. His employer, Princess Cruises, paid him an extra two-month salary after the crisis ended. But now, he has charted a different course. After having been on cruises for ten years, Sarkar has set up his own travel company in Siliguri, West Bengal. He and his brother Tanay also make short horror thrillers for their YouTube channel under the banner of T&B Brothers. It is not that he has shut his mind to cruises. 'The Indian culture is to save money. People think why spend Rs 1-2 lakh on a cruise. I have to change that culture. I will certainly send some people on a cruise once the situation normalizes.'

3

ONE NATION, MANY BOUNDARIES

ON 3 MARCH 2020, the Delhi government held a meeting of a state task force under Chief Minister Arvind Kejriwal. The city had reported its first case of COVID-19 by then. The patient in East Delhi's Mayur Vihar had returned from Italy on 25 February. His eighty-eight contacts were tracked, of which fourteen were in Delhi and seventy-two in Uttar Pradesh. The meeting issued instructions to all the state government wings.[1] For transport entities—airport, railway, metro and bus—sanitization and surveillance measures were suggested. Five days later, on 8 March, in the second meeting of the task force, primary schools were asked to shut down till 31 March, but considering that the decision was taken when cases in Delhi were only three, and in the country only thirty-one, it appeared that the state was needlessly panicking. Surveillance, however, continued to be limited to the airport. Till then, 140,603 passengers had been screened at the Delhi airport.[2] The Union and state governments across the country initially focused only on airports.

By 19 March, things changed dramatically and the Delhi government asked private offices to allow their employees to work from home. People with comorbidities were also asked to stay at home.[3] This drastically reduced the number of people commuting in cities, especially using public transport. The same day, the Delhi Metro Rail Corporation (DMRC) curtailed its services, even though its occupancy was already down by then, since many offices in the National Capital Region (NCR) had instituted work-from-home orders. The DMRC's average daily ridership was over five million in the normal times but the curtailment of service meant that even the smaller numbers of passengers were accommodated in fewer trains.

Three days later, Delhi went in for a complete lockdown starting 23 March. It stopped all public transport and allowed only the Delhi Transport Corporation's (DTC) buses to ferry people engaged in essential services at 25 per cent capacity. 'The motorable and unmotorable borders of NCT of Delhi with the neighbouring states of Haryana and Uttar Pradesh shall be sealed. Movement of interstate buses/trains/metro (DMRC) shall be suspended,' said the order.[4] It was, however, the stopping of all domestic and international flights arriving at Delhi that ruffled feathers, with the Union government asserting its federal powers. The DGCA denied any such ban and tweeted that domestic flights to and from Delhi's Indira Gandhi International Airport would continue to operate and that the airport would remain functional. 'Domestic flights to and from IGIA Delhi shall continue to operate and the Airport shall remain functional,' DGCA said in a tweet within hours of the Delhi government announcing the closure of the city's airport.[5] This, despite the fact that from 22 March, international flights and railway passenger operations had been stopped by the Union government itself. The turf war exposed the lack of coordination between the Union government and the city that seats it, especially since a day later, the Centre itself ordered closure of all domestic commercial passenger operations from midnight of 24 March 2020.[6] The neighbouring Haryana's health and family welfare department imposed a lockdown in the districts of Gurugram, Faridabad, Sonipat, Panipat, Jhajjar, Rohtak, and Panchkula from 9 p.m. on 22 March till 31 March 2020.[7] No public transport, including taxis and autorickshaws, were permitted to ply in the state, except those for essential services or to bus stands, railway stations and airport. All commercial establishments, offices, factories, workshops and godowns were asked to shut operation except for those engaged in essential services and certain notified activities. It also shut down all interstate bus services in the whole state. This, the state government said, was needed because Haryana had in its vicinity two international airports at Delhi and Chandigarh. By then, 6,600 people who had travelled abroad or had contracted COVID-19 were under surveillance in the state.

A scenario similar to Delhi was unfolding in Mumbai, where the municipal commissioner on 20 March ordered the closure of schools, cinema halls, swimming pools, malls, etc., and asked private offices to completely shift to working from home. The Mumbai suburban rail service, which is operated by the Indian Railways, took a more cautious and gradual approach. It first shut air-conditioned services from 20 March, since the COVID-19 infection was more likely to spread in closed surroundings. The total number of trains remained the same, but with the frequent changes in the Union government's approach and the announcement of a national shutdown, this service was discontinued subsequently.

The Maharashtra government went ahead and imposed a lockdown in the entire state from 23 March. In a notification, it said that all state borders would be sealed other than for the movement of essential and perishable commodities. 'All public transport services including inter-city Maharashtra State Road Transport Corporation buses and metro will not be permitted,' said the notification. Even the plying of private vehicles was allowed only for the purpose of procuring essentials. The state borders were sealed, with the operation of all interstate bus and passenger transport services, including private vehicles, suspended.[8] This initial lockdown in the state was till 31 March 2020, but state lockdowns were soon to be overtaken by the national lockdown.

Within seven days of Gurugram shutting down on 21 March 2020, Sanjay Kumar Sharma at around 4 p.m. on 27 March drove back to Dheerpur, his ancestral village in the Alwar district of Rajasthan. The road back home was familiar but tough. Crossing the Haryana–Rajasthan state border was not easy because the national lockdown, too, was into its third day. An Uber taxi driver in Haryana's Millennium City, Sharma, however, has a knack for driving and finding his way, even if it is with the help of a navigation device. He avoided highways and police barricades, and drove through the countryside in a group of about four to five cars. 'It normally takes three hours from Sector 52 in Gurugram to my village, which is about 135 kilometre because the highway is good, but that day it took us five hours,' he says.[9]

Sharma had bought the taxi on a loan from AU Small Finance Bank in October 2019. A Reserve Bank of India relief package, however, allowed him to avail a moratorium on paying a loan instalment of about Rs 13,000 for the taxi.[10] The son of a village priest, he did not have to worry much about two meals for his family, despite the fact that they do not have agricultural landholding. The source of anxiety lay somewhere else. He was expecting his second child. More than the fear of infection for his wife and the child, it was the cost of delivery and an infant's care that made the lockdown days tough for him. He picked up odd jobs and started working as a construction worker during the four months he was in the village. This brought him Rs 300–500 a day; on some days, there was nothing. To meet the additional expenses, he took a personal loan of Rs 50,000 from a sahukar (moneylender) in his village. In September 2021, more than a year after he returned to Gurugram in July 2020, Sharma was still paying off the loan on his taxi as well as the moneylender. 'Despite all the difficulties, I am grateful to God that I have two sons now. My second son was born in a nursing home at Bansur, a town near our village,' he says. In the interim, he drove back again home after he was fined by the local police for driving without adequate supporting documents during the second wave in the summer of 2021. As per the local administration under the Mahamari Alert-Surakshit Haryana (restrictions during the second wave), movement in taxis was allowed for certain designated purposes including for passengers going to or returning from airport or railway stations or bus stations.[11]

Travel by road, whether local or interstate, was the first to see curtailment of operations in 2020. The restrictions were more local in nature, primarily to stop movement within the states and also to prevent an influx of infection from the neighbouring big cities. The Punjab government, for instance, halted all public transport from 20 March, even before the Centre decided to stop railway and airline passenger services. India's fourth COVID-19 casualty was from Punjab. The same day Tamil Nadu closed its border with Kerala. Karnataka did the same, on 22 March. Kerala was the first state to report a COVID-19 positive case in January 2020. By the time the number of countrywide cases reached 151, on 20 March, the Ministry of Road Transport and Highways asked the states to minimize travelling by public transport and consider refunding fares for advance bookings.

Just as in 2020, however, Kerala protested again in 2021 when Karnataka put in place restrictions on arrivals from the state from

16 February 2021.[12] Kerala Chief Minister Pinarayi Vijayan wrote a letter to Prime Minister Narendra Modi on 23 February 2021, complaining about the restrictions. Vijayan said the Karnataka curbs were in violation of Union government guidelines. Karnataka, however, made RT-PCR test report compulsory for drivers and their assistants on 3 March 2021, even for movement of goods from Kerala and Maharashtra on 3 March 2021.[13] The same guidelines requiring a test were imposed additionally on those coming from Punjab and Chandigarh, both by air and train, from 25 March 2021. People travelling due to medical emergency or death in the family, government functionaries and children below two years were, however, exempted, Jawaid Akhtar, additional chief secretary in the Karnataka government, said in a circular.[14] The restrictions in Kerala during the second wave were based on the concept of a 'triple lockdown.' There were three categories of restrictions on localities within the same city or town based on the severity of infection. The Kerala government lockdown measures in 2021 were more severe in many ways than in 2020.

One interesting and relevant indicator of movement within cities and states was devised by Google, which has a navigation service. It started coming out with COVID-19 Community Mobility Report from 3 April 2020, which gave a data set intended to help remediate the impact of COVID-19. Google creates daily reports with aggregated, anonymized sets of data from users who have turned on the location history setting on their phones. Though this can be turned off at any time, Google uses the anonymized data for driving the travel patterns and comparing them with the pre-COVID levels. A disclosure says the Community Mobility Reports were developed to be helpful while adhering to 'stringent privacy protocols and protecting people's privacy.' According to Google, the data is not to be 'used for medical diagnostic, prognostic or treatment purposes' nor is it intended to be used for 'guidance on personal travel plans.'

The data shows how visits to places, such as corner shops and parks, are changing in each geographic region every day.

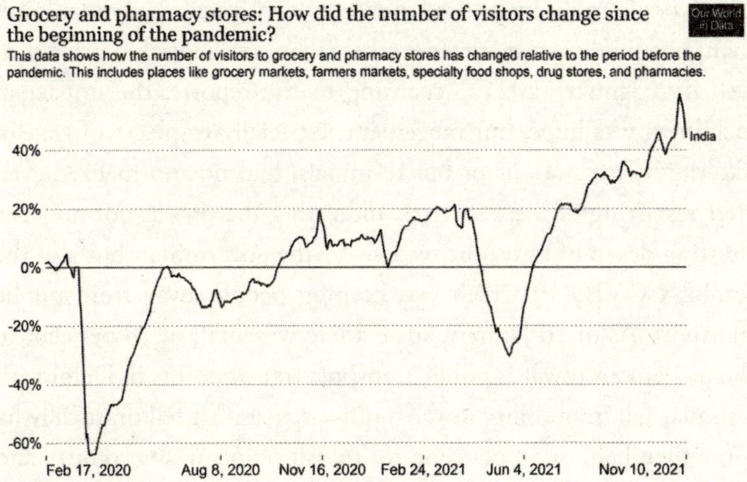
Grocery and pharmacy stores: How did the number of visitors change since the beginning of the pandemic?
Our World in Data
This data shows how the number of visitors to grocery and pharmacy stores has changed relative to the period before the pandemic. This includes places like grocery markets, farmers markets, specialty food shops, drug stores, and pharmacies.
India
40%
20%
0%
-20%
-40%
-60%
Feb 17, 2020
Aug 8, 2020
Nov 16, 2020
Feb 24, 2021
Jun 4, 2021
Nov 10, 2021

Source: Google COVID-19 Community Mobility Trends – Last updated 13 November 2021, 14.54 (London time)

Note: It's not recommended to compare levels across countries; local differences in categories could be misleading.

OurWorldData.org/coronavirus

A Google Mobility Report on how Indians reacted to the first day of lockdown on 25 March throws up some interesting data.[15] According to the mobility report, trips to retail and recreation places, grocery and pharmacy, parks, transit stations and workplaces were all down by 57–76 per cent over the baseline data, and the only place where more people were moving (about 30 per cent more) were to their homes. The baseline is the median value, for the corresponding day of the week, during the five-week period from 3 January to 6 February 2020. This fall continued, and on 25 April, there was a significant fall of 87 per cent in people movement across India for retail and recreation.

The mobility figures continued to be negative for all non-residential purposes till September-end, when the first single-digit increase started to show in the grocery and pharmacy category travel. The Google mobility reports, however, continued to show a lower than baseline movement for other than residential destinations well into January 2021. According to the reports, the impact of lockdown was huge, but movement, especially to places of transit, like the metro stations or bus terminals, had not normalized even after restarting of these services, indicating that it was not only the shutting down of transport systems by the government but also the fear of COVID-19 which was keeping people away from public transport. As of 10 January 2021, there was a fall of 18 per cent in the movement towards public transport transit points in Delhi with a similar fall in mobility towards office spaces.[16] It fell drastically by more than half, or 54 per cent, for transit points in the country and 55 per cent to workplaces on 18 May 2021, when the daily number of official COVID-19 deaths in the country touched 4,529.[17] One reason was the localized lockdowns across states due to the second wave and shutting of metro systems again. The fear factor also played a role, since even movement towards grocery and pharmacy was down about 30 per cent.[18]

State governments had put in place mechanisms to control the movement of people, especially from other cities, even before the Union government announced the national lockdown from 25 March 2020. Punjab, for instance, has a huge number of people going overseas, which was the much-feared reason for the spread of the infection. Since stopping international travel was not in its hand, the state took the strict action of curbing local transport.[19] Similarly, West Bengal first went in for closing of the border with Bhutan and Bangladesh on 14 March and 15 March, and then started intensive screening at the Sikkim and Bhutan borders.[20] Sikkim, too, had sealed its borders with other states by then.

Interestingly, however, though aviation matters were in the hands of the Centre, the Mamata Banerjee government stopped flights from cities, such as Delhi, Mumbai, Pune, Nagpur, Chennai and Ahmedabad, depending upon its assessment of the situation even after partial resumption of domestic flight operations on 25 May 2020.[21]

The restriction by states on people moving within its borders or cities was more governed by the Union home ministry's subsequent guidelines that imposed strict lockdown and curfew timings. Their insistence on cutting off links with other states and cities outside their boundaries had, however, more to do with the pressure that their health services faced because of infection carried in by travellers and passed on to their residents.

This restriction on movement was unprecedented, and its impact was particularly strong in areas such as the NCR. The closure of the Delhi–Gurgaon and Delhi–Noida borders meant traffic snarls and long queues, especially since a lot of movement for work takes place between these cities. When the impact of the lockdown unfolded, the Union government, in fact, relaxed some rules and let specified industrial and commercial activities continue outside of 'hotspots' and 'containment zones' that had a high number of COVID-19 cases and were identified by the district and state administration.[22] All persons travelling to their places of work and back in the exempted categories were allowed. On the ground, however, the situation remained different. Public transport was unavailable and state borders remained closed. The months of April and May were those of strict lockdown and overzealous ground staff creating problems for the common man. 'Any person found violating the containment measures shall be deemed to have committed an offence under section 188 of Indian Penal Code (45 of 1860),' the Haryana government had said in its order of 22 March 2020.

Well into the fourth phase of lockdown in mid-May, industrial units in Gurugram's Udyog Vihar, which borders Delhi, were still finding it difficult to resume operations, despite the relaxations allowed by the government, because owners and employees in these units did not have movement passes to enter Gurugram from Delhi.[23] At some places, labour had to jump walls and stay for the night in open areas to avoid police harassment, because the loss of one day's work meant the loss of one day's wages. Throughout the various phases of lockdown, the confusion at interstate borders continued, with each state asserting that COVID-19 cases were being exported from the adjoining state. Haryana, for instance, saw high cases in districts adjoining Delhi. On 29 May, the state's home minister, Anil Vij, ordered complete sealing of all borders with Delhi, except for essential services.[24] This happened despite a Delhi High Court intervention on 14 May.[25] The court had specifically said, 'The movement of people who man essential services as mentioned in notifications/orders/letters issued by Union of India including but not limited to government as well as private doctors, nurses, paramedics, sanitation workers, staff of Delhi Police, Delhi Transport Corporation, Delhi Jal Board, Municipal Corporations, High Courts, trial courts, etc., shall be allowed between Delhi and Haryana on the production of e-passes and they shall not be quarantined unless and until they test positive for COVID-19 or have been found in contact with COVID-19 patient.'

Days before India locked down on 25 March 2020, there was a shortage of everyday items, with long queues and empty shelves seen at many grocery stores in major cities. Online grocery delivery apps, too, were giving 'late delivery' and 'out of stock' messages. From rumours on the government coming out with some drastic measures and on the announcement of the janata curfew on 22 March, there was an anxiety build-up among consumers. Cargo movers, however, started facing problems at the ground level once the lockdown actually began for an initial phase of twenty-one days. Pick-up and delivery of goods became difficult. Confusion reigned, even though the first Union home ministry guidelines for containment of COVID-19, which came on 24 March 2020, specified that shops, including ration shops under public distribution system, dealing with food, groceries, fruits and vegetables, dairy and milk booths, meat and fish, animal fodder would be exempted from closing down shutters.[26] The guidelines, nonetheless, asked district authorities to 'encourage and facilitate home delivery to minimize the movement of individuals outside their homes.'

The ambiguity came in point six of the guidelines, which said all transport services—air, rail, roadways—would remain suspended except for 'transportation of essential goods only,' and fire, law and order, and emergency services. But what constituted essential was not clear, since government norms do not define essential goods, only essential services. The confusion was specifically around whether app-based home delivery services fell within this ambit or not.

E-commerce player Flipkart temporarily suspended taking orders on the first day of lockdown, stating that it was assessing the possibilities of operating in the lockdown. 'We are prioritising the safety of our delivery executives and seeking the support of the local governments and police authorities to meet the needs of our customers as they stay home during this lockdown,' Rajneesh Kumar, chief corporate affairs officer, Flipkart, said in a statement on 25 March. Amazon, too, stopped taking orders for some of the items, while grocery delivery services BigBasket and Grofers faced logistics issues and suspended services for some time.

As states sealed their borders, many found themselves stuck outside their homes in other states. But the biggest challenge emerged in the movement of goods. The Maharashtra government, for instance, had to clarify through a notification on 15 April that though all state borders remained sealed for passenger movement, movement of all commodities and goods, including non-essential items, was permitted.[27] Its order stated that interstate and intrastate movement of trucks and goods carrier vehicles with one driver and one additional person was allowed with valid documents, irrespective of nature of cargo, whether essential or not. No further approval was required. Empty trucks/goods carriers were also allowed to operate while on way to pick up goods or returning after completion of delivery.

The BJP government in Haryana, which had announced lockdown prior to the Union government in seven districts from 22 March, was clearer in its directive on what constituted essential and said only e-commerce (delivery) of all essential goods, including food, pharmaceuticals and medical equipment, was allowed. Besides, supply chain and related transportation were also permitted. In his order, however, Rajeev Arora, additional chief secretary in the Government of Haryana, left it to the local administration to decide what was essential. 'If there is any doubt as to whether a service is essential or not, the collector and district magistrate shall be the competent authority to decide,' said the order of 22 March 2020.[28]

In the consolidated guidelines issued on 15 April, the MHA had to further clarify that all facilities in the supply chain of essential goods, whether involved in manufacturing, wholesale or retail of such goods through local stores, large brick and mortar stores or e-commerce companies, should be allowed to operate, ensuring strict social distancing without any restriction on their timings. It further said that vehicles of e-commerce operators would be allowed to ply with necessary permissions. The ambiguity on essential and non-essential continued, but the West Bengal government cited this order to say on 27 April 2020 that sale of non-essential items was allowed through 'home delivery mode and all associated activities in the supply chain of these items are also allowed.'[29] Other states, too, started allowing e-commerce companies to deliver non-essentials as well. Since the lockdown lasted more than two months in 2020, this approach was better since people did need non-essentials and buying those could not always be postponed for very long, but physical store operators resented allowing home delivery of non-essential items since they were not allowed to open their stores. The issue again cropped up from March 2021 onwards, with states imposing localized lockdowns during the second wave. Since this wave came with more anxiety due to the lack of adequate medical infrastructure, the movement for buying even essentials, like groceries and pharmaceutical items, was down, according to Google Mobility Reports.

The very next day of issuing the first guidelines on lockdown on 24 March 2020, the MHA had to clarify that operations of railways, airports and seaports for cargo movement, relief and evacuation and their related operational organizations were exempted from the lockdown.[30] It even said there was no restriction on interstate movement of goods/cargo for inland movement and exports. The clarification, however, did not make much of a difference since even by 8 April, 90 per cent of trucks were off the roads.[31] And, well into May 2020, truckers continued to face problems at the checkpoints.

In a 10 May press note, the All India Motor Transport Congress (AIMTC), a representative body of transport associations across the country, said there were cases of corruption and harassment of truckers and transporters across the country. 'We have been receiving distress calls from truckers on roads who are not allowed to proceed by police, beaten, extorted and challaned, if extortion not paid. This is even for vehicles carrying perishable fruits and vegetables and other essential goods,' it claimed. The AIMTC alleged a day earlier that about 300 vehicles carrying fruits and vegetables bound for Delhi were stopped at Behrod (Rajasthan) for four to five hours. But when these moved on after persuading authorities, they were again stopped at the Shahjahanpur border (Rajasthan). 'The police even used lathis on drivers and broke glass panes of some vehicles to divert them back to Rajasthan. Even our late-night efforts could not help them and the haughty police personnel drove away those vehicles back to Rajasthan, which will now spoil the fruits and vegetables anyway, apart from monetary loss to the transporters. It seems that the Rajasthan Government wants scarcity of fruits and vegetables for people of Delhi,' said the AIMTC in its note.

Similar incidents, it claimed, were reported from Madhya Pradesh border checkposts. 'Most notorious of such border checkposts are Sendhwa, Balsamath, Khawasa, Chichola and Hanumana [*sic*],' it said. All this was being reported despite the MHA having clarified that agricultural operations, mandis and procurement, and production of fertilizer and seeds should be allowed to continue.[32] The direction was specifically needed since it was harvest season and annual procurement of wheat in states of Haryana and Punjab had to start.

The apex transporter body also said that the police was forcibly making truckers carry migrant labourers at Indore and Devas checkposts, and yet, they were being fined unless they paid bribes. The strongly worded AIMTC note said:

> Cases have been reported from Mizoram where four trucks carrying goods for BSNL are stopped at Baring Border in Mizoram, Eastern & Western Peripheral. Vehicles have been stopped and drivers beaten and documents taken [*sic*]. The past few days has thrown up stark reality with cases of corruption, harassment and extortion by law enforcers and their agents emanating from various parts of the country. The police, control room numbers from MHA do not help on the ground.

The problem was particularly bad for empty trucks that could not show that they were carting essential commodities. Movement between districts and between states was severely impacted and AIMTC said it received complaints of harassment from truckers in Uttar Pradesh, Rajasthan, Haryana, Bihar, Bengal, Assam, Himachal Pradesh, Mizoram and Madhya Pradesh. 'It seems dry days of lockdown have made the corrupt run amuck for want of easy money. All orders of MHA are thrown to [the] winds. Even senior officials who were earlier supportive are turning a blind eye to the woes of truckers on the ground,' it alleged.

For the Indian Railways, the situation was not so dire. With no passenger earnings, the only option for it to sustain earnings was not to let freight volumes get impacted. Railway Board chairman Vinod Kumar Yadav gave a presentation on 17 July, which showed a lesser loading compared to 2019, for April, May and June 2020.[33] Low coal loading due to reduced demand for the fuel from the power sector was one of the major reasons for the shortfall,[34] though at some places, there was also a shortfall of labour to load and unload cargo from railway premises to trucks. Last-mile connectivity was hit hard during the lockdown period.[35] The advantage of freight trains gaining record speeds due to negligible passenger train movement was being lost to the bottlenecks arising in unloading. Eventually, the Union home ministry stepped in with the formation of a group for coordination with the states.

Compared to 101 million tonne in April 2019, the loading was down to 65 million tonne in April 2020. The gap, however, was closing in by mid-July, when the Indian Railways reported 47 million tonne loading in the first sixteen days of July compared to 51 million tonne in the same period the previous year. Part of the reason that the railways were able to somehow sustain the freight loading was a bumper crop. Grain procurement by the governments reflected in increased foodgrain (rice, wheat, maize, pulses) loading over the previous year from April onwards.

From August 2020 onwards, however, the Indian Railways was able to surpass last year's total monthly loading volumes. The August loading figure was 94.3 million tonne compared to 91 million tonne in the same month in 2019.[36] This had a lot to do with the lifting of lockdown and disposal of inventory that had been lying at the manufacturing centres. Added to this was the railway strategy to offer concessions and quickly work on its freight rates. There were freight incentive schemes, which included giving rebates in the empty load direction or the return journey of wagons after they had been unloaded. Piecemeal load instead of full train load, as part of a host of measures, was also allowed in September 2020.[37]

Cargo movement picked up and the first sixteen days of December showed that the railways had caught up by achieving 110 per cent of loading over the same period the previous year. Cumulatively, however, at 811.49 million tonne, loading was still a notch less or 97 per cent of the last year. According to the Ministry of Railways, the national transporter achieved the highest-ever loading of 1,233.24 million tonne in the twelve months of 2020–21 despite the pandemic. Besides, its approximate earnings surpassed that of 2019–20 by 3 per cent, at Rs 1.17 trillion in 2020–21.[38] It said in a press release on 12 March 2021:[39]

> It is worth mentioning that a number of concessions/discounts are also being given in Indian Railways to make Railways Freight movement very attractive. Strong emergence of Business Development Units in Zones & Divisions, constant dialogue with the industry & logistics service providers, faster speed, etc are adding to the robust growth of freight business for the Railways. It may be noted that COVID-19 has been used

by Indian Railways as an opportunity to improve all-round efficiencies and performances.

Cargo movement at ports, however, had been impacted by the lockdown and also due to global factors. Besides, when there are supply bottlenecks in the hinterland, manufacturing units are shut, and there is a sudden demand slump, it is bound to reflect in cargo volumes handled at a country's ports, unlike in the case of Indian Railways, where a large portion of its freight earnings comes from coal and foodgrain, movement of which was exempted during the lockdown. Port traffic is additionally linked to a pick-up in global trade. According to the Indian Ports Association data, there was an almost 9 per cent fall in the total cargo volume handled at thirteen major ports in India between 1 April and 31 December 2020.[40] Cargo traffic during April-March 2020-21 at India's twelve major ports tracked by the Ministry of Shipping decreased by 4.6 per cent to 671.82 million tonne from 704.56 million tonne during April-March 2019-20. This was the lowest in four years and about 5 per cent lower than the previous year.[41]

Both at the ports and at the airports, cargo clogged warehouses.[42] The Ministry of Civil Aviation (MoCA) and the Directorate General of Shipping, therefore, ordered a cut in demurrage charges since the owners of cargo could not move the stuff out because of the national lockdown, which had created a shortage of both transport and manpower. Five days into the lockdown, the Director-General of Shipping issued an order acknowledging that a delay in evacuation of goods from the ports was inevitable 'due to the disturbance of the downstream services.' It said that some shipping lines, of their own volition, decided to suspend container detention charges to provide relief to importers and exporters, and to maintain proper supply lines at the seaports. The waiver, however, was made mandatory.[43]

Similarly, demurrage charges at the airports, too, were cut by half. This led to a situation where, by mid-April, more than 3,000 tonne of goods, primarily high-value products such as electronic consumer durables and automobile products, were lying at the Delhi airport.[44]

An interesting consequence of only cargo movement was that passenger aircraft were allowed to be used for moving goods. On 1 April 2020, the DGCA allowed scheduled and non-scheduled operators to use the available passenger category aircraft (without configuration change) for carriage of cargo because of 'the extra-ordinary situation the country is facing.' Certain safeguards were later added to this order and fresh guidelines were issued on 11 April.[45] This was an extra source of income for the airlines that were not allowed to carry passengers till the phased reopening of domestic operations on 25 May. Consequently, domestic scheduled carrier SpiceJet said it operated 9,950 flights carrying 77,000 tonne of cargo till 12 November. The previous month, in October, it had become the biggest Indian international cargo operator.[46] Indigo, the market leader in domestic air travel, transported cargo equivalent to the total load carried in 2019-20 within the April–August 2020 period. The airline converted ten of its passenger aircraft into full-time freight carriers, with a capacity to ferry up to 20 tonne of cargo.[47]

The story of cargo movement during the lockdown had at least one lesson for the planners. No amount of effort or relaxations, which were implemented immediately after the first set of lockdown guidelines, can keep the goods moving if the last mile of loading and unloading, done mainly through manual labour, is not sorted out. Transit, after all, is a collection of loose links, timed and well-coordinated to induce a movement.

PART II

THE UNVEILING

4

A THREE-DAY COUNTDOWN TO LOCKDOWN

WHEN PRIME MINISTER NARENDRA Modi delivered his first COVID-19-related address to the nation on 19 March 2020, he called for a people's curfew, or janata curfew, on 22 March from 7 a.m. to 9 p.m.[1] He was watched by 83 million people across 191 television channels.[2] Five days later, when the full lockdown was announced on 24 March, this viewership more than doubled to 197 million, according to Broadcast Audience Research Council. The reason for this was that everyone was anticipating drastic measures for dealing with COVID-19, which could be measures as unsettling as the demonetization of currency notes, announced by the Prime Minister in an 8 p.m. address to the nation on 8 November 2016. As later events proved, Modi through his addresses charted out an equally damaging plan to fight the contagion, albeit the trauma of which was felt for months on, with the government changing the plot every few days or sometimes within a day. It even appeared that the government was just putting out a set of rules without any plan.

In his 19 March address, Modi first prepared the ground for janata curfew by saying that the COVID-19 crisis was greater than the world wars and natural calamities, since this time, all of mankind was in crisis. 'World Wars 1 and 2 did not impact as many countries, as have been affected by Corona today.' The people's curfew, he said, was imposed for the people, by the people and on the people themselves. By saying so, Modi created an impression that the curfew was voluntary and people had a choice not to join it. The question that arose was: did ordinary people want everything to shut down and the transport connectivity to be snapped in one go? If that was not the case, then how was it being imposed 'by people' themselves? The other parts of the speech made it clear that the call for janata curfew was purely a call to do what the Prime Minister was asking to be done. So, all citizens were asked to abide by it on Sunday, 22 March: 'During this curfew, we shall neither leave our homes nor get onto the streets or roam about our localities. Only those associated with emergency and essential services will leave their homes. Friends, 22nd March will be a symbol of our effort, of our self-restraint, and our resolve to fulfil our duty in service of the nation.'

That the janata curfew was a dry run of what was to come in the form of a national lockdown just three days later was evident in the speech itself. 'The success of a people's curfew on 22nd March, and the experience gained from it, will also prepare us for our upcoming challenges. I urge all state governments to take leadership in ensuring compliance of this people's curfew,' said Modi. This clearly indicated that it was not going to be a one-day affair and challenges were coming. Ordinary people, however, did not know what form they would take or how big or wide these would be.

Modi also wanted people to express their gratitude to doctors, nurses, hospital staff, sanitation workers, airlines employees, government staff, police personnel, the media, people associated with trains and buses, autorickshaw services and home delivery agents for selflessly serving others. The seriousness of the impact of a curfew or subsequent lockdown, however, was watered down by the way the Prime Minister wanted them to express this gratitude. 'On Sunday (22 March) at exactly 5 p.m., we all stand at the doors, balconies, windows of our homes, and give them all a five-minute standing ovation. We clap our hands, beat our plates, ring our bells to boost their morale, salute their service. To inform people about this, I request local authorities across the country to ring a siren at 5 p.m. on 22 March,' he said. Perhaps this idea occurred to the Indian Prime Minister from countries such as Spain, Italy and Denmark,[3] where citizens came to their balconies and clapped as part of a social media campaign called Clap for Carers or #AplausoSanitario (I applaud health services)[4] in Spanish. Indians, too, reciprocated to Modi's call by banging and clapping across the country with enthusiasm.

This show of empathy played out false festivities that were in stark contrast to the panic on the ground, since by then, the supply of essential daily items had already started to run out in the markets. Even the Prime Minister in his address acknowledged this. He tried to reassure the citizens that all steps necessary were being taken to ensure there was no shortage of essential items such as milk, groceries and medicines. 'I thus urge all my fellow citizens to make purchases as normal, and not hoard essential items in panic buying,' he said.

Before this mega one-day event, offices had already started asking their employees to work from home. The business continuation departments of large companies had begun to put plans in place to facilitate remote operations. In smaller set-ups, like those of newspapers and other media, however, the decision-makers were averse to giving their employees a work-from-home option. But, forced by the rules of local governments, offices had to function with bare minimum staff. According to a March 2020 report by Gartner, a global research and consultancy service company, a survey of 800 global human resource executives on 17 March 2020 found that 88 per cent of organizations encouraged or required employees to work from home, regardless of whether or not they showed coronavirus-related symptoms. Nearly all organizations (97 per cent) cancelled work-related travel. This figure on work-related travel was more than an 80 per cent increase over similar findings on 3 March.[5]

In India, the IT hub of Gurugram in Haryana had already seen curtailment of operations, with district magistrate Amit Khatri issuing orders for closure of gymnasiums, cinema halls, shopping malls, weekly bazaars, among others, as early as 18 March. This was followed by the Haryana government's health and family welfare department imposing a lockdown in the districts of Gurugram, Faridabad, Sonipat, Panipat, Jhajjar, Rohtak and Panchkula from 9 p.m. on 22 March itself till 31 March 2020 under Section 2 of the Epidemic Disease Act, 1897.[6] All commercial establishments, offices, factories, workshops and godowns were asked to shut operations except for essential services and certain notified activities. No public transport, including taxis and autorickshaws, were permitted to ply except those for essential services or to bus stands, railway stations and the airport. Clearly, the Haryana government, like other state governments, did not know that railways stations, bus stands and airports would be shut too.

The janata curfew marked a total transport shutdown that came without warning and completely snapped physical contact between places, people and families, especially for those in the lower segment of society who did not have their own vehicles. Train and metro services across the country stopped. The country's largest metro system, the DMRC, announced that it had decided to keep its services closed on 22 March. 'The move is aimed at encouraging people to stay indoors and maintain social distancing, which is essential in the fight against COVID-19,' the DMRC said in a tweet on 20 March.[7]

The Indian Railways, too, curtailed services and came out with a statement at 8.14 p.m. on 21 March 2020, saying that it anticipated 'vastly reduced' demand during the janata curfew and asked the zonal railways to therefore cancel services.[8] Strangely, a differential approach was followed for different categories of trains. While all passenger trains starting less than four hours later, or from midnight of 21 March, stood cancelled, all long-distance mail/express and intercity trains, including premium trains, starting between 4 a.m. and 10 p.m. on 22 March, were cancelled. For railway passenger services, this shutting down was to continue well into April. There were, however, no such curbs on domestic air service on the janata curfew day.

Train number 02198, a weekly special from Jabalpur Junction to Coimbatore, and its reverse direction service 02197 from Coimbatore to Jabalpur, may hardly be central to the working of trains in India, but in the railway history, these were the first trains that were cancelled for two weeks on 21 March and 28 March 2020 and on 23 March and 30 March, due to the outbreak of the COVID-19 pandemic in India.[9] The announcement of the cancellation came on 18 March, by when the Indian Railways had already started issuing advisories for meeting any eventuality arising out of COVID-19, including creating quarantine facilities within its premises. Clearly, no one at the Railway Board, the apex body that runs the railway network through zonal wings, knew the magnitude of what was to come just five days later, though four more trains were cancelled on 19 March through another order.[10] How the running of these trains was adding to the spread of COVID-19 no one could tell, but the reason behind their cancellation was commercial. There were low bookings for the trains. People were not willing to travel and even before the government shut the transport lines, many had cut back on their travel plans. At the same time, railway authorities asked passengers to avoid non-essential train journeys and ensure that they did not have fever at the time of commencement of journey. At any point during a journey, if a passenger felt that they had a fever, they were to contact the railway staff for medical attention and further assistance.[11]

As daily advisories from most Union and state government departments started to pour in, the railways was doing their bit to restrict travel. Besides cancelling trains, it decided to withdraw travel concessions as well. It reduced the categories of travellers who were entitled to avail of concessions.[12] Of 55 of them, 23 sub-categories under patients, students and divyangjans (differently abled) were allowed the concessions for both unreserved and reserved segments from 20 March. Those who had already booked tickets availing of the concessions were, however, also allowed the discounted fare. Among those for whom travel concessions were withdrawn were senior citizens, since they were the most vulnerable category of the population. What came on 22 March 2020, nonetheless, was a complete shocker: the Indian Railways stopped all passenger trains, something it had never done before on its own.[13]

A little over forty-six years ago was the only time that the railway services had halted countrywide, though the Indira Gandhi government had roped in the territorial army to run train services. It was on 8 May 1974 that the All India Railwaymen's Federation (AIRF) decided to implement a national rail strike after forty-four-year-old socialist leader and organizer of the strike, George Fernandes, and more than 1,000 other union leaders were arrested.[14]

Just a few days earlier, S. Dhasarathy, a young railway engineer, was asked to move to Erode as divisional mechanical engineer in charge of the railway diesel shed there. It was the evening of 1 May, and his sister's marriage celebrations were going on in his house in Chennai when Dhasarathy received the posting order. With his eight-month pregnant wife, he left the same day for a 400 km journey in a taxi. 'There weren't any trains running so I had to hire the car. It took about nine hours,' he says.[15] The Indian Railways never reimbursed the fare, he rues, adding that it was quite a large amount for those days. On reaching Erode, the task was clear. He had to see that a goods train coming from Punjab found its way to Palakkad in Kerala. 'Two drivers and I, we went and managed to run a goods train around 2 a.m. By the time others woke up and could stop the train, it had gone past.'

Dhasarathy, who had served in the Territorial Army for five years after being enlisted during the 1965 war with Pakistan, when he was barely a month into the Indian Railway service, was against the strike. 'How can a government agency strike for bonus? Bonus is for everybody and not based on actual performance. It can be given to everybody; it is government money, not your money,' he says. The priority was to run goods trains even then, just as in the summer of 2020, since a large number of essentials, such as foodgrain, coal and fertilizer, move by rail. 'Kerala would have starved if we had waited for eight or ten more days. We started running passenger trains within five-six days after that (after running the goods trains).'

For him, it was also crucial to keep the diesel shed operational. 'They told us not to attend to locomotives at the shed. It was not that we were against each other. There were 3,000 people in Erode under my administrative control. I was not a very senior person because I had done just eight or nine years of service (five years in the army and three years in the railways), but railway men generally listen to their boss if they know he is honest and does not mean them ill.' On whether he felt threatened by the supporters of the strike, he said, 'We got an FIR [first information report filed with police] against those four-five people. The Indian Railways also started giving jobs to sons of those employees who did not support the strike.'

It is not, however, entirely true that the railway staff was not largely supportive of the strike. The build-up to the 1974 historic strike, in fact, was disruptive for the Indian Railways. Before the strike, Lalit Narayan Mishra, the then railway minister, lamented frequent disruption of work. 'So far as staff discipline is concerned, this has been a particularly bad year for the Indian Railways. From the very beginning, we have been hit by go-slow, work-to-rule and work-to-designation agitations, mass absenteeism, wildcat strikes, bandhs, squatting on track, etc. While the agitations unconnected with railway operation impeded our working, the effect of employee agitations has been particularly crippling. Among such agitations are the lightning strike of station masters and assistant station masters during April on Western Railway, the successive strikes and agitations by loco running staff in May, July, August and December which affected most of the Zonal Railways and the agitation by staff of Sholapur division on the South Central Railway during August and September,' he noted in his speech of 27 February 1974, more than two months before the strike, while presenting the railway budget for 1974–75.[16] Mishra was killed on 2 January 1975 in a bomb blast at the Samastipur railway station in Bihar, for which four, including three Ananda Margas (members of the Ananda Marga organization), were sentenced to death much later, in 2014.[17]

A month and a half after Mishra's killing, when Kamalapati Tripathi presented the Railway Budget for 1975–76 on 20 February 1975, he assessed the damage caused by the strike. He noted:

> Shortly after the strike was called off, a rapid re-appraisal revealed that in the three months of April to June (1974), 11.8 million tonne of freight traffic had been lost. It was realized that the originating traffic during the year would not exceed 197 million tonne, made up of 173 million tonne of revenue earning traffic and 23.8 million tonne of departmental traffic. Passenger traffic had also declined as the number of passengers carried was nearly 150 million less than in the corresponding period of the previous year. Other coaching earnings had also suffered. Consequently, in the first quarter, railway earnings dropped by Rs 92.45 crore [924.5 million] as compared with the Budget proportion.[18]

Fares and freight rates had to be raised 'to recoup the anticipated deficiency of Rs 140 crore [1,400 million] in earnings.'

If the strike had halted railway operations while it was on, it was the shortage of locomotive coal that led to the curtailment of certain passenger trains afterwards. 'The fall in non-suburban passenger traffic beyond the strike-affected period is mainly due to cancellation of trains. The Hon'ble Members know that faced with the shortage of loco coal, the railway administration had to curtail some of their branch line passenger train services. Now that the production of coal has begun to gather momentum, it should be possible for us to build up our stocks. Subject to this contingency, restoration of cancelled trains will be commenced from the first of March, and progressively increased in the next few months,' said Tripathi in his railway budget speech.[19]

The summer of 2020 was, however, different. Operating trains did not pose a security risk, but a health risk. Besides, it was the government that pulled the chain on passenger trains, even as the Indian Railways kept the freight trains rolling. But the scale of operations is much larger now than at the time of the strike in 1974. The Indian Railways could carry only around 200 million tonne of freight in 1975, compared to 1.21 billion tonne annually in 2019–20. It carried 2.7 billion passengers then and 8.4 billion passengers before COVID-19 struck. During the twelve months leading up to March 2021, however, which included two months of national lockdown, it carried a marginally higher freight volume of 1.23 billion tonne, though passenger traffic fell by about 90 per cent over the normal times.[20]

This time, the Indian Railways first issued instructions to its zones on 21 March that no passenger trains would originate from any railway station in the country from 7 a.m. to 10 p.m. on 22 March because of the janata curfew announced by Prime Minister Narendra Modi.[21] A press release was issued at 8.14 p.m. for the same, but it didn't take even twenty-four hours for the Indian Railways to make another announcement, at 1.48 p.m. on 22 March, that all trains would be stopped till 31 March 2020.

Domestic commercial flights stopped three days later, from 25 March 2020 onwards. This was announced on the evening of 23 March, which meant that unlike in the case of the railways, there was more than a day's notice for air travellers, though it was not much help for those caught away from home, since airlines started bunching flights together and changing schedules at short notice. A three-line statement from the MoCA issued to the media said, 'Airlines have to plan operations so as to land at their destination before 23.59 hours on 24 March 2020.'[22]

There was no clear reason why trains were stopped before domestic air journeys, or why the Union government decided to first pin down the Delhi government by asserting its federal right on aviation matters, overruling the state's decision to shut the Delhi airport on 22 March, and then doing precisely this from 25 March.

This, despite the fact that those travelling by air after a foreign journey or touching down at airports were probably more likely to transmit the infection (because they were coming from outside the country) than those travelling by train. It is true, though, that the number of train travellers and the difficulty of screening passengers at railway stations or in trains was more daunting than at airports.

Opposition leaders claimed that the government wanted to keep running Parliament to make the point that the Madhya Pradesh state assembly could also meet and vote on a no-confidence motion against the Kamal Nath-led Congress government, and that COVID-19 could not come in the way of legislative work. 'It is obvious, Parliament was run only to ensure that the Madhya Pradesh Assembly could run and the Congress government be toppled,' the embittered Nath told media persons later.[23] He said the nationwide lockdown was announced a day after the Shivraj Singh Chauhan-led BJP government was installed in Madhya Pradesh. Airlines needed to operate to ferry politicians and legislators.

On 31 March, a *Business Standard* news analysis said, 'The initial approach followed by the Indian Railways and airlines was to cancel services on those routes where the occupancy was low. For commercial airlines, it did not make sense to fly to, say, China, Italy and Iran, which reported initial COVID-19 casualties, because business travellers had stopped going to these countries anyway. Besides, their staff was risking exposure to the virus by travelling to those destinations.'[24]

The railways, too, had started cancelling low-occupancy trains because of the pandemic. This approach ran contrary to the messages of social distancing, the first rule of which was to avoid crowding. It should not have followed the same approach as the airlines, for two reasons. One, it is the crucial lifeline for long-distance travellers, especially for those who do not have airports in their city or cannot afford flights. Second, it should have ensured that trains were not crowded during the peak period; instead, it could run more trains, just as it does for Holi and Diwali. 'Running two-three trains for four-five days would have saved harassment. It was an unplanned situation,' says Shanti Narain, former member (traffic), Railway Board.[25]

Even the normally efficient the DMRC took decisions that dangerously contradicted social distancing norms. On 19 March, it curtailed its services, even though its occupancy was already down by then, since many offices in the NCR had instituted work-from-home protocols. 'This meant that even the smaller numbers of passengers were accommodated in fewer trains. Delhi Metro's average daily ridership is over 5 million,' says the article.[26] The Mumbai suburban train services, which the Indian Railways runs, took a more cautious and gradual approach, perhaps because of the directions from the state government. It first shut air-conditioned services on 20 March, since the COVID-19 infection was more likely to spread in closed spaces. The total number of trains remained the same.

The other perplexing approach was that the Indian Railways always gave a date till when passenger services would be shut. It first said on 21 March that services would be cancelled for 22 March because of janata curfew but, the very next day, announced the services would remain cancelled till 31 March 2020. Then, on 25 March, it announced that the cancellation had been extended to 14 April, or the end of the first phase of lockdown. In five days, three different end dates had been announced till which passenger services were to remain cancelled. Obviously, the Ministry of Railways (MoR) had no clue what decisions would come from the higher-ups in the government, and so the confusion for the 23 million people on average who travelled on trains daily (prior to the pandemic) in the year leading to 31 March 2019 was immense.

The initial cancellation of train services for passengers for the duration of the first lockdown phase till 14 April 2020 also showed that the government anticipated that trains could be run once the virus transmission chain was broken at the end of the twenty-one-day period.

Even the domestic air travel circulars had this ad hocism about them. The first circular suspended domestic air service till 31 March. On the last day of domestic air travel, 24 March, both airlines and passengers were equally at sea. In a report, news website Moneycontrol.com said airlines had three important tasks at hand: to get their crew back home, to park their aircraft, and to process requests from customers. 'The first two tasks are unprecedented as never have the country's entire fleet been grounded at the same time. All airlines put together have about 660 aircraft,' it said.[27] The last time an airport in the country had parking woes was back in 2010, when the volcano eruption in Iceland forced airlines to ground their fleet. Many international airlines' aircraft were stuck in Delhi's Indira Gandhi International Airport, and its runway twenty-seven became a parking lot, the report recounted.

Sensing that drastic measures were coming, many had reached the places where their families lived by either booking themselves on flights early or narrowly taking the last flight home. But for some who landed at airports in cities such as Delhi and Mumbai, which had already shut down, getting public transport for the last-mile connectivity was a challenge.

An airhostess with Air India explained how she flew from Tokyo on the last day of international flights on 22 March. 'It was a very tense situation because everything was shutting down. While deplaning, some passengers had tears in their eyes and said, "You were our last hope." They clapped for us in appreciation,' she said. Due to the sensitivity of her job, she does not want her name to be printed but recalls how, once back from that last flight, she faced some of the tensest moments of her life for the next two weeks. 'Local authorities put up a poster outside our house, too, since both my husband and I had returned from overseas—I from Tokyo and he from Dubai. The way people looked at these posters was as if we had the disease,' she recollects. She had already sent her mother-in-law and six-year-old daughter to a relative's house. 'Initially, for four-five days, I felt a bit relaxed, but then I started missing them. There was constant surveillance outside our house to ensure that we did not step out.' One day, a policeman, too, knocked at their door, asking if they needed something or wanted to go somewhere. But stocking up essentials at home before this crisis helped them at that point.

She lamented how people accused the airline crew of bringing COVID-19 into their locality during the lockdown in 2020. When the second wave started to build up in February 2021, she asked, 'Aren't those going all over and not behaving responsibly the ones spreading the infection now? A lot of our crew in Mumbai and Delhi were hounded by neighbours with localities not allowing entry to them [during the initial phase of COVID-19 in 2020].'

Air India issued a statement after its staff was harassed in a number of places. 'It is alarming to note that in many localities, vigilante resident welfare associations and neighbours have started ostracizing the crew, obstructing them from performing their duty or even calling in the polices, simply because the crew travelled abroad in the course of their duty ... These vigilantes have conveniently forgotten that many a spouse, parent, sibling, child and near and dear ones have been brought home safe and secure from affected countries, thanks to the heroic efforts of these Air India crew,' said the airline statement.[28]

For the passengers who had not anticipated the scale of the lockdown measures or even the severity and nimbleness of COVID-19, and had booked themselves on trains and flights, the rules of refund were confounding. Even though, unlike trains, airline services are run by private operators as well as public ones, the unprecedented shutting down of services demanded that the government spell out the rules for the refunding of both railway and airline tickets. Left to themselves, these operators who were hit hard by the shutting down of services would not have wanted to return the money. The Indian Railways first said a full refund for all cancelled trains could be claimed till 21 June 2020. To make it more convenient for passengers, it said adequate arrangements would be made to facilitate hassle-free refunds to passengers affected by train cancellations. All rules for e-tickets remained the same, since a passenger did not need to come to a railway station for the refund of their ticket. This relaxation was for the three-month journey period from 21 March to 21 June 2020, said a railways statement dated 21 March 2020,[29] which was issued just about an hour before the announcement of stopping of trains on 22 March. '[The] Indian Railways has advised passengers to avoid non-essential travel and sudden crowding of trains or the refund counters which will only raise [the] possibility of spread of the Corona virus,' said the statement's last line.

Obviously, the Indian Railways had not anticipated that the lockdown and curfew timings would force a further extension of the refund period. So seven days later, on 28 March, a new statement said, 'In view of [the] cancellation of all passenger trains and all passenger ticketing up to 14 April 2020, it has been decided by the Indian Railways to give a full refund for all tickets for journey period from 21st March-14th April 2020. These instructions shall be in addition to and in continuation of the relaxations in refund rules vide instructions dated 21-03-2020.'[30] Refunds for railway tickets were again allowed in two categories: those booked at the counter, and e-tickets. For those who had booked their tickets prior to 27 March 2020, the balance refund amount was to be given, while for those who had booked tickets after that date, a full refund was provided.

The Indian Railways had, in the past, benefitted from waitlisted passengers who had neither undertaken the journey nor claimed a refund. A Press Trust of India report dated 25 February 2020 quoted an RTI query to report that the Indian Railways earned over Rs 9,000 crore from ticket cancellation charges and non-cancellation of waitlisted tickets between 2017 and 2020. The report said:

> The Centre for Railway Information Systems (CRIS), in response to the RTI application filed by Kota-based activist Sujeet Swami, said that in the three-year period from January 1, 2017 to January 31, 2020, there were over 95 million passengers whose wait-listed tickets were not cancelled. Such passengers brought the Indian Railways revenue of over Rs 4,335 crore. In the same period, the Railways earned over Rs 4,684 crore from cancellation fees of confirmed tickets. In both segments, the earnings were maximum from sleeper class tickets, followed by third AC travellers, the RTI response revealed.[31]

Swami filed a plea in the Rajasthan High Court, alleging that the reservation policy of the Indian Railways was discriminatory. He argued a differential policy was adopted for online bookings and for reservations done through booking counters, which created problems for passengers while earning revenue for the Indian Railways. Refund is automatic when booking is done online, while refund for booking done through counters is not automatic if a journey is not undertaken. This argument would have held true even in the lockdown period, though this time, those seeking refunds of tickets booked through the Indian Railway Catering and Tourism Corporation (IRCTC) did not get the convenience fee back.

Since each lockdown guideline was coming with an end date, the Indian Railways continued booking tickets for beyond that date. Railway reservations could be done for 120 days ahead. According to an estimate used by a *Business Line* report, assuming a convenience fee of Rs 15 a ticket, the IRCTC collected at least Rs 14.1 crore on 9.4 million tickets booked for travel between 22 March and 3 May.[32] The convenience fee goes to [the] IRCTC for running the ticketing system, while the rail fare goes to the Indian Railways. '[The] IRCTC incurs a fixed expenditure of Rs 57 lakh per day for running the ticketing system,' an official was quoted as saying. 'That convenience has already been offered in booking a ticket and [the] IRCTC has rendered its service. Since the Railways could not offer the service of transporting a passenger from point A to B during the lockdown, it is giving full refund on the rail fare,' he said.

After such reports started appearing, the Indian Railways decided to correct this by stopping the booking of tickets from 15 April till further orders. A railways statement said:

> No booking of any type of tickets, including E tickets shall be done till further advice. However, facility of online cancellation will remain functional for ticket bookings. All counters for ticket booking for UTS & PRS will remain closed till further orders. Full refund will be given for tickets for the bookings made for the trains cancelled. Full refund will also be there for those cancelling the advance bookings of tickets for trains not yet cancelled.[33]

India had entered the second phase of lockdown, and it was decided that trains would remain cancelled till 3 May. So for trains cancelled up to 3 May 2020, the refunds would be automatically remitted to the customers by the railways online, while those who had booked their tickets physically at counters could take their refunds by 31 July 2020.

For airlines, however, the DGCA issued clear instructions on 16 April 2020 for cases in which refunds could be directly credited to the account of fliers.[34] It asked airlines to refund the entire ticket amount with no cancellation charges within three weeks of receiving the request for cancellation. Till then, the period of travel for which tickets were being cancelled was the first and second phases of lockdown, scheduled to end on 3 May. Prior to these instructions, there was uncertainty, with the Indian Railways continuing to take bookings beyond the first lockdown period or from 15 April onwards, but airlines, barring the government-owned Air India, was more conservative and decided not to sell tickets.[35] 'The government should be more proactive regarding such decisions. If we don't book tickets anticipating a ban we will lose out on revenue. If we sell and then have to cancel flights, we will face passenger ire. Bureaucrats should have some sensitivity to how businesses are done,' an airline executive was quoted in a 13 April 2020 *Business Standard* report. The DGCA eventually decided to issue instructions to airlines on 19 April 2020, asking them not to take future bookings. 'All airlines are hereby directed to refrain from booking tickets as described above. Further the airlines may note that they shall be given sufficient notice and time for restarting of operations,' it said.[36]

Despite instructions from the government, however, airline refunds for many passengers of private airlines came in the form of credit shells that could be availed for later travel. These shells were like wallets in which airlines kept the refunded amount, which could be used for buying tickets later. These credit shells ensured that the airlines did not have any liquidity problems because they did not need to immediately pay cash. On 1 October 2020, however, the Supreme Court issued an order, after clubbing five petitions filed by Pravasi Legal Cell & Others, Colonel (retired) Ashok Prehar, Travel Agents Federation of India and Air Passengers Association of India. Pravasi Legal Cell had argued that though it was obligatory on the part of the respondent—airlines, operating domestic as well as international flights—to refund the full amount collected for the tickets because of the cancellation of flights, they were providing a credit shell with the validity of one year, which was contrary to Civil Aviation Requirements (CAR) of May 2008. 'It is alleged that as per the CAR, the option of holding refund amount in credit shell by the airlines is the prerogative of a passenger and cannot be a default practice of the airline,' said Pravasi Legal in its petition.[37] It quoted the office memorandum of 16 April 2020, issued by the MoCA, while stating that it dealt only with the refund of tickets that were booked during the lockdown period, and left out the majority of passengers who had booked tickets before flights were halted. Col. (retired) Prehar and another petitioner sought the quashing of the same memorandum. He had been denied a refund by Air India for tickets booked by his family on 18 December 2019, to travel to the US on 8 May 2020, with a return ticket to India for 5 June 2020. This, he petitioned, was 'illegal, arbitrary and contrary' to CAR. They sought directions to refund the full amount of Rs 166,434 collected by Air India.

The third petition was filed by the Air Passengers Association of India and the fourth by the Travel Agents Federation of India, pleading the same arguments. The government however, contended that if any enforcement action was initiated by the DGCA for violations of CAR, it would result in 'reduction/suspension of approved schedule of airline, who have already started operating their flights with limited capacity.' In its affidavit, the MoCA stated that any such strict enforcement action against an airline would 'further restrict/reduce their operation and any such strict enforcement action may further jeopardise the possibility of generation of cash by the airline which can further adversely affect/delay the refund cycle.' Clearly, the government didn't want airlines to bleed and shut down because of the ban on flying. The ministry even submitted a refund plan covering domestic travel tickets booked directly through airlines or through a travel agent, and for international tickets on Indian carriers or foreign carriers but ex-India (from India). These were 'formulations arrived at to harmonise the interests of passengers and the viability of airlines to an extent.'

The Supreme Court order of 1 October 2020 laid down the contours of the refund process based on the government's suggestions. It made a distinction between tickets booked prior to lockdown and during the lockdown. For bookings done during the lockdown, when airlines knew that flights might not be able to take off, an immediate refund was to be given. 'In all other cases, the airlines shall make all endeavours to refund the collected amount to the passenger within 15 days from today. If on account of financial distress, any airline/airlines are not able to do so, they shall provide credit shell, equal to the amount of fare collected, in the name of passenger when the booking is done either directly by the passenger or through travel agent so as to consume the same on or before 31 March 2021,' said the order.[38] This option was given to help airlines tide over their financial distress. The credit shells were transferable to other routes or other persons.

The shutting down of services directly hit airlines, the Indian Railways and the IRCTC. Indigo, the country's largest airline by passenger numbers, recorded a loss of Rs 2,849.39 crore for the three months of April, May and June 2020.[39] This quarterly loss was higher than even its highest-ever annual profit of Rs 2,242.3 crore, which it recorded in 2017–18. It carried 32.6 million domestic passengers in the January–December 2020 period, which was less than half of 67.9 million the airline had carried in the year 2019.[40]

For the IRCTC, a railway online booking and catering company, the shutting down of train services translated to a quarterly loss of Rs 24.6 crore in the first year of it being listed on the Bombay

Stock Exchange. This was during the April–June 2020 period. The IRCTC's bread-and-butter business of catering, which accounts for 46 per cent of its revenue in a normal year, took a hit even after some railway services were resumed. 'COVID-19 proved an unanticipated derailment. On average, the company was booking 825,000 tickets daily through its platform in 2019–2020 but in April and May, the lockdown rendered those bookings down to zero. Instead, the company had to refund tickets,' said a *Business Standard* article.[41] The IRCTC chairman and managing director Mahendra Pratap Mall is quoted as saying, 'We were doing an average 850,000 tickets a day just before the lockdown. Now (in December 2020), we are doing 500,000 on an average, but in the last week of November it touched 650,000 since bookings for Holi started 120 days in advance.' Pre-COVID-19, the air-conditioned (AC) class accounted for about 30 per cent of bookings through the IRCTC's platforms, and it earned Rs 40 a ticket. AC class tickets dropped to 10 per cent, since 90 per cent of the IRCTC's bookings in December 2020 were coming from the non-AC class, for which it earns Rs 20 a ticket as commission.

For those people working for these service providers, the impact of the lockdown might not have been as severe as it was for those on the fringes of society, but nonetheless, it came in the form of job losses. The government, too, admitted to this. 'Based on continuous monitoring of the operations of airline carriers since the outbreak of the COVID-19 pandemic and the reports received from airlines, it has been observed that airline carriers have been severely affected due to restrictions on domestic and international passenger movements,' the then Union minister of civil aviation Hardeep Singh Puri said in the Rajya Sabha in reply to a question by Narain Dass Gupta on 10 February 2021.[42] Full-time and contractual employment by the airlines was 74,887 as of 31 March 2020 but it fell 9 per cent to 67,906 by 30 September 2020.

The fall in employment might not appear substantial, but it was accompanied by salary cuts for the remaining employees. While announcing job cuts on 20 July 2020, Indigo, for instance, said:

> From where things stand currently, it is impossible for our company to fly through this economic storm without making some sacrifices, in order to sustain our business operations. Therefore, after carefully assessing and reviewing all possible scenarios, it is clear that we will need to bid a painful adieu to 10 per cent of our workforce. It is for the first time in the history of IndiGo that we have undertaken such a painful measure. This is indeed a very unfortunate turn of events from the optimistic growth trajectory we had carved out for ourselves just six months ago; but this pandemic has forced us to re-evaluate our best laid plans.[43]

Deccan Air even closed down during the lockdown in April 2020.[44] An email by Air Deccan chief executive officer Arun Kumar Singh to employees was quoted in media reports, giving the lockdown as a reason for shutting down of service. 'In view of the recent global and domestic issues and subsequent directive by the Indian regulator (to suspend all commercial passenger flights till 14 April), Air Deccan has no choice but to cease its operations until further notice.' The airline did not restart operations.

To another parliamentary question posed by K.C. Venugopal on 3 February 2021, Puri replied that the employment at airports reduced from 67,760 as of 31 March 2020 to 48,513 on 30 September 2020.[45] This was a 28 per cent drop. Equally drastic was the 34 per cent fall in employment at ground handling agencies, which fell from 37,720 on 31 March 2020 to 25,074 on 30 September 2020. The employment at cargo operators reduced from 9,555 on 31 March 2020 to 9,385 on 30 September 2020.

Alongside, SkyGourmet, an inflight caterer, shut its kitchens at Delhi and Mumbai airports, impacting about 1,300 employees, according to a 19 February 2021 *Times of India* news report.[46] Part of the reason was the non-renewal of its lease, but low traffic, even after a graded resumption of flight operations, had hit the company hard.

According to the minister's reply in the Rajya Sabha, domestic passenger traffic fell from 119.9 million (119,945,632) during March–December 2019 to 37.8 million (37,779,592) during March–December 2020, while international passenger traffic fell from 19.7 million (19,664,179) to 1.9 million (1,855,033). The revenues of major Indian scheduled carriers fell from Rs 46,711 crore during April–September 2019 to about Rs 11,810 crore during April–September 2020. Even though there was no restriction on cargo movement, the handling of domestic air cargo fell from 1.15 million tonne (MT) during March–December 2019 to 0.72 MT during March–December 2020, while international air cargo handled fell from 1.74 MT to 1.19 MT. The revenue of Airports Authority of India (AAI) airports reduced from Rs 12,837 crore during 2019–20 to an estimated revenue of around Rs 4,755 crore in 2020–21.

The pandemic year of 2020–21 saw all Indian airports together handling 1.19 million aircraft movements, which fell by more than half from 2.6 million (2,601,670) in 2019–20. The fall in the number of passengers was even sharper at 67 per cent, with 115.51 million people flying in 2020–21 instead of 346.28 million in 2019–20.

5

A NATION LOCKED DOWN

> Every state of the country, every union territory, every district, every municipality, every village, every [*sic*] street, every locality is being put under lockdown.
>
> —Prime Minister Narendra Modi, 24 March 2020

INDIA WENT INTO LOCKDOWN on 25 March 2020 after less than four hours' notice to its residents. That day, the country's total number of confirmed cases of COVID-19 was 562, and nine had died of the disease, said a WHO situation report.[1] The disease was at the local transmission stage, which, according to the WHO definition, meant the source of infection was within the reporting location. A day earlier, in a speech at 8 p.m. on 24 March, Prime Minister Narendra Modi had announced a twenty-one-day lockdown, which led to some of the worst horrors in the lives of the poorest of the population.

In numbers, the COVID-19 infection and the resultant deaths probably did not look high enough to warrant drastic action, but by then, some states and cities had already gone ahead and announced some form of lockdown. And the Union government was understandably under pressure to contain the spread, which it thought could be best done through a nationwide lockdown. The Prime Minister quoted WHO to say that a person infected with coronavirus could transmit it to hundreds of people within the span of a week to ten days. 'It took sixty-seven days for the count of people infected with corona to reach the first one lakh [100,000] all over the world. After this, it took only eleven days for another one lakh people to get infected. What is even more alarming is that it took only four days for this number to go from two lakh [200,000] to three lakh [300,000] infections. You can imagine how rapidly coronavirus spreads. And once it begins to spread, it is very difficult to contain,' Modi said in his 24 March speech while justifying the need to impose the lockdown.[2]

Modi marvelled at the success of his 22 March curfew, and said, 'Every Indian made janata curfew a success. Through a single day of janata curfew, India proved that when the nation is facing a crisis, when humanity is facing a crisis, every Indian comes together to overcome it. All of you deserve praise for ensuring the success of janata curfew.'[3] Each time the Modi government placed a restriction on its people to contain COVID-19, the Prime Minister made it sound as if it was a people's decision or a matter of choice. Keeping in mind the advice of health-sector experts and the experiences of other countries, 'the nation is about to take a very important decision,' he said. 'From midnight today, the entire country, please listen carefully, the entire country shall go under complete lockdown. In order to protect the country, and each of its citizens, from midnight tonight, a complete ban is being imposed on people from stepping out of their homes.' The lockdown, the Prime Minister said, was a critical step in 'the decisive fight against the corona pandemic.'

On the first of India's lockdown on 25 March, Dr Tedros Adhanom Ghebreyesus, director general, WHO, at around

10 p.m. India time, raised a pertinent point: whether lockdowns were successful would depend on what countries did while they were in place. 'To slow the spread of COVID-19, many countries have introduced unprecedented measures, at significant social and economic cost—closing schools and businesses, cancelling sporting events and asking people to stay home and stay safe. We understand that these countries are now trying to assess when and how they will be able to ease these measures,' he said in his opening remarks to a media briefing.[4]

The answer, he said, depended on what countries did while such population-wide measures were in place. 'Asking people to stay at home and shutting down population movement is buying time and reducing the pressure on health systems. But on their own, these measures will not extinguish epidemics. The point of these actions is to enable the more precise and targeted measures that are needed to stop transmission and save lives. We call on all countries who have introduced so-called "lockdown" measures to use this time to attack the virus.' As the second wave of 2021 showed, however, India had wasted its lockdown period and the hardships that came with it, because it was no better prepared, or prepared to any degree, for the pandemic.

There was a realization even in the government that shutting down everything could mean disaster for the economy. 'There is no doubt the nation will have to pay an economic cost for this lockdown. However, at this moment, my utmost priority, and that of the Government of India, state and local governments, is to protect the life of every Indian. Hence, it is my plea and prayer to you to continue to remain wherever you are right now in the country,' said the Prime Minister in his 24 March 2020 address.

The initial assessment was that a twenty-one-day lockdown would be sufficient, or at least that was what Modi told the people in the historic broadcast. He quoted health experts as advising that a period of at least twenty-one days was critical to break the infection cycle of COVID-19, though the decision in itself was based on pressure from the states that had already shut down or on the experience of other countries. 'In the last two days, several parts of the country have been put under lockdown. These efforts by state governments should be taken very seriously,' said the Prime Minister.

For some seventy-five districts, including those in the national capital, Delhi, the lockdown began earlier, on 22 March itself. According to an MHA status report dated 31 March 2020, submitted to the Supreme Court, most states and Union territories had invoked the provisions of the Epidemic Diseases Act, 1897, Criminal Procedure Code and the Disaster Management Act, 2005 by 24 March to implement complete or partial lockdown orders.[5] 'While the above-mentioned steps were in the right direction, lack of uniformity in the measures adopted as well as in their implementation was not found to fully service the objective of containing the spread of the virus,' said the report. This was cited as the reason for the New Delhi-based National Disaster Management Authority (NDMA) invoking powers under section 6(2) of the Disaster Management Act to issue directions to all Union and state government departments and authorities. The Union Home Secretary was made chairperson of the National Executive Committee, which started issuing orders for effective implementation of the lockdown measures. But the Union government itself abrogated this strategy in 2021 when a deadlier wave gripped the country.

Modi also saw 'a ray of hope' to combat corona in the experiences of 'those countries that have been able to contain corona to some extent.' 'Citizens of these countries have not stepped out of their homes for weeks. Citizens of these countries have fully adhered to the government rules. Hence, these countries are now moving towards overcoming this pandemic,' he said.

By 17 March, there were widespread restrictions in many countries. In Italy, which was third, following China and Iran, in the number of infections, there were severe mobility restrictions, with citizens being asked to stay home, limit social contact as much as possible and only leave home for essential reasons, including going to work and for health reasons. At first, everything in Italy was shut till 3 April. All non-essential service industries, except supermarkets, banks and pharmacies, were closed. All public gatherings were banned. There were travel restrictions throughout Italy, with exceptions only for essential travel (compelling business or health reason, or to return home). In Britain, people with even mild symptoms needed to self-isolate for seven days. People had been asked to work from home where possible and avoid pubs, clubs and theatres. China, the epicentre of COVID-19's first phase, had some of the local governments put restrictions on travellers coming into the country. This was a kind of reverse restriction, since most countries were putting bans on travellers coming from China. All international travellers to Beijing were being asked to undergo the fourteen-day quarantine. The restriction in Shanghai only applied to travellers from countries such as Iran, Korea, and the US.

As of 2 March, over 140 countries had imposed some form of restrictive policy on travellers from China, in the form of entry bans, visa restrictions, health declarations and quarantine.[6] As of 15 March 2020, it was only Iran, among major Asian countries, which had imposed a national lockdown. But by 1 April, Nepal, Malaysia, India, Pakistan, New Zealand, Bangladesh, Uzbekistan, East Timor and Laos had imposed national lockdowns.[7]

The Prime Minister was right in saying that countries had imposed restrictions on citizens' movements, but his claim that these countries were on their way to beating the disease simply fell flat, since infections continued to rise in all countries except in China, where a strict lockdown had been imposed much earlier.

All modes of transport in the Wuhan, Huanggang and Ezhou cities of China were restricted as early as 23 January. By that day, a total of 581 confirmed cases of the novel coronavirus (2019-nCoV) had been reported globally; of this, 571 cases were from China.[8] Cases reported in Thailand, Japan, the Hong Kong Special Administrative Region, Taipei Municipality, China, the Macau Special Administrative Region, the US and the Republic of Korea, all had a history of travel to Wuhan in the Hubei province. Of the 571 confirmed cases in China, 375 cases were confirmed from Hubei. On 24 January, travel restrictions were imposed in twelve more cities in Hubei. On 13 February, the Chinese government issued an extension of the order to shut all non-essential companies, including manufacturing plants, in Hubei province till 20 February. But a few days before India locked down, on 22 March, Wuhan eased its two-month lockdown while the Hubei province lifted the lockdown outside of Wuhan on 25 March, the day India shut down.

On 8 April, while India was struggling with the human crises unleashed by the lockdown, the city of Wuhan, where the coronavirus was believed to have originated, resumed all transportation and lifted the lockdown.[9] A CNN report quoted China's state broadcaster as saying that Wuhan's railway authority estimated more than 55,000 passengers would leave the city by train on the first day of unlocking, with about 40 per cent bound for the Pearl River Delta region, a major manufacturing hub in China.

Nine days into the lockdown in India, Prime Minister Narendra Modi again addressed the nation through a video message. This time, the call was to switch off electric lights, and light candles, lamps and torches at 9 p.m. for nine minutes on 5 April.[10] There was no doubt that this exercise would in no way help in the fight against

COVID-19 or address the issues being faced by those stranded, but it was certainly an emboldened experiment at garnering attention and support after the success of clapping hands and clanging utensils on the janata curfew, 22 March. 'Whether it is the people's curfew, ringing bells, clapping hands or clanging plates, they have all made the nation realize its collective strength in these testing times. It has led to the deepening of the belief that the nation can unite as one in the battle against corona,' Modi said in his video message. 'Some people may also be worried about how they are going to fight such a big battle on their own. Many will be concerned about how many more days they will have to spend like this.'

Modi presented this collective celebration from the balconies of people's houses as some kind of resolve to fight the grimness around them. 'Friends, in our country, the citizenry (janata) is considered a manifestation of God itself. Amid the darkness spread by the corona pandemic, we must continuously progress towards light and hope. We must continuously strive to take those of us most affected, our poor brothers and sisters, from disappointment to hope. We must end the darkness and uncertainty emanating from the crisis, by progressing towards light and certainty. We must defeat the deep darkness of the crisis, by spreading the glory of light in all four directions,' he said. To a nation that celebrates the festival of lights in Diwali each year, Modi was not saying anything new, but the power of light was given an altogether new meaning by asking people to shut electric lights. All of the country's power sector managers, led by Union Power Minister R.K. Singh, had to use their collective might to prevent a potential collapse of the electricity grid because of the sudden drop in power consumption.[11]

All power load dispatch centres started planning for the pan-India lights-off event at 9 p.m. for nine minutes so that 'reliable and secure grid operation' could be ensured during the event. A day earlier, on 4 April 2020, an emergency meeting of the Forum of Load Dispatchers (FOLD) was conducted through video conferencing and the preparedness of all state load dispatch centres was discussed. The nodal power load manager, Power System Operation Corporation Ltd (POSOCO), issued an elaborate advisory on the measures required for generation scheduling, frequency control and voltage control, besides other general guidelines.

All clocks at power generating stations were synchronized and set to the Indian Standard Time. It was a Sunday. Hydropower stations were backed down to reduce generation from 6.10 p.m. to 8 p.m. so that by 9 p.m., they could be used for managing power generation. Power from thermal interstate generating stations was gradually reduced to a near-technical minimum of 60 per cent by 8.55 p.m., five minutes to the crucial 9 p.m., and hydro generation was simultaneously increased to maintain the load generation balances. Since hydro- and gas-based generation units can provide flexibility, hydropower units were asked to ramp down from 8.57 p.m. and roll at 0–10 per cent of their rated capacity and gas stations at their minimum.

It was an unprecedented event that did bring the power sector fraternity together, but for what? It was an unnecessary situation. Clearly, Modi was only using his charisma on the people who were confined inside their homes, or even away from their homes in unfriendly cities and shelters. 'At that time, if you have turned off all the lights of your homes, and each one of us in all directions has lit a diya, we will experience the superpower of light, clearly illuminating the common purpose we are all fighting for. In that light, in that lustre, in that radiance, let us resolve in our minds that we are not alone, that no one is alone,' said Modi, creating an illusion of collective optimism around the crisis that had firmly gripped the country by then.

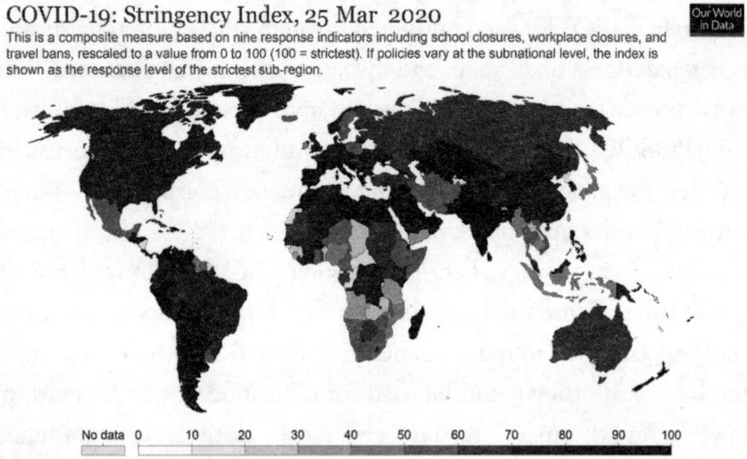

Source: Hale, Webster, Petherick, Phillips and Kira (2020). Oxford COVID-19 Government Response Tracker – Last updated 6 March 2021, 01.00 London time.

Note: The index simply records the number and strictness of government policies, and should not be interpreted as 'scoring' the appropriateness or effectiveness of a country's response. OurWorldInData.org/coronavirus

In India, many thought the confinement would be over in twenty-one days, and so would the virus. 'If we are not able to manage these twenty-one days, the country and your family could be set back twenty-one years. If we are not able to manage these twenty-one days, several families will be devastated forever,' he had said. Even the MHA's status report to the Supreme Court on 31 March 2020 said, 'As the incubation period of coronavirus is for 14 days, it was directed that the lockdown measures shall remain in force for a period of 21 days with effect from March 25, 2020.' Clearly, as later events showed, the government had not foreseen that the twenty-one-day first phase of lockdown, or Lockdown 1.0, as it came to be known, would not be able to break the chain of infection or even prevent the spread of infection.

The Stringency Index of the Oxford COVID-19 Government Response Tracker, put out by the Blavatnik School of Government in the UK, showed India in the most stringent category among all the countries on 25 March 2020, with a score of 100. In comparison, stringency in the US was around 72 at that time, though it had reported 673 deaths due to COVID-19 and 51,914 confirmed cases by then, compared to just seven deaths and 562 cases in India.[12] The index is the mean score of nine metrics (school closure, workplace closure, cancellation of public events, restrictions on public gatherings, closures of public transport, stay-at-home requirements, public information campaigns, restrictions on internal movements, and international travel controls). A higher score indicates a stricter government response (i.e., 100 = strictest response).[13]

Modi did term the twenty-one days of Lockdown 1.0 as 'a long time,' which was essential for the safety of every Indian, but this initial period turned into two long summer months for ordinary Indians. The national lockdown was initially to last twenty-one days,[14] but was extended for nineteen, then fourteen, and then fourteen days again, till 31 May 2020. District-level bureaucrats exercising the power of executive magistrates, such as tehsildars and naib tehsildars, were designated as 'incident commanders' and asked to take action against any lockdown violations.

There were four phases of the lockdown, and each came with a set of gradual measures meant to restart businesses and check the sudden setback to manufacturing in India. Between these phases of lockdown, there were scores of addendums to the MHA guidelines, since the government was on the back foot because of the crisis that the lockdown had unleashed. The twenty-one-day period between Lockdown 1.0 and Lockdown 2.0, for instance, saw five addenda. In addition to these, sometimes there were conflicting orders on migrant labourers. The MHA clamped down on the movement of people by issuing an order to states to ensure strict adherence to lockdown measures and prevent any movement. 'State/Union territory governments shall ensure adequate arrangements of temporary shelters, and provision of food, etc., for the poor and needy people, including migrant labourers, stranded due to lockdown measures in their respective areas. The migrant people, who have moved out to reach their home states/home towns, must be kept in the nearest shelter by the respective state/union territory government quarantine facilities after proper screening for a minimum period of 14 days as per standard health protocol,' said the 29 March 2020 order.[15]

Apart from the states, private citizens and employers were also expected to follow certain guidelines, like paying regular wages to their workers and not collecting rent for one month. Landlords were asked not to force labourers and students to vacate their premises. The same day, the MHA issued orders for disciplinary proceedings against four officers of the Delhi government for 'dereliction of duty' regarding containment of the spread of COVID-19.[16] While the state's additional chief secretary, transport department, and principal secretary of finance (who was also the divisional commissioner) were suspended, show-cause notices were issued to additional chief secretary, home and land buildings departments, and sub-divisional magistrate of Seelampur area in east Delhi. Though the official communication did not mention the charges, the order was issued after there was a large gathering of people at the Anand Vihar bus stand. A video of the desperate crowd wanting to go back to their native places had gone viral. 'It has been brought to the notice of the competent authority that the following officers, who were responsible to ensure strict compliance to the instructions issued by Chairperson, National Executive Committee, formed under Disaster Management Act 2005 regarding containment of [the] spread of COVID-19, have prima facie failed to do so. These officers have failed to ensure public health and safety during the lockdown restrictions to combat COVID-19. Due to the serious lapse in performance of their duties, the competent authority has initiated disciplinary proceedings,' said the ministry order. The movement of the large number of stranded people in big cities did cause a black mark against these officers' names, but did not move the Union government, which continued with a strict enforcement of lockdown rules.

There was, however, another congregation in Delhi before the lockdown, which created a crisis for the Muslim community in India. These weren't people caught in the lockdown, wanting to go home, but a religious gathering by Tablighi Jamaat. Though this Muslim congregation at Delhi's Hazrat Nizamuddin Markaz was a usual event, it took a communal turn after many in a 13–15 March gathering tested positive for COVID-19. There was no lockdown in the country during those days, only a Delhi government order dated 13 March that prohibited sports events involving a gathering of more than 300 people for any kind of activity.[17] After the positive tests, there were reports of Muslims across the country being harassed and of some leaders of the ruling Bharatiya Janata Party upping their communal agenda through social media. Police across the country, including the Delhi Police, registered cases against the Jamaat.[18] According to an MHA report, there were about 1,746 persons staying in Hazrat Nizamuddin Markaz on 21 March, of which 216 were foreigners and 1,530 were Indians.[19] Additionally, about 824 foreigners had been, as of 21 March, doing 'Chilla' (Tabligh) activities in various parts of the country. 'Details of these 824 foreigners had been shared on 21 March with the state police for identifying them, getting them medically screened and quarantining them. Besides, on 28 March, state police were advised to collect the names of Indian Tabligh Jamaat workers from the local coordinators, locate them on the ground, get them medically screened and quarantine them. So far, about 2,137 such persons have been identified in different states. They are being medically examined and quarantined. This process is still on and more such people would be identified and located,' said the ministry report.

On 28 March, the ministry issued a detailed advisory to chief secretaries and director-generals of police of all states, as well as to the commissioner of police, Delhi, to trace the movement of all Tabligh workers in their area, identify their contacts and take steps for their medical screening. 'It is estimated that from January 1 onwards this year, approximately 2,100 foreigners had visited India for Tabligh activities. While approximately 824 of them, as on 21 March, were dispersed in different parts of the country, approximately 216 of them were staying at Nizamuddin Markaz. Others might have left the country before the lockdown,' the advisory said. The foreign nationals were mainly from Indonesia, Malaysia, Thailand, Nepal, Myanmar, Bangladesh, Sri Lanka and Kyrgyzstan. The Nizamuddin Markaz area was cordoned off. It opened for a day more than a year later, on 28 March 2021, for fifty persons to offer Shab-e-Barat prayers.[20]

That the country was passing through a tough phase, because of both a health emergency and a lockdown induced by it, started to reveal almost immediately after the lockdown was put in place. Though the government continued to claim that the lockdown was yielding the desired result of controlling coronavirus infections, it had not anticipated the hardships it was causing to businesses and to ordinary people. The second set of guidelines, for what was to be Lockdown 2.0, came on 14 April[21] and 15 April 2021. 'Completely adhere to the *Lakshman rekha* of lockdown and social distancing. Please also use homemade face covers and masks without fail,' Prime Minister Modi said in his speech on 14 April, while announcing the second phase of lockdown. This extension was to be in place till 3 May 2020. The phase, however, came with some relaxation in rules for industrial activity, with a focus on 'rural and agricultural development, and job creation.'[22] There was no blanket lifting of prohibition in commercial and manufacturing activities, but from 20 April onwards, those in rural areas, industrial estates and export zones were allowed to reopen, provided workers stayed in their premises or nearby. An MHA order said this was being done to mitigate the hardship to the public. The state governments, however, were allowed to impose stricter measures. The transport lockdown continued nationally, with airlines, railways, Metro, buses and taxi aggregators not being allowed to operate for passenger services. The onus of moving the workforce was on employers and incident commanders. The MHA said it expected industrial and manufacturing sectors to revive with these measures and 'create job opportunities while maintaining safety protocols and social distancing.' The Union health ministry had, meanwhile, issued guidelines for containment zones within hotspot districts. State governments were notifying containment zones, in which only essential services were permitted.

The third phase of lockdown was from 4 May 2020 onwards and lasted another fourteen days. This time, the Union government came out with new guidelines that profiled areas based on their risks.[23] The country was divided into green, orange and red zones, with containment areas marked. Green areas were those districts with no cases of COVID-19; red areas were those that had a high number of cases and a high doubling rate of confirmed cases; and orange districts were those that were neither green nor red. The severity of measures continued to be the highest in the containment zones in the red and orange districts, and overall in the red zones. While the MoHFW issued the list of zones, states could add more areas in the danger zones of red and orange, but not reduce the number. Surprisingly, even though the announcement of new guidelines on 1 May came with a reinforcement of the ban on passenger movement by all modes of transport, including interstate movement of individuals, special trains for three categories of passengers – labourers, students and stranded tourists – were started in a somewhat secret operation. The guidelines did not mention any special move to transport stranded people. The order had said 'all passenger movement by trains, except for security purposes or for purposes as permitted by the Ministry of Home affairs,' would continue to remain prohibited across the country, irrespective of the zone, for a period of two weeks with effect from 4 May 2020.

The only relief for common people with no personal vehicle of their own was that taxis and cab aggregators were permitted to operate with one driver and two passengers, and inter-district movement of individuals and vehicles for permitted activities was allowed in the orange zones as long as it was not in any containment areas. This meant that only those who could afford private taxis could commute in the orange zones, while inter-district and intra-district movement of buses was not allowed. For the green zones, however, buses were allowed to be operated at half their seating capacity, along with most other activities.

The guidelines for the third phase of lockdown did ease commuting within cities and districts as long as those areas were not reporting a high number of infections, but the challenge of long-distance travel entered another phase with the start of special trains that were initially unable to manage demand.

The Prime Minister appeared on television screens each time a phase of lockdown was to end. For the fourth phase, Modi's address came on 12 May 2020.[24] The initial part of the speech was full of rhetoric that went into the history of the nation and its greatness and how his government created institutions, such as the International Solar Alliance, to establish the country as a force among global players. Clearly, the initial part of the speech, as always, was of no relevance to the distressed. Modi, however, announced something that was to become the government's flagship programme and around which it pushed its entire propaganda for months to come:

The Atmanirbhar Bharat Abhiyan (Self Reliant India Campaign). Union Finance Minister Nirmala Sitharaman was tasked with formulating economic packages to revive the crisis-ridden economy.

The MHA came out with another set of guidelines on 17 May. The fourth phase of lockdown was to start from 18 May and end on 31 May 2020.[25] This time, states were given the power to divide districts into red, orange and green zones. The chief ministers of many states, in a meeting with the Prime Minister, had asked that the decision to classify districts should be left to them. The MoHFW, however, set some parameters, such as the one that said that an area would be 'critical' if the total number of active cases was higher than 200. Similarly, an active case count of fifteen and above for a population of over a hundred thousand, as well as a fatality rate of more than 6 per cent, was to be considered 'critical.'

The government was confident about 'flattening the curve' of the spread of coronavirus and lauded the lockdown for helping to achieve low infection rates. At the same time, the economy, which had slowed down already, was witnessing plunging indicators. India's services sector, which contributes 55 per cent to the country's gross domestic product (GDP), an indicator of economic growth, declined to its lowest level in over fourteen years in April 2020, the first full month of national lockdown. The services Purchasing Managers' Index (PMI) for India dropped to 5.4 that month, a sharp decline from 49.3 in March. This was the sharpest decline in services output since IHS Markit, a data analytics firm, started collecting data on it in December 2005. A figure above 50 indicates expansion, while a sub-50 number signals contraction. Manufacturing PMI for the same month had dropped to a record low of 27.4 in April from 51.8 in March.[26]

The rationale for the lockdown and the complete shutting down of transport services and many other segments of economic activity was, however, justified even in the Modi government's Economic

Survey for 2020-21, presented on 29 January 2021. 'India has transformed the short-term trade-off between lives and livelihoods into a win-win in the medium to long-term that saves both lives and livelihoods,' it said, though it was not clear how livelihoods were saved.[27] In fact, later in the survey report, it did admit that the economic impact of the lockdowns and closure of economic activity would have adversely impacted the livelihoods of people: 'COVID-19, therefore, posited complex and multi-faceted health and socio-economic trade-offs for policymakers – whether to save "lives" or "livelihoods".'

The survey estimated the natural number of cases and deaths expected across countries based on their population, population density, demographics, tests conducted and the health infrastructure, and compared those with the actual number of deaths in India, to show that India had restricted the spread of COVID-19 by 3.7 million cases and saved more than 1,00,000 lives. 'Uttar Pradesh, Gujarat and Bihar have restricted the case spread the best; Kerala, Telangana and Andhra Pradesh have saved the most lives; Maharashtra has underperformed the most in restricting the spread of cases and in saving lives. The analysis clearly shows that early and more stringent lockdowns have been effective in controlling the spread of the pandemic – both across countries and across states in India,' it said.

Further, the survey claimed that in the absence of both a vaccine and a treatment, failing to impose restrictions on the free movement of individuals during the pandemic would have exposed the population to the threat of contagion, thereby leading to deaths in enormous numbers. Evidence, it claimed, showed that the timing of the intervention was crucial as population density plays a key role in aggravating the spread of disease at the onset of a pandemic and that the speed and the duration of lockdowns help in keeping mortality in check. 'Given the "black swan event" marked by sheer uncertainty and once in a century crisis, Indian policymakers followed an approach similar to the Barbell strategy in finance – hedging for the worst outcome initially, and updating its response step-by-step via feedback. The clear objective of "Jaan Hai to Jahan Hai" (if you have life in you, you have the world) and to "break the chain of spread" before it reaches "community transmission" helped the government face the dilemma of "lives vs livelihood", pace the sequence of policy interventions and adapt its response as per the evolving situation,' said the survey's chapter on lockdown.

The government document presented to the Indian Parliament each year as a report card of economic activity said the stringent lockdown in India from March 25 to May 31 was necessitated by the need to break the chain of the transmission of COVID-19. 'This was based on the humane principle that while GDP growth will come back, human lives once lost cannot be brought back … The 40-day lockdown period was used to scale up the necessary medical and para-medical infrastructure for active surveillance, expanded testing, contact tracing, isolation and management of cases, and educating citizens about social distancing and masks, etc. The lockdown provided the necessary time to put in place the fundamentals of the "5T" strategy – Test, Track, Trace, Treat and Technology,' it said.

Though the government's response through a lockdown was driven more by pressure from the state-level lockdowns and some international examples, the survey claimed that the response drew on 'epidemiological and economic research,' especially research on the Spanish Flu, which highlighted that an early, intense lockdown provided 'a win-win strategy to save lives, and preserve livelihoods via economic recovery in the medium to long-term … The strategy was also motivated by the Nobel-Prize winning research in Hansen & Sargent (2001) that recommends a policy focused on minimizing losses in a worst case scenario when uncertainty is very high. Faced with an unprecedented pandemic and the resultant uncertainty, loss of scores of human lives captured thus the worst case scenario.'

Since the sixty-eight-day national lockdown did enforce social distancing—or cut off people-to-people contact except among those residing in one place—it would have certainly prevented early infections. India's score in the Stringency Index of the Oxford COVID-19 Government Response Tracker of the Blavatnik School of Government showed that from the highest score of 100, India was 79.17 at the end of the lockdown period on 31 May 2020.[28] The following months of staggered unlocking, however, showed that infections started peaking in September 2020, with no abatement, though in theory, the health infrastructure should have been better prepared by then. India reported over 90,000 cases every day at its peak in 2020, with the maximum being 97,894 on 16 September. This was the time when no other country was reporting more than 75,000 cases in a day, which meant that the gains of the lockdown, if any, had been wiped out.

PART III

THE ANGST

6

THE LONG ROAD HOME

'IT IS BETTER TO die at home in our village than stay here and get beaten up by the locals for venturing out,' said thirty-two-year-old Keerat Kori, whose life took an unexpected turn when his employer living in Haryana's Gurugram passed away in February 2020. Kori drove the retired air force officer's car, but a month after his employer's demise, before he could get another job, the national lockdown was imposed. It left him, his wife and their three children with no source of income and Rs 3,600 rent to pay for a room and a common bathroom. Kori lives in Wazirabad village, near his former employer's house. He had just one question. 'When I wanted to go out to buy something for my house, the locals beat me up for coming out of the house, but if I go to deliver essentials at my former employer's house, they let me go. Why this discrimination?'[1]

Angry and faced with uncertainty, he decided to head home to Damoh district in Madhya Pradesh on 12 May 2020 with his whole family on one motorbike. 'A group of ten bikes was leaving, so we all left at 4 a.m. via the Kundli-Manesar-Palwal highway,' he says. He had Rs 20,000 in hand, but it took time for him to reach home because his kids would doze off, making it difficult to drive. The two-day journey had never seemed longer.

Once in his village, he was asked to quarantine in a school, but he decided to do so in his own house since he owned an independent house, not a joint property. 'My brother would hesitate giving even water to us,' he says. They came back to Gurugram in October 2020, and his children started going to a school belonging to Saksham Bal Vikas Sanstha, a charitable organization. 'I still have to pay Rs 50,000 to my landlord. He has assured me that I can pay in instalments,' he said in February 2021. But he did not get another steady job and did odd jobs as a labourer till the local lockdown of 2021, when he set off for his village again, this time, on a train.

Unlike Kori, who returned from his village to the city in October 2020, forty-five-year-old Mohan Paswan, who resided in a slum cluster in the DLF Phase V area of Gurugram, just a few kilometres from where Kori lived, decided not to return from his native Bihar. Paswan, who had lived in the city for seven to eight years, had been bedridden with a fractured leg after an accident in January 2020.[2] A few days before the city shut down in March 2020, he had started to drive an electric rickshaw again, despite unhealed stitches on his leg, so that he could make money and leave for his village. After the accident, his family members from his native village, Sirhulli in Darbhanga district, had come to visit him. Fifteen-year-old Jyoti Kumari, the second of his five children, had stayed back to nurse him. But then, the city shut down on 22 March.

The father-daughter duo lived off their savings for some time, but soon it became clear to them that they could not survive the harsh realities in the city. His landlord threatened to throw him out since he was unable to pay the rent of Rs 1,500 a month. 'One day, Jyoti said, let us leave with Mullahji uncle. Six-seven people, including one woman, were going to Araria in Bihar via Darbhanga on bicycles. At first, I did not want to go, since we did not have a cycle, but she convinced me, saying that since we did not have money or a home, we would not be able to stay (in the city),' says Paswan. The next task was to look for a cycle. One was available for Rs 1,000, but he did not have the money to buy it. 'Jyoti got Rs 500 in her account twice from Pradhan Mantri over two months and then, after filling a form, we got Rs 1,000 from the Bihar government,' he recounts. All together, they were left with Rs 800, of which Rs 500 they gave for the cycle along with a promise to pay the rest later. They decided to go by cycle since motorized vehicle owners would charge Rs 3,000.

The group left for Bihar on the night of 8 May 2020. After crossing Palwal in Haryana, they found that the Uttar Pradesh administration was putting people on trucks so that they did not have to walk or cycle, which also minimized the danger of spreading infection locally, but Paswan and his daughter could not get on a truck because his leg was injured and anyone touching it could create a problem. The entire group decided to be with the father–daughter duo. Jyoti Kumari, who was pedalling, sometimes could not keep pace with the group. Paswan does not know the full name of Mullahji and his family who were going to Araria, but they became his companions for the arduous journey over the next few days. 'However many days it takes, we will not leave you, Mullahji told us,' Paswan says. It took them eight days to reach their village, Sirhulli.

It was both a relief and the beginning of the next stage of their struggle, once they reached their village. 'The villagers were pressurizing our family and insisted that both father and daughter were getting corona,' he says. Some eleven people were quarantined together in the village. His daughter slept on the roof since she was the only female among the quarantined lot. Paswan did make it home successfully, and his daughter won laurels for cycling 1,200 km with her injured father. The family got Rs 7-8 lakh in total as monetary help from a number of sources, including the government. From this fund, Paswan paid off a debt of about Rs 3.5-4 lakh, which he had incurred on marrying off his elder daughter. With some of the money, he constructed a house while the remainder he kept for Jyoti's education. With media and other people pouring in and classes going online, Jyoti Kumari found it hard to focus on her studies. 'She is not good at studies, but I have told her to keep trying,' Paswan says.

Before he drove an e-rickshaw, Paswan had worked as a cook in an Italian restaurant in DT Mega Mall in Gurugram. He says that doing any job in Bihar would be fine since it would be 'home' and he could look after his schoolgoing children. 'I do not know what the politics were, but there was a lockdown and we were helpless. I saw lakhs on the road. If people did not feed us, we would have died. People of all religions were feeding us when were in Uttar Pradesh,' he says. Tough days, however, did not end with his returning to his village. A year after he came back, Paswan died of a heart attack on 31 May 2021.[3]

There has been widespread criticism of the Indian government for giving just Rs 500 in cash transfer, but for people like Paswan and his daughter Jyoti, who received the money in her account, this dole turned out to be a lifesaver when they did not have any source of income or savings. A higher benefit amount, nevertheless, could have addressed many of their woes.

In a June 2021 report titled 'No Country for Workers,' Stranded Workers Action Network (SWAN), a volunteer group, suggested a monthly transfer of Rs 3,000 for six months to 270 million households. This translated to Rs 100 daily or less than one-third of the national minimum wage threshold of Rs 375 a day. This would mean a total spending of Rs 4.86 trillion for the government. After subtracting the PM-KISAN and National Social Assistance

Programme budget for six months, it implied an additional spending of Rs 4.44 trillion.[4]

According to a World Bank document, 277 cash transfer programmes in 131 countries, including India, had been introduced by June 2020 in response to COVID-19. This figure included ninety-eight existing programmes, which were scaled up, and 179 completely new initiatives. The number of countries or territories that had planned or implemented 1,414 social protection measures by 11 December increased to 215.[5] In reply to a question by Karti P. Chidambaram in the Lok Sabha on 8 February 2021, Union Minister of State for Finance Anurag Thakur quoted the Ministry of Rural Development's data to say that a total of 20.64 crore [206.4 million] women Pradhan Mantri Jan Dhan Yojana (PMJDY) account holders were benefitted through the ex-gratia payment under Pradhan Mantri Garib Kalyan Yojana (PMGKY).[6] While PMJDY, which facilitates the opening of zero-balance savings accounts, was launched in August 2014 to increase financial inclusion, PMGKY is a COVID-19 relief package announced by Union Finance Minister Nirmala Sitharaman on the second day of lockdown, 26 March 2020. However, less than half of such account holder beneficiaries received the cash transfer since Thakur in his reply said 417.5 million accounts were opened under PMJDY as of 27 January 2021. This was probably because the government credited Rs 500 a month into the accounts of women beneficiaries of PMJDY only, restricting the benefit as well as access to the dole.

Under the PMGKY, Sitharaman had announced a Rs 1.70 trillion relief package 'to combat the economic impact of COVID-19 on the poor and needy and to help them in the fight against [the] Corona virus.'[7] This included free rations and LPG cylinders, and other benefits including insurance and employment. According to Modi's address to the nation on 30 June 2020, however, a total of about

Rs 1.5 trillion was to be spent towards the scheme, including five extended months.[8] The Prime Minister announced the extension of the scheme to November while also announcing the second phase of unlocking measures. He said that Rs 31,000 crore had been transferred into the Jan Dhan accounts of almost 200 million poor families and Rs 18,000 crore had been transferred into the bank accounts of more than 90 million farmers during April, May and June 2020. The government would spend more than Rs 90,000 crore towards the extension of the scheme, the Prime Minister said, adding that if the amount spent on it in the previous three months was added, it would amount to Rs 1.5 trillion in total. Clearly, the government had not been successful in reaching out to 'the poorest of the poor' to the extent it had announced: not only was the planned spending less than what Sitharaman had announced in March, the period over which it had to be spent was also extended from three to eight months.

The bigger the city, the harder the struggle for those stranded as they ran out of money. 'Stay inside your home, stay inside your home, and do just one thing: stay inside your home,' Modi told people on 24 March while announcing the lockdown, but millions came out onto the roads due to lack of livelihood, food and even shelter. When no transport was available, they just walked.

Five days into the lockdown, Shailendra Singh, a social worker from Patna in Bihar, called up Seemant Kumar Singh, inspector general of police (administration) in Bengaluru on 30 March 2020. He sought help for 400 persons stranded without food at Billanakote in the city's outskirts. 'At first, I told him that it was not possible for 400 people to gather at one place because of social distancing norms. He gave me the number of one Dharmendra Chauhan and asked if I could help those people,' says Singh. Chauhan was one of the stranded labourers.[9] He came from Kharhana village in the Buxar district of Bihar. Dinesh Kumar Singh, a Patna High Court judge, belonged to that village too. Out of helplessness, Chauhan had called the judge who, in turn, asked Shailendra Singh for help.

Seemant Kumar Singh called the number around noon the same day. Chauhan was not convincing enough but as Singh and a team of policemen soon realized, some 400 people really were huddled in a transport colony at Billanakote near the national highway connecting Bengaluru and Mumbai. 'I immediately contacted one of the hotel owners here. The hotel association was doing some charity. They readily agreed to provide packed lunches,' Singh says. Some 400 lunch packets were sent by 3 p.m. through police vehicles, to the relief of those stranded.

The pandemic and the lockdown were unprecedented, and the administration could not anticipate the new challenges they threw up. 'We had not foreseen it, so I thought providing that lunch would be the end of things,' says Singh. Chauhan called again and thanked him, but posed another challenge: What after this? These people had gathered near the highway over the previous four-five days and had tried to run away in trucks since they did not have money to pay for rent. Some people might have managed to leave, but when police became strict and started stopping them, the rest were stranded. 'As an individual, I was in a fix,' says Singh. 'I contacted ISKCON (a religious organization). That day, they had finalized a sample ration box for the Bengaluru district administration: some 5 kg of rice, flour, pulses, oil and other things for twenty-one days. I was aware of that. I asked ISKCON to allow it to be distributed, but they said it was yet to be inaugurated. But after a lot of persuasion, they delivered the boxes by about 8 or 9 p.m. and then we delivered them in two trucks,' he says.

One box of this dry ration would cost roughly Rs 1,000, but ISKCON provided it for free. 'I was a bit worried about social distancing. I kept telling the labourers not to create a stampede and be organized. They listened to me and stood in a line. They took 376 boxes and even wanted to return the remaining twenty-four. I told them to keep the remainder,' says Singh.

This stranded lot told people back home in Bihar how an inspector general helped them. In Patna and Bokhara, some news outlets carried the story along with Seemant Kumar Singh's personal number. 'I had nothing to do with the relief work since I was IG administration, but I did it in my personal capacity. Some people who called me did not know I was an IG; they thought I was a ration shop owner, giving food on behalf of the government. When trains started, they thought I was in charge of train operations. I used to get calls from even Bihar. Once, a lady called asking for a gas cylinder. They just had a number, my number,' he recounts.

According to Singh, there were over a million people stranded in Karnataka alone. These included people from Bihar, Jharkhand, Odisha, Madhya Pradesh, Chhattisgarh, the north-eastern states and Bengal. Since labourers from different states stayed together, they exchanged Singh's number with each other. From 1 April onwards, he started to get 300–400 calls daily. He saved these phone numbers, along with the details of how many people were stranded and in which area. Being a senior officer in the police helped in both verification and delivery.

Bengaluru Police's Hoysala, police control room vans named after the dynasty that ruled most parts of what is now Karnataka, from the tenth to the fourteenth centuries, became chariots of goodwill when they reached the hungry. The city has about 350 such vehicles. 'I used to get calls from people giving me the number of people in their group. Sometimes, they would exaggerate the number or take from me as well as others, so I used to send the food boxes to the concerned SHO in Bengaluru. Maybe 5 to 10 per cent were cases where numbers were exaggerated. Most of them were genuine calls,' Singh says. The police staff in the Hoysalas were told that they did not have to do this work at the cost of their official assignments, but if they were going to the area from where a distress call had come, they should check the number of people and their situation.

Singh said they supplied Rs 6 crore worth of food, translating to 60,000 ration boxes, over April and May 2020. The situation was bad till mid-May, but since an article on this appeared on the front page of the Bengaluru edition of *The Times of India* and on television, he started to get donors. Without involving any financial transaction with Singh, the donors were given the phone numbers of retail shops and the account details of their owners. Donors needed to pay shop owners who prepared the meal box. Twenty-one-day ration boxes, such as those provided by ISKCON, were prepared, costing an amount equivalent to the donation. Many people sitting in the house used to send money electronically. Hoysalas would pick up the boxes, keep them in police lock-ups and then deliver them when they could.

Singh says their handling of the crisis earned them much goodwill. Once, there was a heated argument about whether a train to Jharkhand or Bihar will go first, so the officer-in-charge put the phone on the loudspeaker and made Singh speak to the labourers. The situation calmed down after that. The labourers were confident speaking to Singh, who belongs to the Pakariya village of Banka district in Bihar, because he could understand their dialect.

Before stranded people started to move out in special trains and buses, Singh started getting calls from other states too. 'I got calls from Bihari workers in Kerala and Tamil Nadu as well. They did not know I was in Bengaluru. I would call my batchmates in those states and through them, I arranged food for those callers. So it was that we arranged rations in Tamil Nadu, in Gujarat and in Delhi. In Delhi, the administration was giving them cooked food. The difference is, if you give cooked food, then you have to provide each meal, but giving rations took care of their needs for twenty-one days,' he says.

Food was the need of the hour. Singh had the resources to help, and he got enough donors to supplement his efforts. 'We evolved a flawless system,' he says. Well into March 2021, he still got calls complaining, among other things, about employers who have not paid their workers. 'But now it would be beyond my brief,' he says. 'What we did then could be said to be part of community policing.'

For forty-three-year-old Dharmendra Chauhan, who became the first to seek help from Seemant Singh, the dry rations were very important. He was a daily wage earner at VRL Logistics in Bengaluru, loading and unloading goods on trucks. 'For every tonne loaded, we were paid Rs 90. So suppose we loaded or unloaded 20 tonne, we got Rs 1,800, which we then divided among all those who together handled that load. During the lockdown, the work went down. We earned only about Rs 150 a day, compared to Rs 450 earlier,' he says.[10] Chauhan recalls how many of those he worked with took any vehicle they could to go back to their villages as soon as the lockdown was announced, but once there was a clampdown, they had to stay where they were. Chauhan was able to take the train only on 12 August and decided to stay back in his village since he had injured his leg in Bengaluru.

From 15 May to 1 June 2020, based on 821 distress calls received by SWAN from across the country, 80 per cent did not have access to government rations. These calls corresponded to 5,911 migrant workers. 'About 76 per cent of people who have called us since 15 May have less than Rs 300 left with them and 72 per cent of people have less than Rs 200 left with them. Sixty-three per cent of people have less than Rs 100 left with them. About 57 per cent of the people sent in SOS calls (representing 820 people) with no money or rations left or had skipped the previous meal,' said SWAN in its June 2020 report.[11]

Many of the viral videos that circulated during the lockdown were of people crowding at railway stations and bus stands. Just when the first phase of lockdown was to end, Prime Minister Narendra Modi announced, on 14 April 2020, an extension of the national lockdown to 3 May. But since these announcements of lockdown extensions never came with a warning, those wanting to leave the big cities hoped to board the next train to their homes each time a lockdown phase was ending. Thousands gathered at Mumbai's Thane and Bandra West railway stations in Mumbai on 14 April 2020.[12] What got these people to these stations that were shut after the lockdown but otherwise are buzzing with activity round the clock?

Rumours of special trains being made available were doing the WhatsApp messaging rounds. The Indian Railways, as a monopoly rail-based national transporter, did nothing to quell the rumours or clarify whether passenger operations would remain suspended in the near future. What added to the rumours was the fact that the Indian Railways had continued taking bookings online beyond the end of the first phase of lockdown, which gave hope to people who were desperate to go back home, since they could not make it to the last train on 21 March 2020. The crowd at Mumbai stations, however, was hoping to catch the elusive train to their native place. As the number of people outside the station swelled, the local authorities and police started dispersing the crowd. Police resorted to lathicharging the unarmed persons who were insisting that they wanted to go back home. A similar crowding of Anand Vihar bus station in Delhi had also been reported earlier. In the case of bus stands, people found that private operators were accepting passengers, charging them very high fares.

Following the incidents at Mumbai stations, the local police sprang into action and arrested an ABP Majha journalist, Rahul Kulkarni, who had cited an internal railway document to report that special trains would transport stranded migrant workers back home.[13] This report was taken to be the reason behind crowding at stations, though the news report in itself was not incorrect—internally, the Indian Railways was discussing starting some special trains, which it eventually did in less than a month.

In the normal course of reporting, journalists do put out information on things that are likely to happen. And the availability of some mode of transport was the most sought-after information for many at that point, when the lockdown had taken the vulnerable sections of society by surprise. An *Indian Express* report quoted Kulkarni's Facebook post to say, 'A responsible officer had in the morning sent me a letter detailing the efforts being undertaken by the Railways to ensure that migrants who are stuck can be sent back home. We made a report on the proposed plans of the Railways. At 9 a.m., we aired a report about the proposal and nowhere did it say as to when the trains will start.' Kulkarni had also tweeted a 13 April document saying it was an 'internal Railways note' on the running of Jansadharan Specials for stranded people.[14]

The railways never denied the existence of such a note, but its chief public relations officer for South Central Railway (SCR), Rajesh Chilaka, was quoted as saying that it was a 'preparatory exercise' and that its contents were 'taken out of context.' The newspaper report further quoted Chilaka saying, 'The idea was to gauge how many labourers are stranded within the zone and how many more trains would be needed, as the regular passenger services would not be sufficient once the services resume operations.' Though Kulkarni was later released and cleared of all charges, another person was arrested for rumour-mongering.[15] These incidents, however, showed how rumours thrived simply because there was a lack of official information. People were dangerously close in the crowds at these places, even though the entire nation was purportedly in lockdown.

Such gatherings outside railway and bus stations indicated the sheer desperation of people who did not belong to the city where they were being locked down by the government. The desperation was simply because their sources of income had suddenly vanished. With manufacturing units shut and construction activity halted in cities, there was joblessness, with daily wagers and even those employed informally finding it hard to sustain themselves. As the crisis unfolded, state governments in Delhi, Bihar and Uttar Pradesh started to quibble over taking responsibility for the stranded labourers. Lack of coordination in transportation and decision-making made a mockery of the vital need to contain the spread of COVID-19 and prevent it from spreading to rural areas, where basic medical facilities are absent or poor.

Both the state and the Union governments were aware of the distress caused by the lockdown. As early as 1 April 2020, Union Health Secretary Preeti Sudan issued a letter to all states on the directions of the Supreme Court that 'the anxiety and fear of the migrants should be understood by the police and other authorities and they should deal with the migrants in a humane manner.'[16] Her ministry had issued guidelines for dealing with 'psychosocial issues of migrants.' Local administrations were asked to provide counselling and other health support to those lodged in shelters while also emphasizing 'the importance of their staying in their present location and how mass movement could greatly and adversely affect all efforts to contain the virus.'[17]

The Union government's own status report, filed in the Supreme Court on 31 March 2020, however, said 'a final decision is taken not to permit further movement of such migrant workers and required them to stay wherever they have reached while providing for shelter, food and medical facilities to them while observing social distance norms.'[18] State governments were required to strictly comply with this, enforce the lockdown for the specified period and follow social distancing norms, 'which would mean complete prohibition of inter-district and interstate migration of any population including the migrant workers who are en route.'

Initially, with a view to dispersing large gatherings of such migrant workers at state borders, some state governments did make arrangements for their travel by bus, the apex court was informed. The Union government had a valid argument that the migration of workers on their own in large numbers defeated the very objective of the preventive measures taken by the government. 'Migrant workers travelling bare foot or otherwise in large numbers inevitably and unknowingly defy the social distancing norm which is one of the globally accepted norms for preventing COVID-19 and put their lives and lives of others in danger,' said the status report signed by Union Home Secretary Ajay Bhalla. It feared that if such large groups were permitted to reach their home villages in rural India, they would carry the COVID-19 infection with them and infect the populations of their respective villages, which had remained untouched so far. The government was also aware that many villages had the same apprehension and were resisting the re-entry of migrant workers. 'This migration, therefore, is not only dangerous for the migrant workers who have started on foot themselves but also for rural India for which they have started the journey,' said the report.

The movement of such people prior to the government allowing it was something that bothered the Union and state governments. They had not planned for people, who had helplessness writ large on their faces, walking home or crowding stations. Union Cabinet Secretary Rajiv Gauba and Union Home Secretary Ajay

Kumar Bhalla took a meeting of chief secretaries and directors-general of police from Punjab, Haryana, Maharashtra, Gujarat and Delhi on the morning of 29 March. In the meeting, they expressed alarm and displeasure over the large-scale movement of migrant labourers on foot, followed by the gathering of a large number of people, especially at the Anand Vihar Bus Terminal in New Delhi. To disperse the crowd from this area, buses had to be provided on 27 and 28 March despite the lockdown. During the meeting, state officials were told that their governments were duty-bound to prevent such large-scale movement of people in violation of lockdown guidelines. To implement these directions and ensure there was no movement of people on the roads, the state governments issued directions to district administrations. In one such order, the Haryana government sealed interstate borders. Districts were asked to ensure that no persons, whether travelling in a bus, truck, tractor or trolley, or on foot or on bicycles, should be allowed to cross interstate barriers. 'They should be turned back without exception. The persons who are travelling on foot within the districts on highways/roads should be picked up, placed in buses and left in localities from where they started,' said the Haryana government directive. Directions were also issued by the state's home department to appoint indoor stadiums and other similar facilities as temporary jails, so that people who refused to obey the directions of the district administrations were lodged there.

The road to home may have been long and tiring, but the stranded labourers went on walking despite the summer heat, once restrictions were eased on 29 April 2020, since public transport still remained unavailable across the country. Some workers, who lost their jobs due to the lockdown, started walking towards Madhya Pradesh from Jalna in Maharashtra. They planned to go to Bhusawal in Maharashtra, a 157 km journey, and from where they planned to walk or hitch a ride for another 850 km to reach Umariya and

Shahdol in Madhya Pradesh.[19] But after walking for about 36 km, they felt tired and sat on the railway track between Karnad and Badnapur railway stations of the Nanded railway division in Maharashtra. Tired bodies that perhaps had not had enough to eat, they fell asleep. At 5.22 a.m. on 8 May 2020, when they were deep in sleep, they were hit by a goods train travelling towards Manmad. Of about nineteen persons in the group, fourteen died on the spot while two succumbed to their injuries later.[20]

An independent data collection of non-virus deaths that occurred due to the lockdown puts the number at 991 till 30 July 2020.[21] The highest number of such deaths, recorded by thejeshgn.com on the basis of publicly reported incidents, was 224, all caused due to starvation and financial distress. This was followed by 209 persons killed due to accidents and walking. The Union government, however, does not have any data on labourers dying in accidents. In fact, in reply to a question by Jasbir Singh Gill in the Lok Sabha on 22 September 2020, Union Minister of State for Road Transport and Highways V.K. Singh said, 'As per provisional available information 81,385 accidents occurred on the roads including national highways during the period March-June 2020 with 29,415 fatalities. However, this ministry does not maintain separate data in respect of migrant workers who have died in road accidents during the lockdown.'[22]

The Azim Premji University, along with ten civil society organizations, conducted a detailed phone survey from 13 April 2020 to 20 May 2020 among roughly 5,000 respondents across twelve major states in India, to gauge the impact of the COVID-19 lockdown on employment, livelihoods and access to government relief schemes.[23] The survey covered 161 districts and seven large cities (Ahmedabad, Ajmer, Bengaluru, Bhubaneshwar, Delhi, Jaipur and Pune). Respondents interviewed in urban areas spanned thirty different occupations. 'The respondents were selected through a purposive sampling method to ensure diversity in location and type of work done. The sample is not representative of the country or the states in which interviews were conducted,' says the survey. Its findings, however, showed that 66 per cent of workers lost their employment, 64 per cent saw their earnings fall, while 77 per cent of households were consuming less food than before. Forty-seven per cent of households did not have enough money to buy even a week's worth of essentials, while 77 per cent of vulnerable households received ration and 49 per cent received cash transfer from the government. Households that had a total income of below Rs 10,000 in February were classified as vulnerable. It further said that more than eight in ten migrants (81 per cent) lost their employment during the lockdown, as compared to 64 per cent employment loss among non-migrants or people who worked in their native places.

Seven in ten urban migrants did not have enough money even for a week's worth of essentials. Eighty-eight per cent of migrants reported not being able to pay next month's rent. More than a third (36 per cent) of migrants reported taking loans to cover their expenses during the lockdown. Seventy-seven per cent of households reported that they did not have enough money to buy even a week's worth of essentials. More than eight in ten respondents in urban areas also reported that they did not have money to pay the following month's rent, while 41 per cent of respondents in urban areas reported that they had to take loans to cover daily personal expenses. In rural areas, more than half of the survey respondents were either farmers or casual workers. A majority of workers in urban areas were service providers or construction workers. They worked as ragpickers, domestic help, tailors, sanitation workers, street vendors, plumbers, painters, carpenters, taxi or auto drivers, balloon sellers, cleaners, bidi makers, construction labourers or security guards.

A report on the state of democracy in various countries published a year later by Freedom House, a Washington DC-based non-government organisation, cites the lockdown in India as one of the ways in which the government's policies hit the vulnerable. 'India's internal migrant population endured significant hardships as a result of the government's pandemic-related lockdown, which was imposed in March and gradually eased beginning in May. Many migrant labourers were unable to access basic supplies and services in cities, forcing millions to travel hundreds of miles—often on foot—to their home villages. Harsh restrictions on movement were violently enforced by police and citizen vigilantes, with Muslims often scapegoated as potential spreaders of the virus,' noted the report.[24]

The report's finding that India was 'partly free' was quick to get a rebuttal from the government, which also defended its decision to impose the lockdown in 2020. 'The Freedom House report titled *Democracy under Siege* in which it has been claimed that India's status as a free country has declined to "partly free", is misleading, incorrect and misplaced,' it said in a statement dated 5 March 2021. On the subject of the lockdown, the Union government said that between 16 and 23 March 2020, most state governments and Union territories resorted to partial or full lockdowns based on their assessment of the COVID-19 situation. 'Any mass movement of people would have spread the disease rapidly throughout the country. Taking into consideration these facts, the global experience and need for consistency in the approach and implementation of various containment measures across the country, a nationwide lockdown was announced. The government was fully conscious that during the period of an inevitable lockdown, people should not face undue distress. Aware of this, the government took various measures to address the situation,' said the government statement.[25] It further noted that the lockdown period allowed the government to ramp up the production capacity of masks, ventilators and personal protection equipment (PPE) kits, and thereby effectively prevent the spread of the pandemic. India has, on a per capita basis, registered one of the lowest rates of active COVID-19 cases and COVID-19-related deaths globally, the government contended in its statement. In a few weeks, however, these would prove to be little more than tall claims.

By the Union government's own admission in the Lok Sabha, more than 10.6 million migrant workers, including those who travelled on foot during the lockdown, returned to their home states, according to data compiled by the MoLE.[26] Strangely, the government's reply in Parliament about migrant labourers has been evasive. In one such reply to a question by Mala Roy in the Lok Sabha, Union Minister of State for Home Affairs Nityanand Rai said, 'The migration of [a] large number of migrant workers was triggered by panic created by fake news regarding duration of lockdown, and people, especially migrant labourers, were worried about adequate supply of basic necessities like food, drinking water, health services and shelter.'[27] Though the question specifically asked the government for the reasons that thousands of labourers ended up walking post the lockdown, it did not list financial distress and shutting down of transport services among the reasons. The fact was that the greatest impact of the shutting down of transport services was on the people who needed to travel urgently, after the lockdown had taken away their sources of livelihood and made it difficult for them to survive in big cities. 'The resolve, taken by millions separately and yet in a strange unison of purpose, was to journey home, whatever it took,' says activist Harsh Mander.[28]

7

THREE SETS OF TRAINS AND A BUS BACK HOME

IT WAS THE FIFTH day of the national lockdown. The Union government was categorical that the movement of a large number of migrants in some parts of the country, trying to reach their native places, was 'a violation of the lockdown measures on maintaining social distance.'[1] Therefore, for effective implementation of the lockdown measures and to mitigate the economic hardship of the migrant workers, states were asked to take additional measures while keeping such people in shelters, said a 29 March 2020 order. Exactly a month later, on 29 April, however, the government decided to ease the stringency and allow for the movement of stranded people through special buses.

There had been no dramatic change in the COVID-19 situation in the intervening period. The number of confirmed COVID-19 cases was 979 on 29 March, with 255 new cases and a total of twenty-five deaths.[2] The infection was officially at the local transmission stage. On 29 April, the spread of infection had moved to the 'cluster of cases' stage, with a total of 31,332 cases and the addition of 1,897 new cases. The total number of deaths was 1,007. It can, therefore, be inferred that the humanitarian crisis was causing great anxiety among people, and state governments were not able to handle the situation effectively, forcing a relaxation. States such as Rajasthan, Delhi and Uttar Pradesh had already started bus services to transport people back to their home states. Some controversy inevitably followed.

When about 300 buses set out from Uttar Pradesh on 17 April 2020 to pick up students stranded in Kota in Rajasthan, Bihar Chief Minister Nitish Kumar called it 'injustice', since it looked like states were facilitating the return of students but 'making excuses' when it came to migrants.[3] He said the movement was against the principle of the nationwide lockdown to slow the spread of COVID-19. The state shot off a letter to the MHA when a group of 300 students from Kota came to the state capital, Patna, mostly in taxis. 'This will open up a Pandora's box. If you allow students, on what grounds can you stop migrant labourers who are also stuck?' Bihar Chief Secretary Deepak Kumar was quoted by an NDTV report as saying in a letter asking the Union government to stop special permits being granted by the Rajasthan government.[4]

The chaos went on for more than a month, forcing the MHA to review its lockdown guidelines and allow the interstate movement of stranded persons.[5] It acknowledged that due to the lockdown, migrant workers, pilgrims, tourists, students and other persons were stranded at various places, and that they would be allowed to move. It asked states to use buses with adequate social distancing provisions.

States were to develop standard protocols for receiving and sending the stranded persons. People willing to move were to be registered with nodal authorities. 'In case a group of stranded persons wish to move between one state/union territory and another state/union territory, the sending and receiving states must consult each other and mutually agree to the movement by road,' said the MHA order. States on the transit route were also asked to allow such movements. The persons travelling were to be screened and only those found asymptomatic would be allowed to proceed. On reaching their destination, these persons were to be quarantined.

States readily started registering and moving stranded people. Web portals were created where specified categories of people—migrant workers, pilgrims, tourists, students and others who were stranded—could register their details. Such registration was being done district-wise by the sender states. An *Indian Express* report quoted Assistant Director (Public Services), Jaisalmer, Rajasthan, Bharat Bhushan Goyal, as saying that 150 labourers were to be sent to the neighbouring state of Haryana from Jaisalmer's Nachna district.[6] These labourers had come to Jaisalmer some two to three months back for harvesting, and as soon as the season ended, the lockdown was announced. For about a month, they had been in shelter homes. Haryana, in turn, had people from Bihar and Uttar Pradesh waiting to go home. The Haryana government launched Operation Samvedna, under which 100 special trains and 6,600 buses were arranged for the return of such people to their home states.[7] A total of 432,000 travellers boarded these trains during the lockdown.

In Haryana's most severely impacted district of Gurugram, which has an eclectic mix of residents, ranging from local villagers and affluent corporate employees to labourers and workers from all parts of the country, schools and community centres were first converted to shelter homes to prevent any movement out of the city. Streams of people were, however, walking on the road towards Faridabad for a journey into Uttar Pradesh, and some even farther to Bihar. Usha Kundu, assistant commissioner of police, headquarters, Gurugram, who was the nodal officer for COVID-19, says, 'The population of

Gurugram is diversified. One did not know that so many labourers would come out [onto the roads]. There was great stress and a fear that the situation would turn so bad that there would be no place to cremate [those who died of COVID].'[8] She shared her thoughts in early March 2021, but weeks later, the second wave made her words sound prophetic.

Even police employees, she says, were not allowed to move outside the district and at the same time, if someone was living in Delhi or outside the district, they were asked to stay where they were. 'We shut the districts. Quarantine zones were created.' Kundu says nobody thought that such a situation would arise. 'Otherwise, we could have allowed them to travel, but the government did not have adequate health infrastructure. Even masks were not available, so lockdown gave us that time to create the necessary infrastructure.'

Geofencing was also done to contain infections. 'One has read about the nuclear bomb being dropped at Hiroshima. It was the same feeling—not a soul on the Golf Course Road. Even in times of war, there are people [outside], but here was a situation where everyone was locked inside,' she says. It was felt that the greater the strictness, the lower the number of people who would come out of their houses, Kundu admits. But once the Union government allowed the movement of stranded people, the local administration and police had another task at hand—of arranging for their travel. The first step was to register the labourers. Those in the shelter homes were first in line. They were tested for COVID-19 and their belongings sanitized. If it was a small bus, about twenty-eight to thirty people were accommodated, while forty could go in the bigger buses. Each bus had two to three policemen. 'We sent buses and trains to Bihar, Madhya Pradesh, Uttar Pradesh, Rajasthan and even Telangana. Forty to fifty buses were sent to Uttar Pradesh,' she says.

Kundu narrates the account of a middle-aged person who was unmarried and wanted to go back to his village. He boarded a bus for Uttar Pradesh but when it came to getting down, he said, 'If I get down here, I will die.' So, he kept sitting in the bus and returned to Gurugram. Kundu, who has been in Haryana Police for ten years, says helping people is routine for them, but this time, the situation was different. 'It was not a law and order situation, but a human crisis. Every person had this fear of death,' she says.

Government buses were used for transporting people since the local administration felt private bus operators would start making money by exploiting the situation. State governments created portals where people could register for travel. By 30 May, 1.2 million had been registered on the Haryana government portal e-Disha.[9] Some 350,000 of those were from Gurugram, but official data shows that 49,095, or just 14 per cent, from the district travelled in government-arranged buses and trains. Some 800 buses were used to move 25,707 persons, while another 23,388 were sent in twenty trains. According to a *Times of India* report, a significant number would have left on foot or arranged their own means to go home. Both Mohan Paswan and Keerat Kori (see Chapter 6) left Gurugram after bus and train services had resumed, but they chose to cycle and drive a motorbike, respectively, putting their lives in danger. Even those who died on the railway track on 8 May were walking from Maharashtra to Madhya Pradesh. The reason people used other modes was the long wait for their turn on government trains and buses, even as the financial stress was building up. In many cases, they simply lacked the means to afford a ticket. A Gurugram district administration official was quoted in the *Times of India* report as saying that on many occasions, the mobile numbers registered with the e-Disha portal were either switched off or deactivated.

Lingampalli in Telangana was the site of a secret operation on 1 May 2020. It was 5 a.m. A train full of people who had been stranded in the nearby areas due to the national lockdown left the Lingampalli railway station for Hatia in Jharkhand. Neither Lingampalli nor Hatia is the main railway stations in Hyderabad and Ranchi, respectively, but the secrecy surrounding the operation was such that till a day earlier, the spokespersons of the railway ministry kept denying the news of such special trains. Main city stations were deliberately skipped to prevent crowds. Railway stations, especially in Mumbai, had earlier seen crowds gathering to board trains, even when there were none leaving. The Union government had instructed the states to keep the movement of people under wraps. In fact, so secret was the operation that even the MHA order allowing such special trains only came later in the day.[10] The order said:

> Movement of migrant workers, pilgrims, tourists, students and other persons, stranded at different places, is also allowed by special trains to be operated by (the) ministry of railways (MoR). MoR will designate nodal officer(s) for coordinating with state/UTs (union territories) for their movement. MoR will issue detailed guidelines for (the) sale of tickets; and for social distancing and other safety measures to be observed at train stations, train platforms and within the trains.

After a little over a month since snapping all transport links, forcing people to sneak out of their city homes on foot but then being detained and held captive in shelter homes, what prompted the Union government to allow the stranded people to move out in special buses and trains is not clear. The crucial question is whether rural areas had been better equipped with health infrastructure in that one month to handle the influx of such people from big cities. Two days earlier, on 29 April 2020, the MHA allowed running special buses, but the sheer number of people and the distance that had to be travelled led to the governments of Telangana, Kerala, Tamil Nadu, Maharashtra, Rajasthan, Punjab and Bihar opposing the movement of people only by bus, and instead sought the introduction of special trains.[11]

The day of 1 May was carefully chosen by the government, since it is International Labour Day. This, however, also showed that the timing of these trains had nothing to do with the COVID-19 situation in the country. They could have been started ten days earlier or ten days later; all that was needed was a standard operating procedure to ensure that no infected person boarded the train. The Railway ministry said in a press statement issued in the evening that day:

> As per the guideline issued by the MHA, it has been decided to run Shramik Special trains from Labour Day today, to move migrant workers, pilgrims, tourists, students and other persons stranded at different places due to lock down. These special trains will be run from point to point on the request of both the concerned state governments as per the standard protocols for sending and receiving such stranded persons. The Railways and state governments shall appoint senior officials as nodal officers for coordination and smooth operation of these Shramik Specials.[12]

On the first day, the Indian Railways ran four Shramik Specials with 3,645 passengers. Another ten trains ran the next day. These were all long-distance trains. Moving the same number of people by road would have required over 550 buses and many more days of travel. These non-stop trains mostly had twenty-four coaches, with each coach accommodating fifty-four instead of the usual seventy-two passengers because of social-distancing norms. The total number of passengers travelling on a train was around 1,200.[13] The passengers had to be screened by the sender states and only those found asymptomatic were to be allowed to travel. Sender state governments were asked to bring the passengers in batches to the designated railway station in sanitized buses, following social distancing norms and other precautions. It was mandatory for every passenger to wear a face cover. Meals and drinking water were to be provided to the passengers by the sender states at the originating station. On longer routes, the railways were to provide a meal during the journey.[14] On arrival at the destination, the receiving state was to make all arrangements for screening, for quarantine if necessary, and for further travel from the railway station.

The first Shramik Special from Bengaluru for Bihar left on 3 May. Seemant Kumar Singh, inspector general (headquarters), whose phone had been constantly ringing with requests for food ever since the lockdown started, says that with the start of train operations, the demand for food gradually came down, but requests for getting people out of the city increased. 'I was made the nodal officer for [sending people to] Bihar and Jharkhand. We could send 1,200–1,500 people on one train. Initially, there were hiccups, but there was no violence in Bengaluru because by then, I had established some goodwill among people,' he says.[15]

Singh narrates the account of a man whose wife was eight months pregnant and was desperate to go home. He boarded one of the trains, and once back in Bihar, he sent a photo of his newborn son to Singh. He later called Singh to thank him for helping the family go back home. 'It was systematic. If we were taking persons from one colony, we used one bus. Some fifty buses were required for one train-load of passengers, so they were divided area-wise,' says Singh. Before the departure of a train, there was a night-long procedure for the required medical screening of the registered persons by the local administration. Passengers were given breakfast, but sometimes, the screening process would go on well into the afternoon. 'Trains left from Malur in the Kolar district, around 50 km from Bengaluru city. If we had started trains from inside the city, there would have been a rush, since a city centre is porous. Even outside, people used to come in rickshaws or autos to board trains, so we had adequate security,' he says. Confidentiality was maintained—only some officers knew what time a train would leave. The local administration collaborated with non-governmental organizations to provide morning meals and a meal en route.

In Bengaluru, there were many students and other people who had come for medical treatment, but had gotten stuck in the city. Singh says it was a big challenge to get them out and arrange for their travel. He says:

> We did not have any data on the number of such people. We would give out our number through the media and send our jeeps to pick them up. Their status was different from that of labourers, so we would reserve one or two compartments for such people, which also included women. Some of them came from well-off homes but had run out of money and were staying in lodges where they did not get food.

Though there was a huge rush to board these trains in some places, in others, the local administration had to ensure that trains were occupied. 'Trains ran from the Gurugram station. We had to ensure that these trains were not empty so that resources were not wasted. In places like Ambala and Bhiwani, the number of labourers was small, so routes were sometimes clubbed. But the routes of these trains were kept secret,' says Kundu.

Despite the secrecy, the Indian Railways had to clarify the very next day that the special trains were being run only for migrant workers, pilgrims, tourists, students and other persons stranded at various places, on the request of state governments only, and all other passenger train services remained suspended till 17 May.

A railway ministry press release, dated 2 May 2020, stated:

> The railways is *only* accepting passengers *brought* and *facilitated* by state governments. No other group of traveler or individual are allowed to come to station. No tickets are being sold at any station … All other passenger and suburban trains remain suspended, therefore, *no one* should come to railway station.[16]

Till 3 p.m. on 10 May, a total of 366 Shramik Specials had been operationalized, of which 287 trains had reached their destination and seventy-nine trains were in transit. Of the 287 trains, one terminated in Andhra Pradesh, eighty-seven in Bihar, one in Himachal Pradesh, sixteen in Jharkhand, twenty-four in Madhya Pradesh, three in Maharashtra, twenty in Odisha, four in Rajasthan, two in Telangana, 127 in Uttar Pradesh, and two in West Bengal. 'These trains have ferried migrants to cities like Tiruchirappalli, Titlagarh, Barauni, Khandwa, Jagannathpur, Khurda Road, Prayagraj, Chhapra, Balia, Gaya, Purnia, Varanasi, Darbhanga, Gorakhpur, Lucknow, Jaunpur, Hatia, Basti, Katihar, Danapur, Muzaffarpur, Saharsa etc.'[17]

After running the Shramik Specials for ten days, the government on 11 May announced the start of fifteen pairs of special train services from 12 May. This was part of the 'partial restoration' of train services in a graded manner. These trains were to run in both directions on certain specified routes.[18] These special trains had only air-conditioned coaches of first, second and third classes. All of them were to start from and end at the New Delhi railway station, quite like the Rajdhani trains, with the same fare structure but excluding catering charges. So there were two categories of trains: one for the labourers, which were basic, express trains, and the other for those who could afford air-conditioned travel. But unlike the Shramik Specials, where the local administration decided who would travel after people had registered on a portal, bookings for these special trains were taken through the IRCTC website or through its mobile app. Booking tickets through reservation counters or through travel agents was still not allowed. Reservations could be made up to a maximum of seven days in advance, but the railways extended this period to thirty days on 22 May, when it also allowed the issue of reservation against cancellation and waitlisted tickets. Those with waitlisted tickets, however, were not allowed to board the train.[19] The process of screening, unlike in the case of Shramik Specials, was done at the right at the railway station. Only passengers with confirmed tickets could enter the station, and they were supposed to reach railway stations on their own. The zonal railways were told to ensure separate entry and exit gates at railway stations in order to avoid face-to-face movement of passengers. All passengers were 'advised', but not mandated, to download and use Aarogya Setu, the government's mobile application, which had the data and the geographical location of people infected with COVID-19.

On 11 May, when the IRCTC started booking tickets for these special trains that were to start from 12 May, there was a flood of bookings, and within two hours, all the tickets had been booked. Bookings were to open at 4 p.m., but opened two hours late, at 6 p.m. By 9.15 p.m., approximately 30,000 PNRs had been generated and reservations issued to more than 54,000 passengers.[20] All AC-1 and AC-3 tickets for the Howrah-New Delhi train were sold out within the first ten minutes. The train was to begin its journey the next day at 5.05 p.m. All AC-1 and AC-3 tickets for the Bhubaneswar-New Delhi train were also sold out by 7.30 p.m. 'All trains towards [the] eastern side—Howrah, Bhubaneswar, and Agartala—were fully booked by 7.30 p.m., same was the case with trains from Mumbai,' a *Business Standard* report quoted an official as saying.

Though these special trains were air-conditioned and had a premium fare structure, like those of the Rajdhanis, the railways thought it best that no linen, blankets or curtain be provided inside the train in order to prevent infection. Passengers were asked to carry their own linen for the travel. The temperature inside AC coaches was to be suitably regulated to limit the requirement of a cover. So, by starting these two sets of trains, the government thought it was catering to the needs of those who were stranded and belonged to two different classes.

Despite these two categories of trains, there was such high demand that on 19 May, the railways appealed to migrants not to panic. 'Efforts are being made to ensure that all of them are able to travel to their home states at the earliest. Efforts will be made such that they will be able to board trains from Railway Station Head on main line which is close to their existing location,' a Press Information Bureau (PIB) statement said while announcing the introduction of 200 time-tabled daily trains from 1 June.[21] By then, the Indian Railways had transported more than 2.15 million migrants to their home states through 1,600 Shramik Special trains. The new time-tabled trains were to be non-AC, but passengers could book tickets online and booking counters were also opened. The railways asked state governments to identify and locate migrants who were walking to their home states and transport them to the nearest main line railway station after registering them online at the nearest district headquarters. It also asked states to provide a list of these travellers to the railway authorities so that arrangements could be made for their travel through the Shramik Specials.

The starting of these three sets of trains was a big relief to those stranded and was meant to save governments the embarrassment of the poor walking on foot, in some cases even beyond 1,000 km.

Controversies, however, accompanied the trains right from the beginning. It started with the bickering over who would pay the fare for those travelling on the Shramik Specials, especially since the passengers of these trains were mostly those that had been stuck in big cities for more than a month without livelihood, food and money. Since the fare was equivalent to that of express trains, the charges were exorbitant for the class of people who boarded them: they normally travelled in less expensive trains. A political blame game soon ensued since reports started coming in that some passengers had had to pay for their tickets. On the fourth day of the running of the Shramik Specials, 4 May, Congress president Sonia Gandhi issued a statement saying, '[W]hat is particularly disturbing is that the Central government and the rail ministry are charging them (workers and labourers) for train tickets in this hour of crisis.'[22] This is when the rail ministry had the largesse to donate Rs 151 crore to the PM's Corona Fund, she said. 'Why can't these essential members of our nation's fabric be given a fraction of the same courtesy, especially free travel, at this hour of acute distress?' she wrote. Gandhi also announced that her party had decided that every Pradesh Congress Committee (state-level Congress unit) would bear the cost of rail travel of every needy worker and migrant labourer. Though Sonia and her party were criticized for 'playing politics,' the letter sent the railway brass and the ruling Bharatiya Janata Party into a tizzy. By the latter half of 4 May, the Union government had issued a statement saying travel on the Shramik Specials would be free for the passengers and the cost would be shared between the Centre and the states. Though the Congress scored political points, a government spokesperson, trying to salvage the situation, said later in the day, 'Neither the Government of India, nor the Railways had indicated of charging from the workers.'[23] Of the transportation cost, the railways were to bear 85 per cent, while the states were to bear the remaining 15 per cent. States were only coordinating the movement of these stranded passengers, the spokesperson said. This, however, was clearly an afterthought that ran contrary to the railway ministry's own instructions. A Railway Board note to all the zonal railways, dated 1 May 2020 and signed by Shelly Srivastava, director, passenger marketing, detailed the fare structure. 'In order to facilitate the stranded passengers in different part of the country due to COVID-19 situation, on the request of the state government of the originating/destination stations, it has been decided to run special trains on [the] following fare: Fare of sleeper mail express trains + superfast charge (Rs 30) + additional charge of Rs 20.'[24]

Besides, detailed guidelines issued by the railway ministry on 2 May 2020, in point number 11, had instructions regarding the sale of tickets.[25] Sub-section 'a' said, 'The originating state will indicate the exact number of passengers travelling in train, which should be around 1,200 (or at least 90 per cent) considering the capacity of Shramik Special train.' The railways were to print train tickets to the specified directions, according to the number of passengers indicated by the originating state, and then hand them over to the local state government authority.

Sub-section 'c' said, 'The local state government authority shall handover the tickets to the passengers cleared by them and collect the ticket fare and hand over the total amount to Railway.' For the Indian Railways, therefore, these trains meant restarting of passenger business after forty days, albeit as a very restricted and tense operation. The railway ministry was forced to change tack because of the build-up of political pressure. By then, however, a number of states, including the Opposition-ruled Rajasthan, said they would pay the railways for sending migrant labourers home. Bihar Chief Minister Nitish Kumar, though an ally of the BJP, said the state would pay for the tickets of migrants from his state stuck across the country.[26] He issued a video statement saying that no fare would be charged from students returning to the state by special trains while migrant workers would be fully reimbursed for the expenses they had incurred after they completed the mandatory twenty-one-day quarantine. Each worker was to get a minimum of Rs 1,000. This cash did help people belonging to Bihar. Ekdashi Kumar of Adhwar village in the Kaimur district of Bihar was one such person.

Kumar was initially wary about giving his village's name for fear of caste reprisal. He thinks COVID-19 is a big hoax and was intentionally spread as a rumour by the government in order to curb protests against the National Register of Citizens (NRC) and build the Ram Mandir at Ayodhya in the ensuing chaos. When told there were millions across the world who had contracted the highly contagious disease, he stubbornly says, 'I don't believe this. You don't understand; it was just a rumour (*hawa phelaya hua tha*). They say 10 lakh [100,000] fell ill and then suddenly all of them recover. Where did the medicine come from? Where were all these people admitted? I do not believe that so many people fell ill. All this was done by Modi so that they could build the Ram temple at the cost of poor people.'[27] Kumar even shooed away the village head (pradhan) when he asked Kumar to quarantine in a school after he returned to his village. 'Already we were without food in a foreign land and we would have died without food in the school,' he laments.

The reason Ekdashi Kumar is so bitter despite getting help from the Bihar government is that work suddenly stopped at the granite factory in Bengaluru where he was employed. 'The factory shut on 18 March. I was there for one and a half months during the lockdown. We were not being paid, but I had some savings and I got a Rs 10,000-loan from my village on interest,' he recounts. The experience of demonetization, however, had given rise to a distrust of the government. The sentiment was that any day, suddenly, something could shut down just as currency notes turned into meaningless paper and rendered many cashless in November 2016. Each time Prime Minister Narendra Modi was scheduled to address the nation about COVID, anxiety built up, especially during the last few days of March 2020. Ekdashi Kumar feared that all ATM machines would be closed. 'I withdrew all the money that came from village,' he says. They were eight people living together, paying Rs 5,500 in rent a month for one room, with each person paying Rs 1,300.

Once the Shramik Specials began running, local administrations started registering people for travel. Ekdashi Kumar got a message fifteen days after he had filled up the registration form. He took one of the Shramik Specials to Araria in Bihar on 24 May. From Patna, the state government took them to Gaya. When asked whether the police or the local administration on the outskirts of Bengaluru helped him, he curtly says, 'Nobody helped me. Policemen used to say we will break your hands and legs if you move out. But there was information floating around that some police station was collecting documents. I got to know about the trains this way. I deposited my documents and then I got a message after two weeks. The administration put us on a train. We were a group of ten,' he says, adding that the only way the Karnataka government helped them was by allowing them to fill up the registration form for travel and giving food when they boarded. 'We did not pay any fare. Nitish Kumar said the Bihar government would pay for whoever was stuck. So one ticket was for Rs 1,000, which our state government paid,' he says.

Replying to an RTI application, the Railway Board said that a total fare of Rs 433 crore was collected from state governments and from the representatives of state governments for running the Shramik Special trains between 1 May and 31 August 2020:

> Railways in coordination with the state governments ensured smooth movement of passengers of Shramik Special trains between originating and destination railway stations. Railways

> have not collected any fare for Shramik Special trains from migrant labourer/stranded passengers. The fare at normal rates was collected from the respective state governments/authorized representatives of state governments for running of Shramik Special trains.[28]

The huge number of people wanting to travel by these trains showed the desperation of those impacted by the shutting down of transport services. By 14 May, the Indian Railways crossed the milestone of transporting more than one million passengers, through 800 Shramik Special trains, to Andhra Pradesh, Bihar, Chhattisgarh, Himachal Pradesh, Jammu & Kashmir, Jharkhand, Karnataka, Madhya Pradesh, Maharashtra, Manipur, Mizoram, Odisha, Rajasthan, Tamil Nadu, Telangana, Tripura, Uttar Pradesh, Uttarakhand, West Bengal, among others.[29] The journey on the Shramik Specials, however, was one of the worst memories of many who travelled on them, leading to another set of controversies. As if the human suffering wasn't enough, political controversy arose over the provision of trains by the railway ministry and state governments allowing or hindering such trains. In an interview with the ANI news agency, Union Minister of Railways Piyush Goyal said, on 14 May, 'It pains me that several states such as West Bengal, Rajasthan, Chhattisgarh and Jharkhand, are not giving enough permissions for "Shramik Special trains" to enter their states.'[30] The same day, a railways press statement reiterated that trains were being run only after the concurrence of both, the state sending the passengers and the state receiving them. The very next day, on 16 May, the railways again affirmed that in order to ensure safe and quick transportation of migrants, they were ready to run Shramik Special trains from all the districts connected by rail across the country.

Goyal asked district collectors to identify and prepare a list of stranded labourers and their destinations, and send it to the railways through state nodal officers. 'The Indian Railways has got the capacity to run almost 300 Shramik Specials a day, however, less than half are being presently utilised. Stranded Migrants in various districts across the country can reach home states more conveniently and comfortably,'[31] said a PIB statement. While stating that full capacity operationalization of the railways' rakes would provide significant relief to migrants across the country who were seeking to go to their home states, Goyal's ministry was indicating that it was the states that were dragging their feet in drumming up numbers and facilitating boarding and receipt of stranded people. 'Indian Railways is ready to augment the running of Shramik Special trains as per the actual needs of the districts,' the statement added. 'As of today [16 May], more than 15 lakh [1.5 million] migrants have already been transported by the Railways to their home states and almost 1,150 Shramik Special trains have been operationalised. Indian Railways can easily transport almost double [the] number of migrants per day,' said the railways' statement. But with Shramik Specials becoming a publicity nightmare for the Union government instead of bringing them goodwill, the Centre made the decision to run trains. So three days later, on 19 May, the MHA issued a revised standard operation protocol on the movement of stranded workers by train. Right in the first point, it said, 'Movement of Shramik Special trains shall be permitted by [the] ministry of railways, in consultation with the ministry of home affairs.'[32] This was in contrast to what was said on May 1—that these trains would 'run from point to point on the request of both the concerned state governments as per the standard protocols for sending and receiving such stranded persons.' The MoR was now only to communicate the train schedule, including stoppages and destination, to make adequate arrangements for sending and receiving passengers. The railway decision was to be based on the requirement of states.

The political slugfest, however, continued, especially between the Centre and the Opposition-ruled states of Maharashtra, Rajasthan and West Bengal. In a televised speech on 24 May, Maharashtra Chief Minister Uddhav Thackeray claimed that while his government had been seeking eight trains daily to send migrants back to their respective states, the Centre was sending only thirty to forty trains daily.[33] But the same day, Goyal took to Twitter from 7.14 p.m. onwards till the next day to say that the railways were prepared, but it was the Maharashtra government that was not ready with a list. He even said trains were running empty from Maharashtra since the state government was unable to provide an adequate number of passengers. 'Hope like earlier, train after coming to the station does not return empty. I would like to assure you whatever number of trains you want you will get,' Goyal said in personalized tweets addressed to Thackeray.[34] These Twitter barbs continued till 2.11 a.m. on 25 May. 'Where is the list for 125 trains from Maharashtra? As of 2 a.m., received list of only 46 trains of which 5 are to West Bengal and Odisha which cannot operate due to cyclone Amphan. We are notifying only 41 trains for today despite being prepared for 125,'[35] the Union minister wrote. Clearly, Goyal was angry at how the running of these trains was turning out to be a sore point in his career at this crucial, historic juncture.

While politicians were busy exchanging barbs, the misery of those already wracked by the crisis continued in yet another sign of things going out of hands. On 25 May, a video of a child walking around and trying to wake his dead mother, who had travelled from Gujarat to Katihar in Bihar with her child and relatives on board a Shramik Special, went viral.[36] The video was shot at Muzaffarpur railway station in Bihar. The railways said that the woman, Parbina Khatun, was a heart patient, though the death was widely seen to have been caused due to heat and stress.

The railway administration was terribly shaken by reports coming in that many deaths had taken place aboard these trains, so the ministry came out with an appeal on 29 May, asking people with ill health not to travel. A statement said:

> It has been observed that some people who are availing this service have pre-existing medical conditions which aggravates the risk they face during the COVID-19 pandemic. A few unfortunate cases of deaths related to pre-existing medical conditions while travelling have happened. In order to protect the vulnerable persons from COVID-19, in line with MHA, Order No. 40-3/2020-DM-I(A) dated 17.05.2020, Ministry of Railways makes an appeal that persons with co-morbidities (for example, hypertension, diabetes, cardio-vascular diseases, cancer, immune deficiency conditions), pregnant women, children below the age of 10 years and persons above 65 years of age may avoid travel by rail, except when it is essential.[37]

A *Hindustan Times* report put the total number of deaths on board the Shramik Special trains between 9 May and 27 May at almost eighty, quoting data from the Railway Protection Force.[38] The news report caused a major controversy. Railway Board chairman V.K. Yadav addressed a press conference and said:

> Anyone's death is a big loss ... I can imagine the plight of labourers travelling even in these conditions. In case of deaths, the local zones investigate the reason and without an investigation, there are allegations that they died of hunger when there was no shortage of food. Some deaths occurred and we are compiling the figures ... we will issue the figures in a few days.

The railways had started these trains as a relief measure, but there was no arrangement for food, either on board or at the railway stations. At the sender station, the local administration would give passengers water and some basic provisions, enough for one meal. The railways provided mostly the bare minimum snacks of biscuits and water en route. 'We were living on sips of water. The railways would sometimes give a biscuit packet and then for more than a day, nothing. There was to be no stoppage, but sometimes train would run for ten hours and then suddenly stop for water and biscuits,' says Ekdashi Kumar. When the train he took started from Bengaluru, the administration there gave him some rice and two rasgullas. 'But after it was over, we were so hungry that while drinking water, we did not even know where it flowed into our stomach.'

Shramik Specials were taking longer than the usual time despite express train fares being charged from the states. They, therefore, became a gruelling journey for some passengers. The summer was harsh and the journeys were too long. It took Ekdashi Kumar 125 hours to reach Bihar. 'We sat on the train at 10 p.m. in the night on 24 May and on 29 May, we got down at 12 p.m. I spent over five days on a train and then, after I got down at Araria, the Bihar government provided bus transport to Gaya.' In a widely reported case, a train going to Gorakhpur in Uttar Pradesh from Vasai Road station outside Mumbai ended up at Rourkela railway station in Odisha:[39] a train bound for the northern part of the country, near the border of Nepal, from the western coast of India, went first to east India. There were about 1,398 passengers on that Shramik Special, who waited two and half days to reach their destination instead of just twenty-five hours. Initially, television channels quoted passengers saying that the train lost its way, which was probably unlikely in the Indian Railways, given its modern signalling system. The railways, however, dismissed these suggestions, saying it was a planned diversion because of the congestion on the routes to Bihar and Uttar Pradesh. The Railway Board, which had by then started holding regular press conferences and presentations by its chairman, sprang into action doing damage control. In a press conference on 29 May, Railway Board chairman Vinod Kumar Yadav said that about 80 per cent of the passengers in the special trains run during this period travelled to Uttar Pradesh and Bihar. In these states, local governments faced some problems transporting passengers from the stations to their final destinations. Hence, the railways also provided local trains to take passengers to nearby stations. More than 350 such local trains had been run till then. He claimed:

> Trains were diverted only during May 20–24, 2020. During this time, more than 250 trains were run every day. A record number of 279 Shramik Special trains were provided on May 20, 2020. Ninety per cent of these trains were to Uttar Pradesh and Bihar, resulting in rail route congestion in these states and hence need for diversion in some cases. Out of the total trains run so far, only 1.85 per cent of total 3,840 trains were diverted, and that too for only four days, in order to meet the demand of states for trains.

According to Yadav, out of 3,840 trains run till 28 May, 3,836 trains reached their destinations within seventy-two hours. Ten per cent trains faced a delay of two to five hours. Around 3,500 trains reached their destinations, travelling at an average speed higher than that of mail express trains, he said. He added:

> Even among the four trains which took more than 72 hours, some of them faced a delay, caused by landslide in Assam which led to flooding and hence track had to be closed for safety purpose. The trains were stopped for 12 hours at such stations

> where all facilities were available. This apart, a few trains had to be diverted from their route because of the gas leakage incident.[40]

Whatever the reasons, the fact that passengers did not know about the diversion and what to expect from the long, tiring journey put a question mark on the management of these trains.

When the Indian Railways started a graded restoration of train services from 1 June, the guidelines for the new train services had changed dramatically. This could be due to the lessons learnt from running the Shramik Specials but at the same time, it also exposed the class bias of the railway management since the trains starting from 1 June were for a 'higher category' of passengers. Apart from allowing booking from railway counters, the IRCTC started making provisions for limited eatables and packaged drinking water on payment in some of the trains that had pantry cars attached. Information on this was to be made available to passengers at the time of booking the ticket. Though passengers were encouraged to carry their own food and drinking water, all static catering and vending units (multipurpose stalls, bookstalls, chemists and other stalls) at railway stations were allowed to open. In food plazas and refreshment rooms, cooked items were to be offered as takeaway items only, with no dine-in arrangements. What the railways, however, kept harping on was that it had distributed more than 8.5 million free meals and about 12.5 million free water bottles to nearly 5 million migrants travelling in Shramik Special trains by 28 May.[41] The railways claimed in its press statement:

> This includes meals being prepared by Indian Railways' PSU IRCTC and distributed by zonal railways. Food and water

> bottles are being provided to travelling migrants in all Shramik Special Trains. IRCTC is providing puri vegetable pickle, roti vegetable pickle, banana, biscuits, cake, biscuit namkeen, cake namkeen, veg pulao, pao bhaji, lemon rice pickle, upma, poha pickle etc. kind of meals to travelling migrants along with Rail Neer water bottles.

On the ground, however, the situation was starkly different. There were reports of passengers raiding stalls for food and water at railway stations. According to a *Business Standard* report, passengers of Shramik Specials had raided stalls at various stations, including Kanpur, Jabalpur, Deen Dayal Upadhyay, Jhansi, New Delhi and some stations in the south. At the same time, fewer trains meant little business for over 100,000 stalls that had operated at railway stations before the lockdown across the country. Though the railways asked these stalls to begin operations through a notification dated 21 May, the operators faced a staff crunch. 'Medically fit vendors have migrated to their home states. Getting medical fitness certificates for staff takes 15 days. At this stage, it is not feasible to hire new employees. In addition, only few trains are being operated, mostly one or two trains a day in majority of stations, leading to no sale at our stalls,' Ravinder Gupta, president, Akhil Bhartiya Railway Khan-Pan Licensees Welfare Association, was quoted as saying in the news report. These vendors sought a waiver of licence fees till normal train operations begin.[42]

Exactly how many passengers travelled by rail after the special trains started is difficult to say, even though the PIB, the publicity department of the Union government, gave regular updates. An application filed under RTI with the MoR only got two misleading replies. While the query asked for monthly passenger earnings and numbers, the reply directed the applicant to a railway website with a link to '10-day statement of approximate gross revenue and traffic handled.' On filing an appeal with the Appellate Authority, a reply came on 27 May 2021, which again directed the applicant to a website saying 'the 10-day statement' was inadvertently mentioned in the original reply. It again gave a navigational path for looking up the data, which led to a thirty-six-page statement on goods traffic. On another page on the website, there were monthly evaluation reports, but those had data only till February 2021, even almost three months after the end of the financial year on 31 March 2021. The application had sought data till March 2021.

For a government that was sending out signals that the economy was on a V-shaped recovery path and the estimated real GDP growth for 2021–22 would be 11 per cent, 'the highest since independence,'[43] giving out data that showed a fall was perhaps best avoided, even though old-timers say the Indian Railways' data-keeping has historically been good. How much the Indian Railways' passenger earnings fell was anybody's guess since railway passenger operations were shut during the lockdown. Transporters globally saw their earnings impacted due to the pandemic, so the reluctance in sharing information was unnecessary. The number of passengers who travelled by train fell 87 per cent in the eleven-month period ending February 2021, from 7.7 billion in 2019–20.[44]

With the graded reopening of rail services, travel activities started resuming. For local movement, 705 suburban services (Central Railway–355 and Western Railway–350) were started from 15 June 2020, but these catered mainly to essential service workers. Additional special trains, in coordination with the state governments, were run for the Ganapati festival, for those giving entrance exams to engineering and medical courses, and for armed forces and government jobs.

Addressing a virtual press conference on 23 July 2020, Railway Board chairman Vinod Kumar Yadav said they had operated the last Shramik Special train on 9 July, and all existing demand for such trains was fully met, though if there was more such demand, these services could be resumed. In all, 4,621 Shramik Specials were run.

According to figures given out by the Indian Railways, occupancy on 17 July 2020 was below 30 per cent in thirty-seven trains, between 30 to 50 per cent in twenty-five trains, 50 to 75 per cent in thirty-three trains, 75 to 100 per cent in thirty-four trains and full capacity with demand for more in sixty-eight trains. The overall occupancy level was 75.48 per cent, which showed that people were more confident about travelling again. In fact, the average occupancy level between 12 May 2020 and 31 August 2020 was even higher, at approximately 82 per cent, according to Union Railway Minister Piyush Goyal's reply in the Lok Sabha on 16 September 2020.[45]

The Indian Railways' catering and ticketing arm the IRCTC, however, found its foray into train operations dithering all this while. It had started the operation of its first corporate train, the Lucknow-Delhi-Lucknow the IRCTC Tejas Express, on 4 October 2019, and of the Ahmedabad-Mumbai-Ahmedabad IRCTC Tejas on 19 January 2020. But it had to halt these trains from 19 March 2020 due to the COVID-19 pandemic. It announced the restarting of Lucknow-New Delhi and Ahmedabad-Mumbai Tejas train operations from 17 October. 'Both the trains have been received very well by the rail passengers in terms of quality of services, travel experience and punctuality. [The] IRCTC, through its special complimentary travel insurance being offered to the passengers with the feature of compensating the travelers for late running of the trains had ensured the trains are properly monitored and that they run on time. All these facilities will be available to the passengers after the restart of the operations of these two Tejas Trains,' said the company on 7 October 2020.[46]

A month later, on 23 November, however, it announced the suspension of operations. 'Being aware of the COVID situation, lesser number of persons is travelling in both the Tejas express. Thus IRCTC have [sic] temporarily halted the operation of the Lucknow-Delhi-Lucknow IRCTC Tejas Express Train No. 82501/02 further wef [with effect from] 23.11.2020 and that of Ahmedabad-Mumbai-Ahmedabad IRCTC Tejas Express Train No. 82901/02 wef 24.11.2020,' it said in a press statement.[47] This time, the cessation of the service was not due to the fear of contagion but due to low passenger numbers, which also indicated that travel had not normalized. The situation was to be reviewed in December, but it was only on 29 January 2021 that the IRCTC announced the restarting of the Tejas service 'for catering to the growing passenger demand.'[48] Both the trains restarted operations from 14 February 2021. However, the IRCTC suspended first the Ahmedabad-Mumbai service from 2 April and then the Delhi-Lucknow service from 9 April till 30 June 2021 because of the more devastating second wave of COVID-19.[49]

In February 2021, however, the IRCTC was also gaining the confidence to normalize its traditional tourism offerings. So the announcement of restarting the Tejas trains from 14 February came a day after it came out with a note on the promotion of tourism in line with the government policy. It said in a 28 January note:

> Due to lockdown all commercial activities came to on a halt and tourism industry was also not the exception. Tourism industry was badly hit due to the COVID impact and is still struggling to revive. In this toughest scenario, IRCTC has taken a lead and launched different domestic tour packages by tourists trains as well as air mode from its offices across India.

The IRCTC also claimed it was getting tremendous response from the public and a large number of people were booking its tour packages:

> IRCTC's air tour packages for Kerala, Goa, Kashmir, Andaman, Rann of Kutchh in Gujarat and the North East region launched for February and March months from different cities are fully booked and hence additional tours are being launched. Bharat Darshan train from Varanasi to Jyotirling yatra started on 10th January with 600 booked tourists. Another train from Raxaul, Bihar is scheduled on 31st Jan for south India and more than 500 seats are booked. Pilgrim special train from Jalandhar for Jyotirlinga tour on 27th January booked by more than 600 passengers. Other tours from East, South and Western part, planned by IRCTC are also getting great patronage by public.

It further stated that it had decided to run a deluxe AC tourist train on two different tours, Padharo Rajasthan and Jyotirlinga and Statue of Unity in Gujarat.

> This afresh deluxe tourist train has a host of astounding features including two fine dining restaurants, a modern kitchen, shower cubicles in coaches, sensor based washroom functions, foot massager. The fully air-conditioned train provides two types of accommodation viz. First AC and 2nd AC. The train has enhanced security features in the form of CCTV cameras.

Six days earlier, on 22 January, the IRCTC said it was restarting its e-catering services for the passengers travelling in the operational special trains. The IRCTC had started this service in 2014, whereby passengers could order an array of food of their choice from reputed brands as well as popular regional and local delicacies, on the phone or online, while travelling on trains, and get the same delivered to their seats at railway stations. Pre-COVID, the IRCTC had started clocking 20,000 e-catering orders a day. Due to COVID-19, e-catering services were suspended on 22 March 2020. 'However, with the gradual resumption of passenger train services and amidst the new normal wherein IRCTC is serving only "Ready To Eat" meals to passengers on trains, there has been an increased demand for resumption of e-catering services,' it said. This resumption was conducted in a phased manner, with the company starting the first phase of e-catering services from February 2021, wherein the service commenced in over thirty railway stations catering to approximately 250 trains. It was, however, only on 19 November 2021 that the Indian Railways restored serving of cooked food on Rajdhani, Shatabdi, Duronto, Vande Bharat, Tejas and Gatiman trains.

By 15 January 2021, the Indian Railways, too, was running 65 per cent of its pre-COVID mail express trains again. All the important destinations across the country were connected by these trains. According to data provided by the MoR, restoration of train services had reached a level of 66 per cent as of 1 April 2021, a year after services were shut down. In pre-COVID times, the Indian Railways ran an average of 1,768 mail/express trains a day, including festival specials; 3,634 passenger trains, including the short-distance MEMU, DMU and EMU; and 5,881 suburban trains. The average total number of trains before the pandemic struck, across all categories, was 11,283 a day, while the restoration saw an average of 7,474. Within these categories, the maximum restoration of services, or 91 per cent, was in the suburban category, while only 20 per cent had been restored in the slow-moving passenger category. The total number of trains restored, however, was 9,232. The reason for the difference between the total number and the average number of trains restored is that the total number includes weekly/biweekly trains, which are not in operation on all days. Therefore, the daily average number of trains is less than the total trains in operation. Also, some trains were being approved by the Railway Board and notified by zonal railways to commence within seven to ten days. Once they actually start service and run/terminate in the system, they appear in the daily statistics. The number of trains restored based on trains notified and the daily average number operated, therefore, varied.

Technically, the Indian Railways had not resumed its full passenger operations even in June 2021, more than a year after shutting them down, but this did not stop them from launching new trains and holding inaugurations just as in normal times. Since the graded opening began, the approach was to launch a service wherever there was demand. At the same time, the Indian Railways maintained that it wanted to discourage people from travelling, and in order to do this, it increased both fares for short-distance travel (in some cases, like Delhi-Ghaziabad, by three times to Rs 30) and for platform tickets bought by those who are not travelling, and only visiting stations to drop or pick up passengers.

Further, the February railway statement said there were a large number of second-class sleeper coaches besides other classes in all the trains that were being run. These had the lowest fare in the reserved category. Forty per cent of the passengers travelled in this class in much better traveling conditions than in pre-COVID, unreserved travelling situations.[50]

It maintained that fares had been increased only in short-distance passenger trains, which constitute less than 3 per cent of total trains. Many trains, it said, were being run despite low occupancy, only for the benefit of the passengers. Further, the February railway statement said in all the trains that were being run, besides other classes, the trains had a large number of second-class sleeper coaches, which had the lowest fare in the reserved category and that 40 per cent of the passengers travelled in this class in much better travelling conditions than in pre-COVID, unreserved travelling situations.

On 12 November 2021, a letter from the passenger marketing wing of the Railway Board asked all zonal railways to restore full train services.[51] The railways had seen 344 million passengers boarding trains during the previous month of October 2021, compared to 62 million in October 2020, though it continued to be less than half of 703 million passengers that were booked prior to COVID-19 in October 2019.[52] The special status, given to trains after the partial restoration of services in May 2020, was also removed bringing down the passenger fares in certain categories of trains. The requirement for reservation even for the second-class coaches that was put in place because of COVID-19 in 2020 was, however, not removed. This meant more than 1,700 train services across the country were back on the tracks.

8

TAKING OFF AGAIN WITH A BUBBLE AND MORE

FOR SIXTY-THREE DAYS IN 2020, the Indian skies did not see any passenger operations. It was a complete shutdown, though airlines did move cargo. When the lockdown kicked in, airlines transported some of their own staff stuck in various cities. The COVID-19 pandemic had cleared the skies completely, but domestic passenger operations took off again only after a humanitarian crisis had forced the Union government to allow buses and trains to move people who were at the edge of survival. There was no urgent need to start air operations, though there were people who were stuck in various cities and were waiting for flights to resume for safer movement rather than risking contagion by taking a train, since Indian trains are often crowded and have poor hygiene. Some of these persons had flown hurriedly to wherever their families were a few hours before the shutting down of transport services.

On 17 May 2020, just four days after the domestic passenger flight ban was extended till midnight of 31 May 2020, the MoCA issued another circular upon receiving orders from the MHA. The new circular, dated 21 May, said the ban would be valid till midnight of 24 May only.[1] According to an *Indian Express* report, the change in the government's stand came after the airlines red-flagged their financial health in a meeting on 18 May. The airlines had conveyed that they would be forced to retrench staff.[2] The report quoted airlines as asking: when trains could be allowed, why not airlines?

The resumption of domestic flights, however, led to states raising objections, just as the shutting down of services had the Centre and Delhi governments fighting and the Centre asserting its federal rights. Maharashtra, West Bengal and Tamil Nadu, all hosting big airports, objected to the Centre's announcement of opening up the skies.[3] West Bengal, which had been hit by the cyclone Amphan, wanted the flight ban to continue till at least 30 May.

Air travel came with its own set of controversies and uncertainties around what would happen when the passengers touched down. State governments across the country, especially those with high COVID-19 cases, wanted their borders not to be porous so soon after the pandemic had only settled down in mid-May and would resurface again as soon as people moved out. Unlike the Indian Railways, which left the decision to states on what health protocols they wanted to follow for arriving passengers, there was total confusion for air travellers prior to the resumption—whether the receiving states would quarantine, and for how long, whether it would be a government-owned quarantine facility only or whether it could be a paid facility.

While allowing flight operations was a Central government prerogative, states could always stop boarding and deboarding of passengers through local restrictions. The fact that states did not want people from COVID-19 red zones to enter their borders underscores an important policy learning about the federal structure of India's polity, described in Article 1 of the Indian Constitution as 'India, that is Bharat, shall be a Union of States.' What is a federal or central subject has to be a state government matter in times of crisis, or perhaps even otherwise?

The MHA issued a separate set of guidelines for rail, air and road transport. States did not follow any uniform quarantine protocol. An MHA note dated 10 June, in fact, had ten pages listing the different quarantine requirements of state governments.[4] Delhi, for instance, had seven days of institutional quarantine for international passengers at a government facility at no charge, or paid quarantine at designated hotels, followed by seven days of home quarantine. The neighbouring Haryana, however, had no institutional quarantine but a fourteen-day home quarantine. Bihar, on the other hand, had absolutely no quarantine requirement or any other condition, and required airports to do only thermal screening. Within states, too, different rules were applied for different airports. West Bengal, for instance, had the same fourteen-day home quarantine rule for passengers alighting at Kolkata and Bagdogra airports. Screening was required at the Kolkata airport, which was not required at Bagdogra. Maharashtra had six different sets of rules for airports at Aurangabad, Pune, Shirdi, Nagpur, Mumbai and Kolhapur.

The MoCA, too, was not consistent with its rules. On 29 June, more than a month after the recommencement of domestic air travel, it modified the rule requiring passengers to provide a self-declaration that they had not tested COVID-19 positive in the past two months.[5]

> With regard to evolving COVID-19 situation, where new cases that have been cured are in large numbers, a need has been felt to update this (Para 1(j)(v) of Annexure-II to Order dated 21.05.2020) provision to avoid hardships in the matter of air

> travel to the persons cured/recovered from COVID-19. It has accordingly been decided to update the above provision with the clause 'I/we have not tested COVID-19 positive in the last three weeks' (COVID-19 recovered persons fulfilling this condition will be allowed to travel upon showing a COVID-19 recovered/discharged certificate from any institution dealing with COVID-19 subjects).

The Union government's approach for the two classes of travel—those who travelled by train and buses and those who wanted to fly—had all along been starkly different. Besides, the number of people who were waiting to travel by these modes of transport was vastly different too. Unlike the restarting of train operations, the resumption of flight services twenty-four days later was not shrouded in any secrecy, with Union Aviation Minister Hardeep Singh Puri holding a press conference on 21 May 2020 and announcing the partial resumption of air services four days later, from 25 May onwards: a four-day notice and a public announcement.

The MoCA also issued a detailed standard operating procedure to be followed by airlines and passengers in-flight and at the airports.[6] Airlines were permitted to operate at only one-third of their capacity.[7] But, when the first flight was to take off at 12.40 a.m. on 15 May, it had to be cancelled. The Indigo flight 6E-2625 from Bengaluru to Delhi did not get enough bookings. Airlines were not required to take off even without an adequate number of passengers since even in normal times, they cancelled or bunched flights due to low occupancy. There were clear instructions from the MoR, however, to not let any train go empty, and so the local officials of the sender states had to ensure that enough passengers were available. A list of passengers, in fact, was handed to the railway nodal officers, and routes were clubbed to ensure an adequate number.

The first day's flight traffic was already one-third of normal times, but it was further halved, to 532 flights operating with 39,231 passengers to various destinations. 'Whereas it is necessary to ensure that airlines do not charge excessive fare on the one hand and also to ensure that journey is performed only for essential purposes; it is, therefore, necessary to fix a fare band within which the airlines should charge fare,' said a circular signed by Satyendra Kumar Mishra, joint secretary in MoCA.[8] The sectors were classified on the basis of approximate duration of the flight, and the minimum and maximum fares for such classes were fixed. The minimum fare was Rs 2,000 on forty-six routes of sector A, while the maximum was three times that, at Rs 6,000. Eighteen more routes were added to the A category on 25 May keeping in mind the demand from these sectors.[9] These were short-distance routes. The farthest sector, G, comprising six routes, had a minimum fare of Rs 6,500 and a maximum of Rs 18,600. The fare band was not applicable to business class.

Many of these flights reportedly had rows of empty seats, while thousands could not board planes due to last-minute flight cancellations. The day passenger air operations resumed on 25 May, thirty to forty trains had to be diverted because of congestion on railway routes. So while flights were not getting enough passengers, trains were being diverted because of congestion. This was not surprising since the class and the number of people who travel by air are different from those of passengers who travel by train. Besides, air travellers could afford to stay wherever they were stuck, while low-income rail travellers were in economic distress and could not sustain themselves in big cities.

The number of people travelling by air took some time to increase. On 23 August, Puri said that the number of domestic passengers had more than tripled from 30,550 on 26 May to 97,662 on 22 August

2020, nearly three months after the recommencement of domestic civil aviation operations. The number of flights doubled from 418 to 968 during this period and the footfall at Indian airports stood at 194,205. 'It is an encouraging sign that we are now at 33 per cent mark as compared to the pre-COVID domestic civil aviation numbers. We will now move towards 150,000 daily passengers mark by further opening up the sector & adding more flights,' he tweeted.[10] In other words, it took three months for airlines to reach the government-approved capacity.

Domestic passenger operations had resumed in May 2020 with 33 per cent of the original summer 2020 schedule permitted. This was increased to 45 per cent on 26 June 2020, to 60 per cent on 2 September 2020 and to 80 per cent on 3 December 2020.[11] Though this 80 per cent cap was to remain in force till 31 March 2021, the MoCA decided to bring down the cap on seating capacity to 50 per cent from 1 June when the second wave was already weaning off.[12] This order was not only late but also unnecessary, because the number of passengers had already fallen to an average of 40,193 in May 2021; people decided not to take undertake travel on their own.[13] This was just 13 per cent of the 313,668 passengers who had flown on 28 February 2021.[14]

In reply to a question by Hema Malini in the Lok Sabha on 25 March 2021, however, Puri said:

> There is an immense possibility for growth of aviation sector in India. During 2019-20, Indian airports reported a total throughput (arrivals and departures, domestic and international) of approximately 34 crore [340 million] passengers. (The) Indian aviation sector has witnessed compound annual growth rate (CAGR) of 12.4 per cent in total passenger traffic during the last five years in the pre-COVID period.[15]

But the growth suffered due to COVID-19. 'However, it has also shown rapid recovery. The total number of domestic passengers increased from approximately 2 million in June 2020 to over 7.3 million in December 2020.' He also quoted AAI estimates to say that Indian airports taken together would handle a total throughput of around 400 million passengers by 2024–25.

To another question raised in the Lok Sabha by D.M. Kathir Anand on the same day, the minister replied that the domestic traffic contracted from approximately 108 million during April–December 2019 to approximately 30 million during April–December 2020, while international traffic went down from approximately 52.1 million during April–December in 2019 to approximately 5.59 million during April–December 2020.[16] The financial loss that Indian carriers incurred during April-December 2020 is approximately Rs 16,000 crore, while that of airports is Rs 3,000 crore.

According to the data released by the DGCA, a total of 143,736,256 (143.74 million) passengers travelled on scheduled domestic flights during January–December 2019, with airlines recording 87.2 per cent passenger load factor. This came down to less than half at 62,858,348 (62.86 million), with a passenger load factor of 74.3 per cent, in 2020. Non-scheduled domestic service flights carried 245,399 domestic passengers in 2020, as against 438,934 in 2019.

As for international travel, 24,287,654 (24.29 million) passengers flew on scheduled airlines that recorded a passenger load factor of 81.7 per cent in 2019. This fell drastically to 6,101,666 (6.1 million) passengers, with airlines recording a 74.9 per cent passenger load factor in 2020. The number of people who availed of non-scheduled international services, however, rose dramatically to 2,133,539 (2.13 million) in 2020 as against just 3,479 in 2019 because of special flight operations on international routes that fell in this category.

The government allowed domestic operations of passenger services at full capacity only from 18 October 2021, which was seventeen months after domestic passenger air service had resumed in May 2020.[17] It was intriguing that the government continued to impose a cap on the number of seats being offered by airlines even after the economic activity had started to normalise in other sectors. Nonetheless, the restoration of full service coincided with the commencement of the festival season for 2021.

Private-sector airlines are the dominant players in domestic flight operations, though the state-run Air India and its subsidiary, Alliance Air, also offer flight services. The private airlines were waiting to restart operations when the government decided to partially open up the skies. Initially, however, only the Air India group was allowed to operate overseas repatriation flights. In fact, those started earlier than domestic flights, on 7 May 2020, which was also just six days after the starting of Shramik Special trains.

These were called the Vande Bharat Mission flights. 'Initially when Vande Bharat flights started, we were nervous though the travel later became relaxed. We had to take COVID test before going on the flight,' says an Air India hostess who flew on these special mission flights. The crew was provided everything for their safety: a personal protection (PPE) kit that included gown, caps, gloves, N95 masks, covers for the feet and eye protection, so that they were fully covered. Only after the crew wore everything did boarding begin. Passengers were asked to board three to four rows each at a time, not continuously. So around twenty passengers would board, and only when they were seated would others be allowed on the plane. According to government regulations for both domestic and international flights, the person in the middle seat had to wear a PPE kit while masks were mandatory for all passengers all throughout the flight. 'We have to make COVID-specific announcements in intervals where we ask people to wash and sanitise hands, do not touch face, limit movement. Only one passenger should wait outside the bathroom,' the airhostess explained. Toilets would have a large and a small sanitizer bottle. People were asked to sanitize after using the toilet. The crew sanitized the lavatory every forty minutes.

On-flight services were reduced to the bare minimum, even if international flights were long-haul journeys. Food boxes were pre-placed on the seats for passengers. They would contain sufficient food for a nine-to ten-hour flight. For longer flights, there were two boxes. After use, passengers were supposed to put them in a plastic bag and put the bag under the seat in front. The idea was to minimize crew interaction and limit it to only to safety-related issues. Designated areas were provided in the planes to isolate passengers who were suspected COVID cases. She says there were cases of people feeling unwell in some of the flights she served on, but later, those cases did not test positive.

> We used to keep an eye on passengers who were feeling unwell. During flight, you cannot tell whether they have infection or not but tests were carried out after the flight. Once back from international flight, the crew, too, had to undergo another COVID test and till the results were known, they were put up in a hotel. Earlier, all flights returned because there were no layovers, but sometime in August 2020, layovers started in London, Sydney and Paris but crew mostly confined to hotels. We were supposed to be inside the hotel, not that anyone wanted to go out because of fear of corona. Though India has strictest protocol, Sydney was also very strict. Police escorted crew to

their hotel. Rules were tightened there after someone broke the norms and went partying.

Things started to relax a bit from October onwards, with passengers starting to move in the gallery, though flight crews still had to keep reminding passengers that the infection was not yet gone. People who travel with children don't necessarily take precautions. 'We have to keep reminding them to make the child wear a mask. Sometimes, people request a change of seat, but then you have to tell them that it is not possible since the plane is sanitized only once before the flight,' she recounts. She remembers an Ahmedabad to London flight where there were many elderly people, most of them diabetic. It was difficult to persuade them. It led to increased movement in the cabin. 'Elderly passengers will listen once but then again do the same thing. Maybe they were diabetic, so they felt hungrier and kept asking for food,' she says. This flight returned from London to Delhi with passengers, but there were flights to Nairobi and Sydney that had passengers only one way.

Though Air India did not give any special allowance to staff flying on these planes, it was not compulsory for everyone to go on them. Only those willing to do the flight flew. They were allowed quarantine leave. 'In June and July, when we flew people, they were grateful and wished us good luck. We are the only airline that flew during the lockdown and it is a matter of pride for us. Having our jobs is something we should be grateful for,' she says. Air India is a loss-making company, which the government has privatized and agreed to sell to the Tata group.

Vande Bharat Mission flights, however, were not the first repatriation flights during the pandemic. Earlier, the Indian Air Force (IAF) had brought back citizens stranded outside the country. These were called 'evacuation' flights and were not charged to the passengers. In February, an IAF plane evacuated seventy-six Indians and thirty-six foreign nationals from Wuhan in China. The C-17 Globemaster III transport aircraft carried 15 tonne of medical supplies for China and brought back people stranded there on its return.[18] These included twenty-three citizens from Bangladesh, six from China, two each from Myanmar and the Maldives, and one each from South Africa, the US and Madagascar. Earlier, Air India had evacuated around 650 Indians from Wuhan in two flights. An Air India flight had also brought back 119 Indians who were on board the cruise ship *Diamond Princess* but were stranded in Japan.

Countries across the world were repatriating their citizens. On 30 March 2020, American Airlines operated a repatriation flight between Lima, Peru and Miami International Airport. Flight 9441 was a chartered flight coordinated by the US Department of State. It took off from a Peruvian military base adjacent to Jorge Chavez International Airport and brought more than 200 Americans back to the US. This charter was one of six repatriation fights that American Airlines flew from Peru. There were eighty-eight missions from Latin America and the Caribbean.

The Vande Bharat Mission launched by India facilitated the repatriation of people through land, sea and air routes. Two special flights from the UAE with 363 Indians on board, including nine infants, came to Kerala. The first Air India Express flight IX 452 brought 177 passengers and four infants from Abu Dhabi to Kochi. It took off at 5.07 p.m. on 7 May. A little later, the Dubai-Kozhikode flight IX 344 with 177 passengers and five infants took off at 5.46 p.m.[19]

Till 16 September 2020, three evacuation flights and five repatriation flights under the Vande Bharat Mission had been operated from China to bring back stranded Indians, including students. Through these flights, a total of 820 students and 658 other Indians were brought back to India. In addition, forty-seven foreigners were also flown at the request of their respective countries.[20]

The International Civil Aviation Organization, an agency of the United Nations, encouraged repatriation flights, and in a letter dated 15 April 2020, asked its member countries to grant speedy authorization to such flights.[21] It defined repatriation flights as those organized by member states for 'the sole purpose of repatriating their nationals and other eligible persons from other states, with no embarkation or disembarkation of other passengers for "remuneration or hire". This would ensure that necessary authorizations for the entry, departure and transit of aircraft carrying out such repatriation flights are granted expeditiously.' Similar speedy clearances were also sought for 'repatriation flights' carried out on a commercial basis. Member countries of ICAO were asked to review their authorization procedures and exercise flexibility in their approaches 'for granting all necessary authorizations for the entry, departure and transit of aircraft carrying out such operations whether by State aircraft, humanitarian flights or chartered commercial flights.'

While announcing a systematic repatriation mission, the MHA said that many Indian nationals who had travelled to different countries before the lockdown, for various purposes such as employment, studies/internships, tourism, business, etc, were stranded abroad. 'Due to their prolonged stay abroad, they are facing distress and are desirous of returning to India urgently. Apart from the above cases, there are other Indian nationals who need to visit India in medical emergencies or death of a family member,' said the ministry, while laying down a standard operating protocol for the mission.[22] Indians were required to register themselves with the Indian missions in the countries where they were stranded. Their return was to be on non-scheduled commercial flights arranged by the MoCA and on naval ships to be arranged by the Department of Military Affairs. Details of the passengers were to be shared with the states where these flights were to land. The passengers had to carry a negative RT-PCR test result for COVID-19 and undergo a fourteen-day institutional quarantine at their own cost. A repeat test was to be conducted after fourteen days. People entering through land borders were also to follow the same protocol. The quarantine requirements, however, were changed on 24 May, when the government sought to 'harmonise health related instruction' during travel across all modes of travel.[23] The new guidelines said that the travellers would give an undertaking that they would undergo mandatory quarantine for fourteen days—seven days' paid institutional quarantine, followed by isolation at home. Those wanting to travel out of India were asked to register with the MoCA. Only those persons who were citizens of the country they wanted to travel to, or held at least a one-year visa for that country, or Indians with a six-month visa but facing some emergency, could travel. An institutional mechanism was to be created to allow the travel of eligible persons on the non-scheduled commercial flights that were being arranged to bring back stranded Indians from abroad.[24] The MoCA, therefore, designated Air India as the nodal agency to facilitate the process.

The MHA, through an order dated 24 May 2020, also permitted international charter operations and operations by private aircraft to bring back stranded Indians. Certain categories of Overseas Citizens of India were allowed to come to India. The protocol for persons arriving on chartered flights was almost the same as that for those coming on Air India and Alliance Air flights. They, too, had to register with the Indian missions and the details had to be given to the states where the flights were to land.

A similar registration process was followed for Shramik Special trains, where those wanting to travel had to apply to the state or local governments, but the Union government's handling of this category of special trains was found wanting on the human quotient, adding to the distress of those who were stranded for over a month. The running of these trains was in contrast to the high-profile Vande Bharat air service, which got publicity and good media coverage, possibly because of the involvement of the MEA. Tragedy, however, struck one of the Vande Bharat Mission flights when an Air India Express plane with 190 on board was landing in bad weather conditions. It overshot and fell 50 m off the end of a runway at the Kozhikode airport in Kerala on 7 August 2020. The plane broke into two, killing at least twenty people, including the pilot and the co-pilot. This was termed the deadliest commercial aviation disaster in India in ten years.[25]

The Vande Bharat flights were, however, just the beginning of a graded resumption of international passenger operations. So, just as the government started another set of trains after the Shramik Specials, it also came out with 'transport bubbles' for international passengers. These bubbles are temporary transport arrangements between two countries aimed at restarting commercial passenger services while regular international flights continued to remain suspended. The service is reciprocal in nature: airlines from both countries enjoy similar benefits.[26] Compared to Vande Bharat, where transportation of people could be just one way, the transport bubbles help in commercial operations on both sides. For instance, passengers to the UAE, whether nationals or not, would not be allowed on the Vande Bharat Mission repatriation flights, and if anyone wanted to travel, they would require special permission from the UAE's foreign ministry. This it said while seeking India's permission to operate its charter flights, which would fly only with crew and take passengers from India.[27] This created the need for bubble arrangements between countries.

The announcement of transport bubbles on 17 July came after more than 227,000 people had been evacuated on Vande Bharat flights, and more than 89,000 flown out of India. Overall 687,000 Indians had returned under the mission, including on domestic and foreign charters, naval ships and through land borders.[28] In a tweet on 17 July, Puri said air bubble arrangements were being put in place for the US, the UAE, France and Germany to begin with, and similar arrangements were being worked out with other countries. This was being done to further revive international civil aviation operations.[29]

The concept of bubble flights took off from the Baltic region when three former Soviet states, Latvia, Lithuania and Estonia, agreed to open up travel among the three countries. Estonian President Jüri Ratas announced in a tweet that after a video call with Krišjānis Kariņš, the Prime Minister of Latvia, and Saulius Skvernelis, the Prime Minister of Lithuania, internal borders among the three countries were being opened up from 15 May. 'It's a big step towards life as normal,' he said.[30] Though persons travelling on Indian transport bubbles were required to quarantine, citizens from these three Baltic States could travel freely without self-isolating or quarantine requirements provided they had not travelled outside the Baltic States in the previous fourteen days and had no respiratory illness.[31] Though this bubble was the first one in the twenty-seven-member European Union, it fell apart after working for four months. Latvia said those coming from Estonia needed to self-quarantine themselves starting 12 September for two weeks, because of increased infection in Estonia. Truck drivers, diplomats and certain other people who travelled for work were given an exemption.[32]

Singapore and Hong Kong also entered into an agreement on 11 November for an air travel bubble (ATB) starting from 22 November.[33] Edward Yau Tang-wah, secretary for commerce and economic development, Government of Hong Kong, said, 'This is the very first ATB for Hong Kong. It matters not only for cross-border travel between the two places, but also reflects the Government's hope to progressively restore the city's economic activities amid the long-drawn battle against COVID-19.' Hong Kong and Singapore, he noted, are similar in terms of epidemic control; both are regional aviation hubs and international cities, enjoying strong trade, investment, finance, tourism and people-to-people ties. 'The revival of cross-border air travel between the two places is of utmost importance. We hope that aviation, tourism, hotel, retail and catering businesses can benefit from it, thereby enabling Hong Kong's economy to recover gradually,' he said in a statement. Under the arrangement, travellers between the two cities were not to be subject to any quarantine arrangements upon arrival, nor were there any restrictions on their travel purposes or itineraries, on the condition that they complied with a set of anti-epidemic protocols.

On 21 November, a day before the first flight was to start, Hong Kong and Singapore decided to postpone it. 'If the ATB (air transport bubble) is to be launched as scheduled tomorrow, chances of making immediate adjustment are high. The deferral of the inaugural flights is a suitable and responsible arrangement to minimise the inconvenience caused to the ATB travellers and reduce the uncertainty in their itineraries,' said a statement.[34] Golden and silver balloons that had been put up at the Hong Kong airport to welcome the launch of the travel arrangement were taken off and burst. Pictures of the deflated balloons strewn across the airport went viral, symbolizing the sorry situation when an intent to normalize operations could not be translated into action because of the pandemic. The bubble arrangement did not start even six months later, though Edward Yau Tang-wah said his government had sent a new proposal to Singapore to restore the planned travel bubble. He also wrote to six other countries about resuming talks on such plans. The countries he wrote to included Australia and New

Zealand. This time around, the vaccination of Hong Kong residents was cited as one of the grounds for pushing the arrangement.[35]

Meanwhile, on 6 April 2021, New Zealand announced quarantine-free travel with Australia from 19 April. New Zealand Prime Minister Jacinda Ardern said the conditions for starting to open up quarantine-free travel with Australia had been met. 'Our team's success in managing COVID-19 and keeping it out over the past 12 months now opens up the opportunity to reconnect with loved ones and resume Trans-Tasman travel,' she said in a news conference.[36] This announcement came even as two days later, on 8 April, Ardern announced that New Zealand was temporarily suspending entry for all travellers, including its own citizens, from India, from 11 April till 28 April, due to a surge in COVID-19 cases. Of the twenty-three COVID-19 positive cases in insolation, seventeen were from India.[37]

The response of India, however, was not as cautious. In a reply to a question raised in the Rajya Sabha by Phulo Devi Netam, Minister of State for External Affairs V. Muraleedharan said, on 17 September 2020, that the total number of passengers found COVID-19 positive on arrival in India was 3,248 till then. This was when the total number of Indian citizens brought back to India was 1.4 million (1,412,835), of which around 56,874 were students.[38] The number of positive cases among those coming to India could have risen further considering that till 21 June 2021, 2.05 million passengers had come to India in 13,596 Air India group flights that were part of eleven phases of the Vande Bharat Mission.[39]

India, however, did put in place some temporary measures, stopping flights from certain countries. For instance, it stopped flights from the UK from 22 December 2020 till 7 January 2021, when a new and more infectious strain of the coronavirus was found in that country.[40] Subsequently, only thirty flights were permitted to operate between the two countries from 8 January till 23 January

2021 – fifteen flights in each direction. This cap on the number of flights was extended into mid-April 2021.

More than a year after the phased reopening of international travel, India was not sure if it wanted to throw open its skies for international passengers. On 26 November 2021, the DGCA issued a circular that allowed resumption of scheduled commercial international services from 15 December 2021.[41] Countries were, however, categorized into three: those enlisted 'at risk' but had air bubble arrangement with 75 per cent pre-COVID operations; those enlisted 'at risk' but did not have bubble arrangement were allowed with 50 per cent of pre-COVID operations; and countries other than 'at risk' were allowed full entitlements.

Just two days earlier on 24 November, South Africa had reported a new COVID variant B.1.1.529. WHO's Technical Advisory Group on SARS-CoV-2 Virus Evolution met to assess the new variant the day India decided to open up the skies. The group designated it as a variant of concern and named it Omicron.[42] A day later on 27 November, Prime Minister Narendra Modi took a meeting to gauge the threat of the new variant, and asked for a review of the decision to reopen international travel.[43] On 1 December 2021, the decision to resume normal international operations was put on hold.[44]

Many countries suspended international flights even after the resumption of air services whenever the risk of contagion appeared great. Oman and Kuwait, for instance, suspended international flights from 21 December 2020 for a few days. But how far the infection could be contained by suspending international travel was not clear since, unlike 2020, when infections were said to be imported, the COVID-19 pandemic entered its second year with a bigger challenge of stopping the contagion within the country.

PART IV

THE UNLOCKING

9

THE WEB OF INTERSTATE TRAVEL

INDIA WAS AT 75.46 on the Stringency Index of the Oxford COVID-19 Government Response Tracker on 1 June 2020.[1] A day earlier, the score had been 79.17. It was stricter, at 76.39, when there was no national lockdown on 21 March 2020. A score of 100 is the strictest on the index, which has been devised by the Blavatnik School of Government in the UK. The reason that the 1 June score was lower was that the Indian government had begun a phased reopening under what came to be known as Guidelines Unlock 1. A lot had already been relaxed by then—restricted movement by train and by air, resumption of industrial and commercial activity had happened—but from that day onwards, there was to be no lockdown except in the containment zones. According to the government's PIB COVID bulletin for that day, there were 93,322 active cases in the country during the previous twenty-four hours, while a total of 91,818 patients had recovered from COVID-19. 'The recovery rate in the country is progressively increasing and has reached 48.19

per cent amongst Covid-19 patients. The recovery rate on 18 May was 38.29 per cent. On 3 May, it was 26.59 per cent. On 15 April, it was 11.42 per cent,' said the bulletin.[2] The next day's bulletin reported 97,581 active cases. A total of 3,708 COVID-19 patients had recovered during the past twenty-four hours, taking the total of those cured to 95,526. But it also showed that the fresh cases added on 1 June were 7,967, if one factors in the differential between active cases on the two days after subtracting the day's recovered cases. The WHO's situation report of 2 June 2020, however, put the number of fresh cases in India in the previous twenty-four hours at 8,171.[3]

This unlocking was happening at a time when many people from big cities were moving to their home towns on trains and buses and air passenger services had also been partially resumed. Under the new guidelines, movement during the day was allowed except in the containment zones, but a night curfew between 9 p.m. and 5 a.m. was imposed throughout the country. Essential activities were, however, exempted.[4] The new guidelines also spelt out the next steps in the opening up of activities that had been barred during the lockdown. Clause 6 of the guidelines specifically said that there would be unrestricted movement of persons and goods, with no restriction on interstate and intrastate movement, and no requirement of separate permission/approval/e-permit for such movement. But the very next subclause gave states the freedom to regulate the movement of persons based on their assessment of the public health situation. This is why movement continued to be restricted even after the lockdown was lifted.

State governments put in place their own regulations. West Bengal, for instance, decided to continue with the lockdown measures. The state had received particular attention from the Union government since COVID-19 cases were rising there, and the Centre claimed there was a violation of the lockdown measures, posing 'a serious health hazard.' On 19 April 2020, an MHA order

Public transport closures during the COVID-19 pandemic, 25 Mar 2020

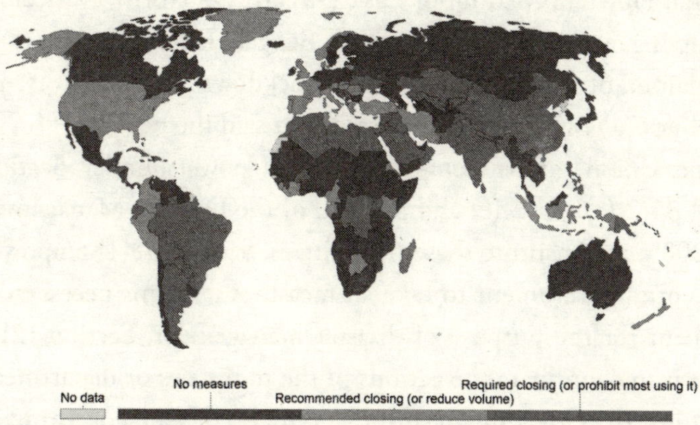

Source: Hale, Webster, Petherick, Phillips and Kira (2020). Oxford COVID-19 Government Response Tracker – Last updated 6 March 2021, 01.00 London time.
Note: The policies shown may not apply at all sub-national levels. A country is coded as having these restrictions if at least some sub-national regions have implemented them.
OurWorldInData.org/coronavirus

said these violations included incidents of violence perpetrated upon frontline healthcare professionals; complete disregard for social distancing norms outside banks, public distribution system shops and in marketplaces; and movement of private and commercial vehicles and passengers in urban areas.[5] 'After analyzing the prevalence of such violations in major hotspot districts, it is clear to the Central government that the situation is especially serious in Kolkata, Howrah, Medinipur East, 24 Parganas North, Darjeeling, Kalimpong and Jalpaiguri districts in the state of West Bengal,' said the order. The Centre constituted six inter-ministerial central teams (IMCTs), two each for West Bengal and Maharashtra and one each for Madhya Pradesh and Rajasthan, to make spot assessments of the situation, issue the necessary directions to the state authorities and submit reports to the Central government 'in larger interest of general public.' 'Situation is specially serious in Indore (Madhya

Pradesh), Mumbai and Pune (Maharashtra), Jaipur (Rajasthan) and Kolkata, Howrah, Medinipur East, 24 Parganas North, Darjeeling, Kalimpong and Jalpaiguri in West Bengal. IMCTs to focus on complaints of implementation of lockdown measures as per guidelines,' a government press statement said the next day.[6]

The Union government exercised its powers under Sections 35(1), 35(2)(a), 35(2)(e) and 35(2)(i) of the Disaster Management Act, 2005, to constitute these committees. Section 35(1) empowers the Central government to take all measures it deems necessary or expedient for the purpose of disaster management. Section (2)(a) allows it to coordinate the actions of the ministries or departments of not just the Government of India, but also of state governments, national authorities, state authorities, and governmental and non-governmental organizations, for the purpose of disaster management. Section (2)(e) talks about cooperation and assistance to state governments, whether it is requested by them or 'otherwise deemed appropriate' by the Central government. Section (2)(i) makes the provision all-encompassing by saying the Centre can exercise power in all matters as it 'deems necessary or expedient for the purpose of securing effective implementation' of the act.

The press statement of 20 April also reiterated that state governments and Union territories had been advised that while they could impose stricter measures than those outlined in the lockdown guidelines, they could not dilute those guidelines issued under the Disaster Management Act, 2005. Though West Bengal locked horns with the Centre during the lockdown, it exercised this option of levying stricter measures by continuing to impose the lockdown till 15 June, even after the Centre started the unlocking process.[7] It, however, allowed inter-district movement of public and private buses from 1 June, with not more than the actual seating capacity of the vehicle. No passengers were allowed to travel standing.

West Bengal had also been following its own nomenclature, designating areas as Category A, which were 'affected' areas; Category B, which were 'buffer' areas; and Category C, which were 'clear' areas. While affected areas continued to see restrictions on movement, such as those imposed by the Union government in containment zones, in Category C or clear areas, restrictions were eased. On 20 July, the state announced a different approach to the lockdown by shutting everything on two days per week, starting with 23 July and 25 July.[8] This lockdown was more stringent, with complete closure of everything, including government offices. It was called 'a complete lockdown' and saw public and private transport, including trains and flights, being inoperative on the two days.

West Bengal, however, was not the only big state to continue with the lockdown. While Uttar Pradesh lifted the lockdown in line with the Union government's guidelines, Bihar, Tamil Nadu and Maharashtra continued to impose strict lockdown measures even as the Union government started the unlocking process. The reason was that the number of COVID-19 cases continued to be high, and the states were not willing to take the risk of allowing free movement.

Tamil Nadu followed the policy of full lockdown, like that of West Bengal, in certain districts. It decided to continue with the state-wide lockdown, though relaxations were added. Some of these relaxations were rescinded in April 2021 during the second wave as part of 'a dynamic response' system. After the Union government's unlocking order was announced, Tamil Nadu came up with a complicated web of instructions for public transport for its new lockdown guidelines on 31 May 2020.[9] The state was divided into eight zones for the purpose of opening up public transport, with the police commissionerate limit of the state capital Chennai in the VIII category. The operation of public transport buses, including stage carriers, was permitted within regions in all the regions except in VII and VIII categories. Transporters were asked to operate 50 per cent of their fleet, and at 60 per cent seating capacity. No travel pass or e-pass was required within zones, but inter-zone and interstate operation of public transport was prohibited. Public transport carriers were allowed to charge 50 per cent additional fare over and above the existing fare for all types of operations as a temporary measure to compensate for the loss incurred from operating at a lower capacity. But this also showed that the government was discouraging travel and despite the more than two months of lockdown, there was no intention of facilitating intercity travel. Rental taxis and cabs could operate with a maximum of three passengers [and the driver], while autorickshaws could carry a maximum of two passengers. On 31 July, the Tamil Nadu government issued another order extending the state-wide lockdown till 31 August, but with more relaxations.[10] However, it stopped the operation of both private and government buses within districts throughout the state in the month of August. Tourist travel to the Nilgiri district, Kodaikanal and Yercaud was prohibited. The state implemented a complete lockdown with no relaxations on all Sundays. 'No other activity except milk distribution, hospitals, pharmaceutical shops, hospital vehicle, ambulance and hearse vehicle service may be permitted during the Sundays and that the private vehicles will be allowed to ply only for medical emergencies,' said the order.

Restrictions in smaller states were equally stringent. Himachal Pradesh, which gets 7 per cent of its GDP from tourism and is aiming to take this number to 8.5 per cent, was severely affected by the shutting down of transport services. According to the state's Economic Survey for 2020–21, there was a mere 4.63 per cent growth in both foreign and domestic tourist arrivals in 2019 as compared to 2018, when it had witnessed a fall of 16.08 per cent.

Foreign and domestic tourist arrivals showed a severe contraction of 81.33 per cent in 2020. The state survey said:

> Trade, hotel and restaurant sector showed a contraction of 9.2 per cent during 2020-21 as against a growth of 4.6 per cent in 2019-20. Transport by other means, namely, road transport [mechanised and non-mechanised], water transport, air transport and services incidental to transport, too showed a negative growth of 28 per cent during 2020–21 as against 5.6 per cent growth during 2018-19.[11]

However, the document was tabled on 5 March 2021 in the state assembly, which implies that the 2020–21 figures were an estimation.

According to the survey, the arrival of tourists sees a variation in the year-on-year growth rate. 'However, a large variation in the growth rate is seen in the time of countrywide lockdown which not only forced domestic tourists to stay locked in their homes, but led to foreign tourists staying back in their countries due to ban on international flights.' The year 2020 saw the sharpest (81.33 per cent) contraction in the arrival of tourists compared to the previous years. In 2020, the arrival of tourists was just 24.22 per cent of the tourist arrival ten years ago, in 2010. In other words, there was a 75.88 per cent contraction in tourist arrivals in 2020, compared to tourist arrivals in 2010. The arrival of foreign tourists saw the highest contraction of 90.59 per cent in 2020 as compared to the numbers in 2010.

Still, the state allowed movement only through select interstate checkposts in order to regulate the movement of individuals, even after the national lockdown was lifted. Entry timings were staggered to avoid crowding at these interstate checkposts. So stringent was this directive that a person entering the state from anywhere other than the checkpost indicated at the time of application of e-pass for entry was to be prosecuted. The order said:

> There might be instances that a person enters the state through the checkpost on a valid permit but fails to arrive at the destination indicated while applying for the e-pass. To prevent such occurrence, the district to which the person was destined to go, shall keep matching the data made available by the integrated permit software with the actual data of persons on surveillance in their jurisdictions. In case, any person fails to reach the indicated destination, the authorities concerned shall track him/her and the latter shall be proceeded against under the Himachal Pradesh Epidemic Disease (Covid-19) Regulation, 2020 and any other applicable laws/acts.[12]

While those travelling to other states from Himachal Pradesh for less than forty-eight hours for medical/business/official purposes were exempted from quarantine requirements, they were to be put under surveillance and tested. All other interstate travellers had to mandatorily undergo a fourteen-day quarantine, and those travelling from cities with high caseloads had to compulsorily go through institutional quarantine. This did not deter people from big cities from travelling to the state, especially for tourism; the risk of contracting the infection on public transport could be avoided by travelling in private vehicles. Destinations in Himachal Pradesh and Uttarakhand are at motorable distances from Uttar Pradesh, Punjab, Haryana and Delhi. The state government, however, was wary of the rising number of infections and clearly did not want to promote tourism. Subsequently, the state allowed the opening up of tourism units in accordance with certain norms.[13] Interstate movement of public transport buses, however, continued to be prohibited. Taxis could ply but required permission from the deputy commissioner.

Pass-free inter-district movement of public transport buses, private vehicles, taxis and autos was allowed.

The neighbouring Uttarakhand decided to shut all shops and establishments on Saturdays and Sundays in the municipal limits of the state capital, Dehradun, through a 4 June order.[14] According to that day's 2 p.m. state health bulletin, thirty-four fresh positive cases out of the state's total of fifty-nine were from Dehradun district.[15] The district had a total of 258 cases by then, though Nainital had more, at 308. The state's first set of unlocking guidelines, issued on 8 June, asked all persons entering Uttarakhand, irrespective of their mode of travel, to register on a portal.[16] They would also have to mandatorily download and update the Aarogya Setu mobile application, though there was no such directive from the Union government, which owned the application. A fourteen-day home quarantine was mandatory, though persons coming from identified high caseload COVID-19 cities had to undergo an additional seven days of institutional quarantine. Even those moving within the state from one district to another had to register themselves online.

Additionally, Uttarakhand imposed a curfew for four more hours from 7 p.m. to 7 a.m., when all non-essential activities and movement of people were prohibited across the state. The Union government had imposed curfew only from 9 p.m. to 5 a.m. Tourists coming to the state had to stay for at least two nights and upload and carry a COVID-19 negative report from a test done no earlier than ninety-six hours before arrival. If they came without test reports, they were to be tested at the border or get tested at the hotel.[17] The conditions of minimum stay and testing, however, were removed on 1 October under the state's Unlock 5 guidelines.[18]

After lifting the national lockdown, the MHA asked states to impose a curfew prohibiting the movement of people in the night hours. How far a 9 p.m.-to-5 a.m. curfew was helpful was being debated well into 2021, when the second wave of COVID-19 led to states resorting to it. The ministry, in a 12 June 2020 letter to the states, clarified that the purpose of restricting the movement of individuals after sundown, except for essential activities, was to prevent congregations and to ensure social distancing.[19] The restriction, however, did not apply 'to instances of loading/unloading of goods (as part supply chains and logistics); buses carrying persons and trucks and goods carriers plying on state and national highways; or persons travelling to their destination after disembarking from buses, trains and flights.' States were asked not to prevent such movement and issue instructions to that effect to the local authorities. While the entire lockdown period was of complete closure, with some relaxations coming in later, Unlock 1 evidently started with a confusing web of regulations, restrictions and relaxations across the states.

The Union government kept emphasizing the need for minimal restrictions outside containment zones, but states preferred to be strict. So when the second set of guidelines for unlocking was announced, the MHA, in the fifth section, specifically said that while states and Union territories could prohibit certain activities outside the containment zones, or impose such restrictions as deemed necessary, 'there shall be no restriction on interstate and intrastate movement of persons and goods including those for cross land-border trade.'[20] It said no separate permission/approval/e-permit would be required for such movements.

The lockdown was to continue in the containment zones, but Unlock 2 guidelines, issued on 29 June, permitted all activities, except five specified ones, in other areas from 1 July onwards. The five prohibited activities included school, colleges and educational institutions; international air travel of passengers except on the permitted special flights; Metro rail; cinema halls, gymnasiums, among others; and social, political, entertainment and other such gatherings. Night curfew timings were also reduced to between 10 p.m. and 5 a.m. Among the modes of transport, it was only Metro links that were to remain shut. In a letter to the states on 29 June, Union Home Secretary Ajay Bhalla said that while domestic flights and passenger trains had already been allowed in a limited manner, their operation would be further expanded in a calibrated manner.[21] 'Further, dates for opening up of the remaining prohibited activities will be decided separately, based on the assessment of the situation,' said the letter.

Unlock 3 guidelines were issued on 29 July with two changes.[22] Yoga centres and gymnasiums were allowed to open from 5 August. It lifted the night curfew completely. The new guidelines that came into effect from 1 August continued the lockdown in the containment zones. Following the monthly cycle of guidelines, the MHA issued Unlock 4 guidelines on 29 August, which came with further relaxations,[23] such as the operation of Metro trains from 7 September onwards in a graded manner. It also allowed half the staff to be called to schools. Students of classes nine to twelve and those in higher education institutions for research or in technical and professional programmes requiring the use of laboratories were permitted. Even social, religious, political and other such gatherings were permitted from 21 September, but with a cap of 100 people.

States that decided not to allow local bus transport, or only selectively opened bus services but opened other activities, such as schools and production units, glossed over the need to have a means of transport. Over 100 girls studying at Government Girls Senior Secondary School in Pinangwan in the Nuh district of Haryana had to wait for hours on the road to get a ride to school, since they could not afford private vehicles. State transport buses in that area had stopped during the 2020 lockdown. According to a March 2021 *Times of India* report, the bus service was stopped owing to low ridership.[24]

When the fifth set of guidelines for unlocking was announced on 30 September, they were simply called guidelines for reopening. It allowed gatherings with more than 100 people and reopening of cinema halls with 50 per cent capacity from 15 October. Subsequent orders just extended the same guidelines for the following month. By November, they were called guidelines for surveillance, containment and caution and contained directives for only containment zones, apart from reiterating the COVID-appropriate behaviour of wearing masks and maintaining social distancing.[25]

These measures were to remain unchanged till 31 March 2021, but there was a fresh surge in COVID cases in March, prompting the MHA to write a letter to the states on 19 March. It said:

> After the steady decline in COVID-19 cases for about five months, for the last few weeks, the number of COVID cases are showing an increasing trend in several parts of the country. It has been observed that it is largely due to laxity in the observance of Covid appropriate behaviour by the people, especially in the crowded places.[26]

The second wave of COVID-19 had started, but this time, the Union government did not impose any restriction. All it asked states to do was to widely disseminate orders/guidelines to the public and to the field functionaries. Even in a 26 March letter to the states, it emphasized on creating public awareness and regulating crowds in view of upcoming festivals such as Holi, Shab-e-Barat, harvesting festivals, Easter and Eid-ul-Fitr.[27] That the MHA was banking only on creating public awareness one year after the Union government had imposed a complete lockdown was strange, to say the least. Perhaps it showed that the ministry either did not have confidence in its own lockdown guidelines, imposed in March 2020, or had no willingness to implement even part of those in March 2021.

10

LIFTING OF THE METRO GATES

IT WAS 8 AUGUST 2020. The lockdown had been lifted, and all modes of transport were operational. The DTC was running its buses on Delhi roads, but the DMRC, just like all other metro services in the country, was not running its trains. The country's largest metro network, which runs across the capital and connects Delhi with neighbouring Ghaziabad, Noida, Faridabad and Gurugram, came out with an office order. Titled 'Rationalisation of Perks and Allowances due to Covid-19 Pandemic,' the order said, 'In view of the extreme adverse financial condition due to non-operation of metro services, it has been decided that the perks and allowances would be reduced by 50 per cent from August 2020 till further orders.'[1] All sanctions of advances for house building, laptop, festival etc. were on hold, though sanctions of advances for medical treatment and certain travel allowances were continued.

It was not just the Delhi Metro that was facing this financial challenge because of the halting of operations. Across the country, metros had not been permitted to operate, whether it was Mumbai Metro, Hyderabad Metro, Chennai Metro or Kolkata Metro. The fear was that these mass rapid transit systems, moving people from one end of the city to another in closed settings, increased the risk of contagion. People undertaking these daily journeys could not be quarantined since they were mostly daily commuters. The result was that people could fly to anywhere in the country and even abroad through limited air operations, but they could not travel within the city in the comfort of the metro systems.

The DMRC suffered a roughly Rs 10 crore loss for each day it was shut. In an interview with *Business Standard*, its managing director, Mangu Singh, said his metro system had touched around 6 million journeys a day, roughly translating to Rs 10 crore in daily revenue, before the lockdown was announced.[2] According to its 2019–20 annual report, the DMRC generated a revenue of Rs 7,015 crore, of which fare box collection, or money earned through passengers commuting on its system, was Rs 3,389 crore.[3] The previous year, in 2018–19, it had clocked Rs 6,462 crore in revenue, including income from traffic operations, real estate, consultancy and external projects. Traffic operations had given it Rs 3,583 crore. This meant that the collection from passengers had begun to fall even before train operations were shut on 22 March 2020. An RTI application revealed that Delhi Metro recorded 175.5 million rides in February 2020, which was a 7 per cent fall over the previous month of January, but it fell a further 44 per cent in March 2020 to 91 million.[4] There were multiple reasons for this. For ten days in the month, the Delhi Metro was inoperative because of the shutdown on 22 March. It had also curtailed its services from 19 March onwards and many regular commuters had stopped taking the metro as a precaution against the contagion from February onwards.

When its services continued to be shut even as late as 6 September 2020, the DMRC, in desperation, requested the Union government to defer its loan payment or allow the corporation some relaxations in the payment of debt amounting to Rs 1,100 crore. The Union government merely sat on the request while the DMRC continued to pay. A joint venture of the Union and Delhi state governments, the company has an ongoing loan from Japan International Cooperation Agency (JICA), a multilateral lending entity. It repaid Rs 765 crore of the JICA loan and an interest of almost Rs 430 crore on it, to the Union government during 2019-20. A total of Rs 6,826.97 crore, which includes Rs 3,489.73 crore in interest had been paid till 31 March 2020. The total amount of JICA loan the end of 2019-20 stood at Rs 31,834.65 crore.

The operations of the Delhi Metro, however, did not reach even the March 2020 level a year later. The number of rides or how many times a person took a metro train was 82 million in March 2021. On 10 May 2021, the DMRC operations were shut again for twenty-two days, to reopen on 7 June, with only half the seating capacity allowed.

The state of private metro systems run by Larsen & Toubro (L&T) and Reliance Infrastructure was equally bad. These companies operate metro systems in Hyderabad and Mumbai. It became tougher for them because they were smaller and new operators, with no government support. Metro operators depend heavily on non-fare box revenue, which is the revenue they earn from renting out their premises and from advertising, so it was a double whammy—not earning rents because of tenants invoking force majeure conditions, even as they themselves were losing fare collection revenue. Private operator Reliance Infrastructure's estimated daily revenue from regular operations prior to COVID was Rs 90 lakh, while L&T's revenue from operations was Rs 587.28 crore in 2019–20.[5]

The metro network became the last transport mode to be opened up, with the MHA giving permission to resume operations as part of Unlock 4 guidelines. Operations were allowed from 7 September 2020. Till then, even though some private offices and all government offices were functional, passengers were commuting either through cabs, local buses or pooled vehicles. Metros saw a graded reopening, with the Ministry of Housing and Urban Affairs issuing a standard operating procedure. While Delhi, Hyderabad and Chennai metros started operations immediately, on 7 September, Mumbai opted for a later date. Kolkata Metro, run by the Indian Railways, resumed operations after two weeks, on 14 September, with health protocols in place. It was to remain close on Sundays. While passengers could use only smart cards, since tokens are reused and carry the risk of passing on the infection, the Kolkata Metro insisted on the additional requirement of e-passes for entry into stations.[6] The requirement of an e-pass was finally removed only in January 2021. There was a cap of 400 passengers that could enter a train at a time to prevent crowding. Before the lockdown, the Kolkata Metro carried about 500,000 people every day.

The country's largest metro, which runs through the Delhi and NCR, with a 389 km network and 285 stations, reopened in a graded manner, too, after being shut for 169 days and incurring a loss of about Rs 1,690 crore, if a daily loss of Rs 10 crore is taken as a benchmark. Union Minister of State for Housing and Urban Affairs Hardeep Singh Puri, however, in a reply to a question by four members of Lok Sabha on 17 September 2020, said the loss of revenue due to closure of metro services due to the COVID-19 pandemic was around Rs 1,609 crore.[7]

DMRC's longest line, coded Yellow (Samaypur Badli to HUDA City Centre) and running 49 km, covering thirty-seven stations, was the first one to open on 7 September.[8] For the first two days, only this line was operational for a period of four hours each, from 7 a.m. to 11 a.m. and from 4 p.m. to 8 p.m. Some fifty-seven trains were run on around 462 trips. Operations were resumed in a graded manner from 9 to 12 September on other lines. The DMRC said in a press statement:

> Over a period of next five days, i.e., by 12th September, rest of the lines will also be made operational with all safety measures in place to check the spread of Covid-19 in the metro premises which requires everyone to follow a new normal of social distancing, face mask and hand sanitization.

Commuters were advised to download the Union government's Aarogya Setu application, but it was not mandatory. Wearing of masks or face covers was compulsory. Passengers could carry hand sanitizers in quantities only up to 30 ml, perhaps because of the security risk involved. The DMRC advisory included travelling with minimum luggage and avoiding carrying metallic items. It also asked the public to keep an extra ten to fifteen minutes in hand for their daily commute. With the opening of metro gates, shops and outlets inside the stations were permitted to operate according to the government's guidelines and subject to social distancing norms.

Entry and exit of passengers were initially permitted only through one or two identified gates at each station, and passengers were required to undergo thermal screening and hand sanitization at the entry point at the time of frisking for security. The DMRC also started auto thermal screening-cum-hand sanitization machines at forty-five major stations, where incoming passengers were automatically scanned. In other stations, there were regular sanitizer dispensers for hand sanitization and thermal screening was done manually by 'thermal guns.'

A team of around 800 officials and staff was initially deployed at all stations to ensure cleanliness and orderliness inside stations during operating hours. In addition, they were to regulate and stop the entry of passengers to the station in case of crowd build-up and violation of social distancing norms. CCTV cameras were installed at stations and in trains for crowd monitoring and management. Inside trains, passengers were asked to sit on alternate seats only or to stand, maintaining adequate distance. Stickers saying 'Do not sit here' were affixed to alternate seats. The dwell time or stoppage of trains at each station was increased by 10 seconds, from the earlier 10–15 seconds to 20–25 seconds, so that passengers had sufficient time to board and alight. At interchange stations, the dwell time was increased by 20 seconds, from the earlier 35–40 seconds to 55–60 seconds. As in other metro systems, tokens were discontinued to minimize human interface and prevent the transmission of the virus through frequent touching/handling. Only smart card holders, including QR code users on Airport Express Line, were allowed to travel.

In the three days between 7 and 10 September, resuming services on most of its network under Stage 1 of the graded resumption, the DMRC ran trains for four hours each in the morning and evening. Thereafter, it announced the resumption of services on its last major line, coded Magenta, from Janakpuri West to Botanical Garden. This line runs 37.5 km, touching twenty-five stations. The Grey Line from Dwarka to Najafgarh, spanning 4.3 km and three stations, also resumed operations on 11 September 2020 under Stage 2.[9] The timings of train services were extended to six hours in the morning and in the evening, from 7 a.m. to 1 p.m. and from 4 p.m. to 10 p.m., with broadly the same frequency as before the lockdown. Normal timings of train services throughout the day, from 6 a.m. to 11 p.m., were resumed from 12 September, which is when the Airport Express Line from New Delhi to Dwarka Sector 21, running 22.7 km and touching six stations, also became operational under Stage 3, the last stage under the DMRC's graded resumption plan of the DMRC services.

Not many, however, resumed travelling by metro, even though the Delhi Metro is a lifeline for commuters in Delhi. The reasons were many—some people were yet to resume travel to office, while others preferred to take their own vehicle or a taxi because commuting with strangers in a closed environment on public transport systems was not the preferred option. This reflected in metro ridership figures, which, according to a news report in *Business Standard*, stood at 8,300 passengers in the first few hours of restarting operations on 7 September.[10] It rose to 250,000 rides on 14 September, a week after it resumed operations, and two days after it started service on all lines throughout the day. Prior to the lockdown on 25 March, the average ridership was 6 million.

Despite being the largest metro system in the country, the DMRC did not get back to its March 2020 ridership levels. For October 2020, the first full month of operations after the reopening of the metro gates, there were just 3.75 million rides, or a little more than one-third of the 9 million it saw in March 2020. This meant that the metro was carrying half of a pre-lockdown day's ridership in a whole month post-lockdown.

When the air pollution level in Delhi touched dangerous levels in November 2021, the Delhi Disaster Management Authority revised COVID restrictions for public transport so that more people use it rather than private vehicles. The Delhi metro was permitted to carry thirty persons standing in a coach while buses were allowed standing equal to 50 per cent of the seating capacity.[11] But a month later when the spread of Omicron variant led to a yellow alert in Delhi, DMRC had to again cut down the number of passengers on train to 50 per cent of the seating capacity.[12]

Metro services in Mumbai were the last to resume, on 19 October 2021, more than a month after the Union government had allowed such a resumption.[13] It restarted with a cap of 300 passengers on one train. By December, it was carrying 50,000 passengers daily.[14] By March 2021, it decided to increase its service by twenty-four trains to carry more passengers while ensuring the cap remained. With this, it was to run around 280 train trips instead of 256.

Railway suburban services, a lifeline for the city of Mumbai, were among the first ones to resume operations on 15 June 2020, but till January 2021, the service was limited to essential workers notified by the government. One of the reasons was that curbs by the Maharashtra government continued, since COVID cases in the city just kept bouncing back after some intervening days of a lull. Another was that the railways were adopting a graded resumption approach. The Mumbai services were gradually increased, but the idea was to avoid crowding and to maintain social distancing. Women passengers were allowed to travel between 11 a.m. and 3 p.m. and after 7 p.m., and so were practising lawyers and registered clerks of lawyers.[15] It was a different sort of graded resumption, governed by the travel needs of particular individuals. The priority was decided by the nature of the profession they practised. Suburban services were opened to all passengers on 1 February 2021, but the restriction on the number of people continued. With the second wave, however, train services were again restricted to essential category workers.

In Chennai, the general public was allowed to travel in suburban trains during non-peak hours from 23 December 2020. The Southern Railway had been running suburban train services only for railway employees as 'workmen's special' in the Chennai region after the COVID-19 lockdown was enforced. The service was slowly opened up when the unlocking started. Just as in Mumbai, employees rendering essential services were allowed to board in the first phase. Then, it was opened up to women passengers in the non-peak hours in the second phase. 'I am happy to announce that Railways will allow women to travel on suburban trains from 21 October between 11 a.m. to 3 p.m. and after 7 p.m. We were always ready and with the receipt of letter from Maharashtra Government today, we have allowed this travel,' Union Railway Minister Piyush Goyal said in a tweet on 20 October.[16]

From 23 December, the Indian Railways allowed the general public to travel by suburban train services in Chennai during non-peak hours. 'With adequate safety measures in place, this will greatly enhance ease of movement and passenger convenience,' Goyal said in another tweet. The non-peak hours are from the early hours of the day to 7 a.m., 9.30 a.m. to 4.30 p.m. and from 7 p.m. to the closing hours of the day. The intervening timings were considered 'peak hours'—7 a.m. to 9.30 a.m. and 4.30 p.m. to 7 p.m. At that time, the number of trains running in the Chennai suburban sector was 410, about 65 per cent of the normal number. Later, on 12 February, students were also allowed to travel.[17]

The suburban train service in West Bengal began operations on 11 November. The service had remained suspended since March, but when the approval to operate these services was given by the railways, it started with 696 suburban services.[18] The second wave changed the course yet again. The Delhi Metro again stopped its services, as it did in March 2020, but this time, it first curtailed the hours of operation and allowed only essential service workers to board the trains from 19 April 2021.[19] It, however, shut down operations completely on 10 May 2021 till 6 June 2021.[20]

Most of the woes of intercity travel in cities such as Delhi and Mumbai are resolved if rail-based mass rapid transport systems function. Though a limited number of offices were functional and the ridership numbers picked up slowly, crowds did return to metro and suburban trains, underscoring the importance of these systems in a city's professional life.

PART V

THE SECOND WAVE

11

THIS TIME NO ONE WALKING

THE TASK OF OPENING up and starting on the road to normalcy from a phase of complete lockdown was quite aptly termed by the Maharashtra government as 'Mission Begin Again'. This, however, turned out to be a 'mission halted' when the state had to come out with a 'Break the Chain' order on 4 April 2021. COVID-19 infections had surged again, and the lockdown was back. Just a week earlier, on 28 March, the Uddhav Thackeray government had imposed a night curfew across the state. Unlike the 2020 state curfews, and later the national lockdown, however, the Break the Chain order did not snap transport connectivity.[1] While there was a cap of five people on group movements from 7 a.m. to 8 p.m., Monday to Friday, no one was allowed to move in a public place without valid reason or permission during weeknights, from 8 p.m. to 7 a.m., and during the entire weekend, from 8 p.m. on Friday to 7 a.m. on Monday.

There was no restriction on public transport—autorickshaws were permitted to carry a driver and two passengers, taxis and four-wheelers could have the driver and only 50 per cent vehicle capacity, and buses could operate at full seating capacity with no passenger allowed to stand. Since, by then, vaccination against COVID-19 was available, the state asked drivers and other staff coming into contact with the public to get vaccinated at the earliest, though the Union government had opened up vaccinations only to people above forty-five years of age and a defined set of frontline workers and medical professionals. The state, however, said that till vaccination was completed, vehicle staff should carry negative COVID test result certificates, valid up to fifteen days. This condition was to come into effect from 10 April 2021. The order said:

> For taxis and autos, however, if driver isolated himself or herself through a plastic sheet or otherwise he or she may be exempted from this requirement. In case, if any of the above are found to be without negative RT-PCR certificate/without being vaccinated as above, a fine of Rs 1,000/- will be levied.

The stringency of the lockdown, however, was much less than that in 2020. Maharashtra counted trains, taxis, autos and public buses as essential services. Even the Mumbai suburban train services, run by the Central and Western zonal railways, continued operations.

As the news of Maharashtra locking down went around, there was a rush of people at railway stations, primarily in Mumbai, not so much in other parts of the country. Railway stations were not shut this time, but there was a widespread fear of being left in the lurch again. *The Indian Express* newspaper spoke to Sonu Patel, a ready-mix concrete vehicle driver from Mahape, Turbhe, Navi Mumbai, who reached Lokmanya Tilak Terminus. Patel and his colleagues had walked all the way to Uttar Pradesh in the summer of 2020 when there was a nationwide lockdown, with all transport connections snapped. Patel told the newspaper:

> Last year, I reached my home in Jaunpur on foot. This time, I don't want to be stuck in a similar situation. The [ready-mix concrete] vehicle owner told us that there will be no further work as new restrictions have been imposed by the government. I don't have work now. It's better to leave before they stop the trains again.[2]

The rise of COVID-19 cases did create anxiety among workers staying in big cities, but many of them were on their planned visits to their villages. With state assembly elections underway in Bengal and panchayat elections in Uttar Pradesh, many headed to their native places to exercise their franchise. Besides, the start of summer is the usual time for marriages and for the harvest, and so of labourers heading home. The situation in the northern part of the country, where lockdown had not yet returned, was different. Station superintendent of Gurugram railway station, S.L. Meena, for instance, was quoted in *The Hindu* newspaper as saying that there was no unusual rush of passengers to suggest an exodus of migrants fearing lockdown.[3] Gurugram had witnessed a huge number of labourers walking to their native places during the national lockdown in 2020. A religious fair had, however, reversed the situation. 'We have more than the usual rush today [Monday] because of a large number of devotees reaching Gurugram from the neighbouring States for Sheetla Mata fair. But the number of devotees too is far less compared to pre-pandemic days,' Meena told the newspaper. The number of trains passing the Gurugram railway station was reduced to forty-six from ninety-eight before the lockdown, including six local trains. Meena said:

> The footfall at the railway station has drastically reduced from 60,000 a day before the outbreak to just 5,000 now. Many daily passengers on local trains lost their jobs due to the pandemic,

reducing the footfall. This is why the number of passengers remains low despite some trains being restored.

In neighbouring Delhi, where night curfew and a lockdown came a little later, the rush at the railway stations was initially not very high. Part of the reason was that the Indian Railways did not allow non-reserved passengers to board trains, though such people could enter railway stations merely by buying a platform ticket. Delhi, too, had followed the Maharashtra government by first imposing a night curfew from 10 p.m. to 5 a.m., beginning 6 April 2021, followed by a weekend curfew from 10 p.m. on Friday, 16 April, till 5 a.m. on Monday, 19 April.[4] Public transport, like the Delhi Metro, state transport buses, autos and taxis were allowed to operate within their stipulated time, but they were to ferry only the exempted categories of individuals. The curfew restrictions, however, were extended first for one week, till 26 April, and then again for a week till 3 May, and then again till 5 a.m. of 10 May. The 19 April order of the Delhi Disaster Management Authority, however, shut malls, cinema halls and other such establishments which were permitted to operate at half their capacity till then.[5] While there was no restriction on the interstate and intrastate movement and transportation of essential goods and no separate permission or e-pass was required for such movement, public transport, such as metro and buses, were allowed with half of their seating capacity, autos, e-rickshaws and taxis with two passengers, maxi cab with up to five passengers and RTV with up to eleven passengers.

With restrictions being reimposed, however, many people started gathering at the Anand Vihar bus terminus in east Delhi to go back home. While announcing the initial six-day lockdown hours before it was to start from 10 p.m. on 19 April, Delhi Chief Minister Arvind Kejriwal asked migrant workers not to leave, while assuring them that the lockdown would be a relatively 'short' one, and promised that the government would 'take care' of them through this crisis.[6] He assured them that his government was working hard to ensure adequate medical facilities, and he was hopeful that the lockdown would not need to be extended. This was, however, not to be—neither did the medical facilities prove to be adequate, nor was the lockdown a short one.

Though both railways and airlines had not returned to their full pre-COVID capacity, the passenger numbers had started to come down as people decided to avoid travel. The Northern Railway and the Southern Railway, for instance, cancelled trains on 6 May 2021 because of low occupancy and a surge in COVID-19 cases. While the Northern Railway cancelled twenty-eight pairs of trains, including the premium Rajdhanis, Shatabdis and Duronto, the Southern Railway cancelled another twenty-eight trains running within Tamil Nadu and twenty-two interstate trains. Passengers who had booked tickets on these trains were intimated through text messages on their mobile phones, and frequent announcements made through public address systems at stations.

Both industry and officials continued to fear that March-end and April of 2021 could be a repeat of the summer of 2020. *The Indian Express* reported on 19 April that the Special Branch of Delhi Police had asked all fifteen district police officials in the city to counsel migrant workers and send them back to their homes or shelters if they were found roaming around without authorization.[7] The Special Branch felt there was a possibility of migrant labourers trying to move out of Delhi-NCR fearing a sudden lockdown, and 'if any mass movement is observed, local police should assist them with adequate deployment to speed up the process.' The branch also feared a sudden rush at major interstate bus terminals and railway stations owing to 'rumours' about a lockdown, the newspaper reported. It further quoted from the advisory:

> The labourers are very anxious to return to their native places and they may turn aggressive and violent. They may also block the roads and damage private and public property. But these labourers may be dealt with tactfully. The behaviour of all police personnel should be polite while dealing with the labourers and if it is found that they are hungry, then it may be coordinated with civil authorities to arrange food and water so that peace is maintained.

None of these fears of violent behaviour proved to be correct, though there were crowds at bus stations. The primary reason for the absence of unruly scenes was that there was no restriction on long-distance or intercity travel. Though lockdowns across various states barred people from coming out of their homes, transport links continued to function. On 29 April 2021, however, the Madhya Pradesh government stopped bus services to Uttar Pradesh. Both buses from and to Uttar Pradesh were discontinued under an order from the Madhya Pradesh transport department.[8] Eleven districts of Uttar Pradesh (Agra, Etawah, Jalna, Jhansi, Lalitpur, Mahomba, Banda, Chitrakoot, Allahabad, Mirzapur and Sonbhadra) border Madhya Pradesh. The decision to stop bus services was not just because Madhya Pradesh wanted to stop any influx of COVID-19 cases, but because Uttar Pradesh had imposed a lockdown.

Exactly a year before, in 2020, when labourers travelled on foot or by whatever vehicle they could find back to their villages, sometimes more than a thousand kilometres away, Uttar Pradesh had stopped their entry into the state. Neighbouring Madhya Pradesh, which lies in the heart of the country, witnessed hordes of people entering the state. Sometimes, their destinations were in the state, but many times, they were just transiting. Thousands of workers got stranded in Madhya Pradesh districts bordering Gujarat, Maharashtra and

Uttar Pradesh. Uttar Pradesh had sealed its borders to prevent further movement of stranded workers, throwing into disarray the social distancing protocol.[9]

Jitendra Yadav, who was working at VRL Logistics in Bengaluru, decided to come back to his village in the Ballia district of Uttar Pradesh.[10] He boarded his company's truck, which was bringing some supplies to Varanasi, on 7 April 2021. The previous year, he had taken a Shramik Special from Bengaluru to Buxar in Bihar, which is about two hours away from his village. In 2021, his family wanted him home because they heard about people dying in and around their village. He narrates:

> Near our village, one person had a fever. He was admitted to hospital and the next day, he was dead. Hospital gave a certificate saying that he was corona positive. My family told me to come back and said if you fall ill there [Bengaluru], who will look after you?

About three or four people have died in his village. 'They give some medicine and people just die,' he says.

In Yadav's village, there are no hospitals, but there are a few private doctors. 'They ask us to sit at a distance from them. If we have body ache, they give medicine and for fever, they give a different medicine,' he says. Yadav, however, does not believe that there is any pandemic, though he knows people are dying. 'Yeah, we hear that people are dying. I do not believe there is anything like Corona. We stayed back with 400 people in one place [in Bengaluru] last year and nothing happened to anyone. Then I came home and later went back to Bengaluru. We have only heard about Corona, not seen it happen,' he says.

Yadav had witnessed the 2020 lockdown and says he faced many problems initially, but he stayed in Bengaluru. Once trains started, he came back to his village and stayed for four months. Work never stopped in his company, though, because it is in the business of transportation:

> The company told us that they would give us a minimum of Rs 600 a day. We were able to make Rs 700–800 daily. Even now [May 2021], there are about thirty to forty persons from north India still there. The company has told them that if you earn less than Rs 400, then it will compensate them.

At VRL Logistics, he says, their temperature was checked daily and they were tested for COVID. 'They put a pipe in our mouth and checked for corona,' he says, adding that he has no complaints from his company. But he is clear about one thing: there should be no lockdown. 'It does not help. When everything was open, it was the same and now when there is a lockdown, it is the same.' His dismissal of COVID and of the need for people to stay home stems from his cynicism about politics. He thinks all the talk around COVID and lockdowns is only for elections. 'Once the elections are over, everything will be fine. This time, the trains are running. If they close everything, poor people will die. In Bengal, there is a problem because everything is shut there,' he says.

State lockdowns did impact workers, especially daily wagers, in 2021 as well, since a number of units and construction sites saw their operations halted. Automobile manufacturers such as Hero MotoCorp, MG Motors and Maruti Suzuki, for instance, were among those that had a shutdown from mid-April to May 2021.[11] A *Hindustan Times* report dated 15 May quoted thirty-three-year-old Arvind Kumar, a worker who came to Manesar, a hub of manufacturing activity in Haryana near to Delhi, eight years back. He said:

> All these years were smooth and I used to save Rs 5,000 a month. But since last year [when the first lockdown was announced in March and lasted sixty-eight days], it is becoming tough to make ends meet. There are no jobs and factories have reduced manpower. Many companies have shut their operations permanently. I sleep under a tree and roam around in search of a free meal.[12]

The reports said the worst affected were daily wagers at small construction sites in Gurugram, while in Manesar and Udyog Vihar, it was the employees of small auto companies and garment export units. 'Naveen Kumar, thirty-eight, had to vacate his rented room in a Manesar village on 3 May, after he failed to pay rent. Although getting new work was unlikely in the lockdown, he decided that heading back home in Bihar would not solve his problem as his family had no money there either,' said the report. Kumar said he used to unload consignments but with no work for over a month, he had no money left to return home. 'We get free food from the police and sleep on the pavement waiting for the lockdown to get over,' he said.

After what was witnessed during the 2020 lockdown, state governments were better prepared to handle the movement of people towards their native places in 2021. A Delhi government report showed that during the first week of lockdown, starting 19 April, travel arrangements for 379,604 people were made through interstate buses. This number came down to less than one-third in the third week, ending 10 May, when 122,490 people were moved.[13]

Under a suo moto writ petition being heard since 2020, the Supreme Court on 13 May 2021 asked the governments of Delhi, Uttar Pradesh and Haryana to utilize the public distribution system to give dry rations to migrant labourers from May 2021.[14] While providing dry rations, the court said the authorities should not insist on checking the identity cards of those who did not have any, and instead accept a self-declaration. They were also asked to open community kitchens at well-advertised places so that labourers and their families could get two meals a day. Since workers had complained of overcharging by transport operators, the court also said:

> NCT of Delhi, state of UP and state of Haryana (for the districts included in the NCR) shall ensure that adequate transport is provided to stranded migrant labourers (in the National Capital Region) who want to return to their home. The District Administration in coordination with Police Administration may identify such stranded migrant labourers and facilitate their transport either by road transport or train. The Union of India may also issue necessary instructions to [the] Ministry of Railways to take necessary and adequate measures to cater [to] the need of migrant labourers.

The Delhi government report, however, claimed there was no complaint of overcharging as the interstate buses were owned and operated by state governments. 'Train travel was a preferred mode by migrants in the current lockdown as trains were/ are operational in the current lockdown period. It may be mentioned that the said mode was not available during [the] first lockdown due to Covid-19 during March 2020,' said the report.[15]

States, however, discouraged travel anyway and were checking people coming from other states throughout the unlocking months, though how far it helped check transmission of the infection was not really clear. Delhi, for instance, came out with a directive on

6 May 2021, when a new strain of the coronavirus was reported. The order of the Delhi Disaster Management Authority said:

> A virulent variant of Covid-19 is reported to have been found recently in the state of Andhra Pradesh and Telangana and this new strain of Covid-19 has a shorter incubation period with high transmission rate and the progress of disease is much more rapid in this strain and therefore, additional precautionary measures in respect of the persons coming from the states of Andhra Pradesh and Telangana to NCT of Delhi through airlines/trains/buses/cars/trucks or any other mode of transportation are required to be taken in public interest with the objective that this new virulent strain of Covid-19 should not enter and transmit into the territory of NCT of Delhi.[16]

All persons arriving from the two states had to undergo mandatory government institutional quarantine or paid quarantine for fourteen days. A person who had received two doses of the vaccine and produced a certificate to that effect, or had a negative RT-PCR report not older than seventy-two hours prior to undertaking the journey, was allowed home quarantine for seven days. 'If no suitable facility for home quarantine is available with the person, he/ she may opt for institutional / paid quarantine in identified facilities for seven days,' it said. Government officials and functionaries were, however, exempted from these requirements if they were asymptomatic.

What Delhi did was just an example of how states were trying to discourage interstate travel at a time when the Union government had shown no intent of curbing travel. However, during the second wave in April and May 2021, the rising number of deaths and an unhindered increase in COVID-19 cases were more because of shortcomings of the Union and state governments, and their inability to prepare for the overwhelming numbers, rather than a simple import of cases from outside a state. On the ground, it meant a huge section of the workforce being impacted by the pandemic, either because they or someone around them fell ill.

An *Economic Times* report quoted Hari Menon, founder and CEO at BigBasket, as saying, 'This year people are falling ill and that's causing a bit of a problem for us. The moment someone shows any signs of illness they're supposed to report to us, and now so many people are calling in sick ... It's madness.'[17] The report further quoted unnamed executives at online marketplace Flipkart as saying they were 'seeing a lot of people fall sick and also a lot of absenteeism' but due to the 'relatively younger age of such workers most are exhibiting milder symptoms.'

Clearly, the euphoria created around 'winning the battle' against COVID-19 in January 2021, with Prime Minister Narendra Modi claiming that a country that was home to 18 per cent of the world's population had 'saved humanity from a big disaster by containing corona effectively,' was too early.[18] Modi was addressing a global audience through the World Economic Forum. But a country as vast as India, on the contrary, had neither learnt lessons on COVID-appropriate behaviour nor built a robust medical infrastructure, including a sound vaccination policy even one year after the national lockdown. The crowing about a victory over the deadly virus from the Union government came without them realizing that the disease would resurrect itself and beat all previous records of infections and deaths. So if it was the humanitarian crisis of hunger and joblessness that had gripped the county in the summer of 2020, it was the sheer number of deaths the next year that showed how the government had failed its people.

12

NOT SO LOCKED DOWN

ON 20 APRIL 2021, Prime Minister Narendra Modi delivered an address to the nation on national television after a long gap. Not that he had been silent, but his recent addresses had been election or inauguration speeches. Only three phases of polling in an eight-phase West Bengal assembly election were left. Elections in three other states and in Puducherry were over by the time Modi decided to address the nation. The Election Commission of India had, on 26 February, announced polls to 294 seats in West Bengal, 234 in Tamil Nadu, 140 seats in Kerala, 125 seats in Assam and thirty seats in the Union territory of Puducherry.[1]

Apart from elections rallies and meetings, the Hindu festival of Kumbh had begun in Uttarakhand's Haridwar, leading to the congregation of a large number of devotees and seers from all over the country. 'I invite all devotees across the world to come to Haridwar and take a holy dip in the Ganga during Mahakumbh. Nobody will be stopped in the name of Covid-19 as we are sure the faith in God will overcome the fear of the virus,' Uttarakhand Chief Minister and BJP leader Tirath Singh Rawat had said on 20 March.[2]

Meanwhile, another wave was sweeping the country. It was the second wave of COVID-19, when deaths due to the disease added to deaths due to lack of oxygen and hospital beds. According to the WHO's situation report of 21 April, India reported another high of daily COVID cases at 233,091, which was over 25 per cent of cases reported in the world that day.[3]

Modi was fully aware of the crisis that had unfolded. 'The situation was under control till a few weeks ago, but the second wave of corona has hit like a storm,' he said in the address.[4] Yet, ruling out any possibility of a repeat of the 2020 lockdown, which was widely criticized for the humanitarian crisis it caused, he said:

> In today's situation, we have to save the country from lockdowns. I would also request the states to use lockdown as the last option. We have to try our best to avoid lockdown and focus on the micro-containment zones. We will also improve the health of our economy and take care of the health of our countrymen.

While the fight was with a deadly virus that was claiming many more lives than it did in 2020, he requested 'young colleagues' to create small committees in their societies, localities and apartments and help others in maintaining the COVID discipline. 'If we do this, then governments will not need to create containment zones, impose curfew or lockdown. There is no question of lockdown.' Was he giving the responsibility of containment to mohalla or neighbourhood committees? Even if this was reading too much into the suggestion, one thing was clear: it was up to states to impose their own version of lockdown, though the Union government was advising against it.

Not that the states were waiting for a signal from the Prime Minister or the Union government. They had already started imposing restrictions, first as night curfews and then as lockdowns.

In 2020 as well, states had gone ahead and imposed restrictions before the national lockdown was announced on 24 March. By 20 April 2021, when Modi addressed the nation, Maharashtra and Delhi, the two important hubs of economic activity, were already locked down. Maharashtra had, in fact, imposed a night curfew from 28 March, followed by a lockdown announcement on 4 April. It began as a weekend lockdown, with restrictions on the movement of people in the night and during the weekdays, but from 15 April onwards, restrictions were imposed on the movement of people outside their houses except for notified essential services.[5]

In Uttar Pradesh, where COVID-19 cases were surging rapidly, the Allahabad High Court had ordered a lockdown from 19 April, just a day before the Prime Minister's address to the nation. The court had reprimanded the state government for not coming up with any concrete plan after the court had made observations six days earlier. Though the court acknowledged:

> [enforcing] a lockdown to public activities is a matter purely in the nature of policy decision by the concerned government and it was in keeping with this principle that we in our last order [dated 13.04.2021], had directed the government to think about restricting public movement to break the chain of Covid infection. However, in the affidavit filed today nothing concrete has been placed before us.[6]

The court said it understood the limitation of the government in creating infrastructure to meet the challenge of COVID-19. But before all efforts could translate into action, much water would have flown under the bridge to 'the utter dismay of a large population of have nots.' This underscored the need for urgent action. It came down heavily on the Yogi Adityanath government on all aspects of health infrastructure, be it provision of beds, medicines or even test results. 'One would only laugh at us that we have enough to spend on elections and very little to spend on public health,' observed the court. Citing the dismal situation as the reason, the court said:

> The night curfew in the name of Corona Curfew and the weekend curfew are nothing else but a mere eyewash. It was probably an effort to show that our last order had been taken care of. We are, however, not satisfied at all. We see people are largely not following our order for putting masks on their faces nor, the police could ensure 100% masking till date.

It even recorded its displeasure with the way the state government and the state Election Commission proceeded to hold local elections, forcing teachers and other government staff to perform duties that exposed them to the threat of contracting the disease. Almost the entire police force was shifted to polling booths, giving priority to elections above public health, it observed.

The court ruled:

> If popular government has its own political compulsions in not checking public movements during this pandemic, we cannot remain mere passive spectators. Public health is the top most priority and call of the moment and any complacency of any degree today will cause havoc to people. We can't shirk away from our constitutional duty to save innocent people from the pandemic which is spreading due to the negligence of a few. Thus in the larger public interest, we are called upon to pass orders to break the chain of the pandemic Covid-19.

For a state such as Uttar Pradesh, which has the highest population in the country, it was the high court that first felt that if people were restrained from going outside their homes for a week, as a first measure, the current chain of the spread of COVID could be broken, and it would give some respite to frontline medical and health workers, who would be able to pay more attention to the patients who were already admitted. Accordingly, for the cities of Prayagraj (Allahabad), Lucknow, Varanasi, Kanpur Nagar and Gorakhpur, it asked the government to strictly enforce certain measures. It ordered the closure of all establishments, government or private, from midnight of 19 April till 26 April 2021. It exempted financial institutions and financial departments, medical and health services, industrial and scientific establishments, essential services including municipal functions, and public transport. The state government, however, stubbornly decided not to go by the court order. Instead, Additional Chief Secretary (Information) Navneet Sehgal issued a press release the same day, stating the government would not be ordering a complete lockdown. The press release said:

> The Uttar Pradesh government has taken several steps and is going to take more steps to contain the situation but it is necessary to protect the livelihood of poor people as well. Thus, the cities will not be going under complete lockdown right away. People have been closing down functions in many places of their own volition as it is.[7]

The very next day, the Uttar Pradesh government appealed to the Supreme Court against the high court, citing various steps being taken to contain the spread of the virus. The Supreme Court granted the state government a stay on imposition of the lockdown.[8] The state government had announced a thirty-five-hour 'Corona Curfew' on 16 April. Though this announcement did not cut much ice with the Allahabad High Court, it had to be extended till 4 May. Later, the curfew was made a 'partial' curfew with certain exemptions.[9] Home delivery services, including food delivery through Zomato and

Swiggy, were allowed during curfew hours from 30 April, the order specifically mentioned.[10] What the state government was calling a curfew was actually the lockdown of everything except essential and transport services.

Uttar Pradesh was not the only state using the word 'curfew' instead of 'lockdown.' The Madhya Pradesh government also imposed a corona curfew in the capital city of Bhopal and in the Berasia municipal area from 9 p.m. on 12 April till 6 a.m. on 19 April. This form of lockdown was, in fact, more stringent, with only home delivery of groceries and medicines being allowed.

While Uttarakhand saw an explosion in COVID cases due to the Mahakumbh, with many seers themselves dying during and after the festival,[11] in neighbouring Uttar Pradesh, the panchayat (rural local body) elections caused the deaths of many teachers.[12] Though the Uttar Pradesh government denied the claims of teacher deaths, the Uttar Pradesh Primary Teachers' Association had sent a list of the victims to the chief minister along with their demands, including financial assistance to family members of the teachers who had died.

While announcing the poll dates for 824 assembly constituencies in a press conference, Sunil Arora, chief election commissioner (CEC), had said that the vaccination drive had made the situation more conducive for elections and that everyone on poll duty had been declared a frontline worker for vaccination purposes.[13] Arora's tenure ended on 13 April 2021, so it was left to the subsequent election commissioners to get a lashing from the Madras High Court just thirteen days later on the conduct of the elections.

On 26 April, the Madras High Court blamed the Election Commission for not stopping political parties from violating COVID protocols during election campaigns in the four states and a Union territory. The court said murder charges should probably be imposed on the panel for being 'the only institution responsible for the situation that we are in today.'[14] 'You have been singularly lacking any kind of exercise of authority. You have not taken measures against political parties holding rallies despite every order of this court saying "maintain Covid protocol, maintain Covid protocol",' the Madras High Court bench of Chief Justice Sanjib Banerjee and Justice Senthilkumar Ramamoorthy said while hearing a petition filed by AIADMK leader and Tamil Nadu transport minister M.R. Vijayabhaskar. The petition sought directions to the Election Commission to implement strict measures during counting on 2 May in his Karur constituency.

A day later, on 27 April 2021, an individual filed a complaint against Sudip Jain, deputy election commissioner, and other officials of the Election Commission, under Sections 269, 270 and 304 read with Section 120-B of the Indian Penal Code, 1860, in Khardah Police Station of Kolkata. He, however, did not make any reference to the 26 April 2021 order of the Madras High Court. Meanwhile, the Election Commission approached the Supreme Court, where it said the high court had made 'disparaging oral observations without proof or material.' It contended

> The remarks made by the High Court were widely reported in the media and have tarnished the image of the EC as an independent constitutional authority. These remarks have reduced the faith of the people in the EC and undermined the sanctity of its constitutional authority; The scope of judicial review over the EC in matters pertaining to the conduct of elections is limited and courts should exercise restraint while making observations about the EC or the electoral process, as it falls within the domain of another expert constitutional authority.[15]

The Election Commission also sought that media reporting be restricted to the material that formed a part of the judicial record before the Madras High Court, not the oral observations of the judges. Besides, they asked that a direction be issued so that no coercive action could be taken against the officials of the Election Commission on the complaint filed before the Khardah police station in Kolkata.

The Supreme Court, however, disposed of the petition, saying the oral remarks were not a part of the official judicial record and, therefore, the question of expunging them did not arise.

> It is trite to say that a formal opinion of a judicial institution is reflected through its judgments and orders, and not its oral observations during the hearing. Hence, in view of the above discussion, we find no substance in the prayer of the EC for restraining the media from reporting on court proceedings. This court stands as a staunch proponent of the freedom of the media to report court proceedings. This we believe is integral to the freedom of speech and expression of those who speak, of those who wish to hear and to be heard and above all, in holding the judiciary accountable to the values which justify its existence as a constitutional institution.[16]

Days before the disparaging comments of the Madras High Court, Prime Minister Modi had decided to cancel his rally in West Bengal and instead take a meeting of chief ministers on the COVID situation. This was when six phases of polling had already taken place in the state. 'Tomorrow, will be chairing high-level meetings to review the prevailing COVID-19 situation. Due to that, I would not be going to West Bengal,' he tweeted on 22 April.[17] Earlier, on 17 April, Modi had spoken to top seer and Hindu Dharma Acharya Sabha President Swami Avdheshanand Giri Ji Maharaj over the phone, making an appeal about the Kumbh in Haridwar, asking people to make it a symbolic affair.[18] Much damage had already been done by then.

Tamil Nadu, West Bengal and Kerala, the states that went through assembly elections, imposed restrictions or lockdowns at different points. In Tamil Nadu, it came immediately after voting in elections ended on 6 April. The state government brought in some restrictions from 10 April through a notification on 8 April.[19] It acknowledged that there was a considerable increase in the number of COVID-19 cases 'day by day across the state in the recent days and the very reason for the increase in the number of positive cases is due to non-adherence of Covid-19 appropriate behaviour,' including wearing of masks and maintaining social distancing. Industrial and commercial activities were still allowed with a restriction on the number of people. Both public and private intrastate bus transport and metropolitan buses were allowed, but in the Greater Chennai limits, the number of passengers was limited to seating capacity. Buses to Puducherry, Andhra Pradesh and Karnataka continued. The state imposed a night curfew from 10 p.m. to 4 a.m. on weekdays and a complete lockdown on Sundays. Through a notification issued on 3 May, public transport capacity was reduced to 50 per cent.[20]

West Bengal, which went through eight phases of elections, with the last phase of polling on 29 April, imposed some restrictions from 30 April onwards but on 15 May, it decided to become stricter. Though it allowed sweets, sari and jewellery shops to remain open, it prohibited all intrastate local trains, Metro railway and intrastate bus services and inland water transport except for emergency and essential services personnel.[21] Strangely, intrastate movement of trucks and goods carriers was also closed, except those relating to medical supplies, oxygen, essential food and fuel.

In Kerala, where COVID had not retreated right from the start of the pandemic, the lockdown during the second wave of COVID started from 8 May, six days after the assembly elections results were announced on 2 May.[22] The state-wide lockdown was complete, with all offices and industrial establishments shut, except some such as those manufacturing essential commodities and engaged in continuous process industry. A large part of the transport network was also shut, unlike in other states. All roadways, waterways and Metro transport services, for instance, were suspended. Air and rail services, which are in the domain of the Union government, continued operations. Only goods transport was allowed to continue. The use of taxis and autorickshaws, including Uber and Ola, was permitted only for procurement of essential commodities, medicines and for attending to medical emergencies as well as transport from/to airports and railway stations. Similarly, the plying of private vehicles was allowed only to the extent of procuring essential commodities, medicines, vaccination and for other such activities. Movement of persons from other states and those coming from other countries from railway stations and airports with proof of ticket was also permitted, but interstate road transport was allowed only for goods and emergency services. For interstate road transport of individuals for emergency purposes, the registration on COVID-19 Jagratha portal was made mandatory.

The state, however, implemented a 'triple lockdown' concept across Malappuram, Thrissur, Ernakulam and Thiruvananthapuram from 26 May 2021. It had tried the concept in the state capital, Thiruvananthapuram, in July 2020. The first degree of lockdown applied to an entire municipal area or district, into which entry or exit was not permitted. The second was to lock down colonies with high infection rates, a bit like containment zones. Inside these clusters, the houses of infected persons were also locked down so that close contacts of the person could also not move out. The remaining districts were under general lockdown.

Long-distance travel, however, was open, and limited intracity and intrastate travel across the country was allowed during the second-wave lockdowns in 2021. They were, therefore, milder than the 2020 national lockdown. Besides, the acceptability of this second phase of lockdowns was higher because Indians had already experienced one the previous year and the stringency in 2021 was lower. Nonetheless, it was the scare of contagion and the fear of falling ill and dying of lack of basic medical infrastructure that kept people locked up inside their homes in 2021.

13

THE LONG HAUL FOR OXYGEN

IT WAS 22 APRIL 2021. Delphin Massey was turning sixty-one. A short video call brought her closer to her children, but she could only gesture. It was not possible to speak. Delphin, who had always loved the innumerable colours of life, was in the midst of deep grey of her life that was running on oxygen support. Down with COVID-19, she had been at Jaipur Golden Hospital for a week. Her daughter and an elder son were admitted to a different hospital.

Her youngest son, Erick Massey, who had the deadly infection too, though it was mild, says:

> Things were going wrong from the very beginning because of the lockdown and also because the government website that would have shown our test results was down, so there was a delay in getting the reports. Initially, she was doing fine and her oxygen saturation level was above 95. But when it started fluctuating between 78 and 83, we started panicking.[1]

This was on 14 April, two days after his mother tested positive for COVID-19, though his own test produced a negative result. Hospital beds were, however, not available.

Delphin had a swelling on her face by 15 April. In desperation, Erick turned to friends and contacts to get her a hospital bed. He says:

> There was no ICU bed available and her situation was deteriorating rapidly, so it was difficult to shift to another building. We had the option of one or two more hospitals, but people said Jaipur Golden was better. We did not have much time. When she was at home, she was still able to talk. She did not panic when we took her in an ambulance to the emergency room

With oxygenation, her SpO2 (peripheral capillary oxygen saturation or the level of haemoglobin containing oxygen in the blood) would rise to above 90 but without the support, it was often between 65 and 75.

By the evening of 22 April, Erick had developed a fever and had all the symptoms of COVID-19, so it was his sister who took a health update on their mother the next day, around 4 p.m. The same day, his sister was discharged from the nearby Rajiv Gandhi Hospital, and Erick went to pick her up. Tired and unwell, he fell asleep once he was home, but his phone rang around 2.30 a.m., in the dead of the night. A doctor on the other end of the line told him his mother had suffered a heart attack and was no more. It was unusual for a doctor to call up and deliver such news, but he was told to come in the morning, since the discharge process would take time. The news was more grievous than Erick's own struggle with COVID-19 all alone at home. He went to the hospital on the morning of 24 April, where he found agitated family members of other patients at the reception. It was only then that he realized what exactly had happened. 'I was not following the news because my family was unwell and hospitalized. But something terrible had happened in the night. My mother died because of a lack of oxygen. There was [a] lot of chaos, and about fifteen to twenty policemen were there,' he narrates.

Delphin was in the hospital's Respiratory Intensive Care Unit where the family could not meet her, so the only way they could get an update on her was through nurses and video calls. Some of the patients who had died were in the Medical Intensive Care Unit, where families could meet them and bring food, but within a few hours of meeting their kin, they received news of their death, says Erick. That the hospital did not inform relatives about the depleting oxygen stock is a grudge Erick and others still have against Jaipur Golden. He says:

> One patient's family had an oxygen cylinder in their car. Maybe if they had told us, we would have gotten together and [done something, so that the] authorities would have taken note of it, because that is how it happens in India. No one listens to you unless you are in large numbers.

It is not that the Union and state governments were unaware of the crisis developing in Delhi and across the country. The Government of the National Capital Territory of Delhi (GNCTD), on 15 April 2021, projected an oxygen demand of 300 tonne per day (TPD) for 20 April 2021, 349 TPD for 25 April 2021, and 445 TPD for 30 April 2021. Three days later, on 18 April, it revised the projected demand to 700 TPD due to a surge in COVID-19 cases and communicated this to the Union government. This meant that from a 48 per cent expected increase in fifteen days, it was anticipating an over 133 per cent increase in oxygen demand.

Despite the increase in projected demand, however, 'the supply of oxygen to GNCTD has continued in terms of the allocation order dated 25 April 2021, in which 490 TPD were allocated. As against this as well, the manufacturers have only been able to supply 445 TPD,' Rahul Mehra, senior counsel appearing for the Delhi government, told the Supreme Court in a case relating to essential supplies and service during the pandemic.[2]

Mehra further said the required volume could increase to 976 TPD since the state government planned to increase medical infrastructure, including beds with oxygen cylinders and beds for patients in intensive care units. The apex court, on 30 April 2021, ordered the Centre to supply 700 TPD oxygen to Delhi by midnight of 3 May. But this did not happen. The Delhi High Court, where a parallel case filed by a host of hospitals and other entities for the supply of oxygen was going on, took this as a contempt of court directions. On 4 May, it asked the Union government to show cause as to why contempt action should not be initiated for 'not only non-compliance of our short order dated 01.05.2021, but also of the order passed by the Supreme Court dated 30.04.2021.'[3] It ordered the presence of Piyush Goyal, additional secretary in the MHA, and Sumita Dawra, additional secretary in the Department of Promotion of Industry and Internal Trade, before the court the next day. The contempt proceedings were later struck down by the Supreme Court, but it upheld the order asking the Union government to supply 700 TPD of oxygen to Delhi. The apex court observed in its order dated 5 May:

> It needs to be clarified that the reason why this [Supreme] Court has been persuaded to take up these proceedings during the pendency of the contempt proceedings in the High Court is because recourse to the contempt jurisdiction against two officers (one of whom, Ms Dawra, has tested Covid-19 positive

> but continues to attend to her duties while in isolation) will not in itself resolve the problem which is confronting NCT of Delhi.[4]

'At this stage, when the country is faced with a serious pandemic, the effort of the court must be to facilitate problem solving by the active engagement and cooperation of all stake holders ... The contempt notice is an expression of its anguish.' In fact, the Supreme Court took note that its order dated 30 April 2021 directed the allocation of 700 MT of oxygen per day to NCT of Delhi, but there were efforts to persuade the High Court that there was, in fact, no such direction by the court. This, it said, was an evident attempt at legal 'disingenuity.'

From 18 April till 5 May, when Delhi finally received 730 TPD, sixteen days had lapsed. In the interim, Jaipur Golden Hospital in west Delhi's Rohini told the Delhi High Court on 24 April that twenty-five patients admitted to its critical care unit had died the previous night due to the shortage of oxygen. 'Twenty-five patients lost their lives yesterday due to shortage of oxygen. We are literally gasping for breath,' the hospital said in its plea.[5] Dr D.K. Baluja, medical director, Jaipur Golden Hospital, was quoted in media reports as saying, 'Yesterday, we were supposed to get 3,600 tonne of oxygen, but we received only 1,500 litres.' Batra Hospital, in the southern part of the city, reported the death of twelve COVID patients, including that of the hospital's gastroenteritis head Dr R.K. Himthani, on the afternoon of 1 May.[6] Both Batra Hospital and Jaipur Golden Hospital had petitioned the Delhi High Court against the Union government, asking for adequate oxygen supply. Though the Delhi government later submitted to the High Court that deaths in the Jaipur Golden Hospital were not due to lack of oxygen,[7] both these hospitals are tertiary care hospitals, which had adequate health infrastructure in place, but could not save lives because those critical care beds were devoid of oxygen. When existing facilities were inadequately equipped in the nation's capital, what purpose would the creation of additional facilities for COVID-19 treatment serve? Without oxygen, there is no human life.

Simultaneously, another legal battle was being fought for Karnataka, first in the state's high court and then in the Supreme Court. The oxygen allotment for the state stood at 802 TPD prior to 30 April 2021, which was increased to 856 TPD from 1 May 2021 and to 965 TPD from 5 May 2021. The minimum requirement of oxygen, as projected by the Karnataka government on 5 May 2021, was 1,162 TPD.[8] In the state's Chamarajanagar district, twenty-three patients died on 2 May, and their families alleged it was because of a shortage of medical oxygen at the facility. The state government, however, claimed that only three of the deaths occurred due to the shortage.[9]

In any country with adequate medical infrastructure, the courts of law should not be the ones resolving how much oxygen should be going to which state. The hearings, issuing of orders and eventual compliance mean nothing to a person in the middle of a medical emergency.

The Supreme Court observed in its 30 April 2021 order:

> Recriminations between the Central Government (which contends that GNCTD has not lifted its allocated quantity) and GNCTD (which contends that despite its projected demand the quantity allocated has not been enhanced) can furnish no solace to citizens whose lives depend on a thin thread of oxygen being available ... In the battle of shifting responsibility of supplying/offtaking of oxygen, lives of citizens cannot be put in jeopardy.

> The protection of the lives of citizens is paramount in times of a national crisis and the responsibility falls on both the Central Government and the GNCTD to cooperate with each other to ensure that all possible measures are taken to resolve the situation.[10]

The reason, however, these issues landed up in court was that the Union government had assumed the power to manage oxygen supply in the country. By an order dated 11 September 2020, the MHA exercised its powers under Section 10(2)(h) of the Disaster Management Act to constitute an Empowered Group-II as an inter-ministerial body to ensure the availability of essential medical equipment and oxygen management. According to the Union government's plea in the Supreme Court, oxygen is not produced evenly in India. 'While some states may be oxygen producing states such as Maharashtra, Rajasthan and Jharkhand; other States/UTs such as Delhi, Goa and Madhya Pradesh, do not have production capacity and rely on supply of oxygen from oxygen producing states,' it said.[11]

For an estimation of the required oxygen supply, an expert group categorized patients into three sets: Class I, comprising 80 per cent of the cases, which were mild and did not require oxygen; Class II, comprising 17 per cent cases, which were moderate and could be managed on non-ICU beds, and of which 50 per cent may require oxygen at the rate of 10 litres a minute; and Class III, comprising 3 per cent of cases, which were severe ICU cases requiring approximately 24 litres oxygen a minute. These calculations were worked out by an expert group comprising V.K. Paul, member, NITI Aayog; Dr Randeep Guleria, director, AIIMS; and Balram Bhargava, director-general, ICMR, and director-general health services, and their calculations formed the basis of computing the pan-India requirement of oxygen based on the number of such beds.

The Union government estimated that the total oxygen requirement of the states, calculated on the basis of the categorization and the number of active cases, was around 8,462 TPD in the second week of April 2021. It was, however, this calculation that formed the basis of the Union government's contention that Delhi was asking for oxygen that it did not need. Solicitor General Tushar Mehta argued in the Supreme Court that the optimal demand of the Delhi government should be 415 tonne and not 707 tonne as demanded by the Delhi government. The consequent tussle between the two sides was nothing short of cheap bargaining that wasted a lot of time. 'It is not like GST [goods and service tax] compensation that the Centre and state should bargain upon. It was a matter of life and death,' says Massey.

The Union government also undertook an exercise in matching the sources of supplies with the demand for medical oxygen across states. Nearer the source of production, the faster it could reach the demand centre. States were asked to indicate their projections of the requirement of medical oxygen based on the expected active caseload. These projections were to be given as they were on 20 April, 25 April and 30 April 2021, and an indicative mapping framework was drawn up and approved by an order dated 15 April 2021. This order provided the name of the supply point, the state to which supply was allocated and the quantity to be supplied. A revised projection was also issued, following which a revised supply plan for medical oxygen to fifteen states was issued on 18 April 2021, but the orders had to be revised several times subsequently since the situation changed. The Union government also claimed that the major principles that governed these changes included the allotment of the projected requirement of liquid medical oxygen (LMO), allocated sources being located within the state or closest to the state while balancing requirements from states that had no or low internal manufacturing capacity, feasible transportation, and minimum disruptions in existing supply chains.

According to the Union government's dispositions in the Supreme Court, states such as Delhi, Rajasthan, Punjab, Uttar Pradesh, Uttarakhand and Madhya Pradesh faced challenges despite the allocation made to them. There were issues such as logistical bottlenecks in transportation and incidents of local authorities disrupting supplies to other states. On 22 April 2021, Union Home Secretary A.K. Bhalla had to issue an order that said, 'No restriction shall be imposed on the movement of medical oxygen between the states and transport authorities shall be instructed to accordingly allow free interstate movement of oxygen carrying vehicles.' The instruction followed reports that the Haryana and Uttar Pradesh administrations were preventing the movement of oxygen tankers to Delhi. States and union territories were asked to abide by the supply plan of medical oxygen prepared by the empowered group.

The Union government was procuring and allocating medical oxygen to each state while it left it to the state governments to arrange transportation of the allotted quantity from the supply point. There were still logistical bottlenecks preventing smooth movement, which put a question mark on the purpose the 'virtual central control room' was serving. The room consisted of senior officers of additional and joint secretary ranks and chief secretaries of all states and union territories. Though the basic issue of logistical support was not being resolved, the Supreme Court, in its order of 30 April 2021, asked the Union government to open information from the virtual control room to citizens. It said:

> We understand that the Virtual Central Control Room of the Central Government displays the allocation of supply of oxygen by the Central Government to each State/UT. By extension of this, a mechanism for displaying real time updates of supply

> of oxygen from each state to hospitals in each district, along with the remaining stock of oxygen with the hospitals may be maintained and shared with the citizens to ensure transparency. This will also ensure that citizens can easily identify the hospitals where medical aid can be availed.

The two factors in the availability of medical oxygen were production and supply. Production was easily ramped up with just two directives from the Government of India. On 7 April 2020, the Drug Controller General of India ordered that licences for making medical oxygen be issued to industrial gas manufacturers within twenty-four hours of receipt of the application.[12] The suggestion for this came from the industry, or All India Industrial Gases Manufacturer's Association, itself. That the need to have more medical oxygen was felt in 2020 itself shows that at least the industry had anticipated an increase in demand and saw a market in it. Obviously, it also wanted to exploit the commercial opportunity. But this order left it to the manufacturers to take a call. One year later, the supply of oxygen for all industrial use was completely prohibited from 22 April 2021 onwards, except for certain industries such as ampoules and vials, pharmaceuticals, petroleum refineries, oxygen cylinder manufacturers and others.[13] This, according to the Union government, added 1,000 TPD to the medical oxygen capacity. Additionally, steel plants increased the production of LMO while reducing the production of other liquid products, argon and nitrogen, required for manufacturing steel.

The ramp-up in supply was substantial, considering that these companies supplied an average of 1,500–1,700 TPD in mid-April and then 3,131.84 MT on 25 April.[14] By 4 May 2021, they were producing 3,680.30 TPA of LMO and were supplying (some part from their earlier stocks as well) 4,076.65 tonne. Since the total supply of medical oxygen that day was 8,862 TPD, the steel sector alone was meeting 46 per cent of the medical oxygen supply. There were other companies, such as Indian Oil Corporation and Reliance Industries Ltd, that started to produce LMO. At the public-sector company Bharat Heavy Electricals Limited's (BHEL) Bhopal unit, people queued up in large numbers every day to get oxygen cylinders refilled.[15] 'The queue of people and hospital representatives with cylinders is so long that they have to wait for six to seven hours for their turn to come,' one eyewitness was quoted as saying in a Press Trust of India 24 April report. Bhopal BHEL's general manager Raghvendra Shukla told the news agency that its oxygen plant had been operating at its full capacity of about 5,000 cubic metres a day for over a week following a Madhya Pradesh government's request. 'On April 10, we had told the state government that we can arrange only 1,800 cubic metres a day, but after the requirement increased, we have been running our plant round the clock in full capacity of more than 5,000 cubic metres a day starting April 18,' he said.

When the pressure of public criticism and judicial oversight grew, the Union government's publicity wing, PIB, came up with regular updates on medical oxygen supply, but none of those gave an estimate of the total nationwide demand and how much of it was being met. On 10 May, for instance, it issued a press release on behalf of the Ministry of Commerce and Industry that said:

> Commensurate with the increase in production and demand, LMO sale in the country has also increased from about 1,300 MT/day [metric ton per day] in March' 21 to 8,920 MT/day on 6 May. During the first wave of COVID-19, the maximum sale of 3,095 MT/day of LMO was seen on 29 September 2020. The sale of LMO grew more than five-fold from 1559 MT/day on 31 March 2021 to over 8,000 MT mark by 3 May 2021.[16]

The 1,822-word press release did not mention any estimation of demand; whether the government did not have an idea of the demand and was delivering as is basis or whether it was blanking out this information was not known. The reason it was important to know the total demand was that lack of oxygen was causing deaths even in established medical facilities, leading to hospitals turning away patients even though they had beds available. Additionally, as Delhi counsel Mehra said in the Supreme Court, new medical facilities could not be used due to the lack of oxygen.

> The daily requirement of 700 MT for NCTD has been computed on the basis of the formula adopted by the Union Government, without factoring in an additional requirement of 256 tonne consequent upon setting up of new facilities (including a facility being set up by DRDO); The additional facilities cannot be put to use for want of oxygen; The additional requirement of NCTD (from 490 tonne to 700 tonne) is only 210 tonne, which is a small fraction of the pan-India availability of oxygen, estimated at 8,410 tonne by the Union Government. Further, the actual oxygen lifted by the respective States/UTs (as on 28 April 2021), out of their allocated quantity, was only 7,334.53 tonne.[17]

Given that the Central and state governments had failed to anticipate a second wave and there was unprecedented stress on the medical infrastructure, the creation of additional medical facilities was important and for that, availability of oxygen was the foremost requirement.

With the formula for the allocation of oxygen coming under scrutiny, the Supreme Court ordered the formation of a new taskforce.

> It is necessary that an effective and transparent mechanism is set up within the Union government for the purpose of allocating medical oxygen to all states and union territories for being used during the Covid-19 pandemic. The Union government has agreed to set up a National Task Force to streamline the process. This Task Force would be tasked inter alia with formulating a methodology for the scientific allocation of oxygen.[18]

Based on the Union government's suggestions, the court ordered the appointment of Dr Bhabatosh Biswas, former vice-chancellor, West Bengal University of Health Sciences, Kolkata; Dr Devender Singh Rana, chairperson, board of management, Sir Ganga Ram Hospital, Delhi; Dr Devi Prasad Shetty, chairperson and executive director, Narayana Healthcare, Bengaluru; Dr Gagandeep Kang, professor, Christian Medical College, Vellore, Tamil Nadu; Dr J.V. Peter, director, Christian Medical College, Vellore, Tamil Nadu; Dr Naresh Trehan, chairperson and managing director, Medanta Hospital and Heart Institute, Gurugram; Dr Rahul Pandit, director, critical care medicine and ICU, Fortis Hospital, Mulund (Mumbai, Maharashtra) and Kalyan (Maharashtra); Dr Saumitra Rawat, chairman and head, department of surgical gastroenterology and liver transplant, Sir Ganga Ram Hospital, Delhi; Dr Shiv Kumar Sarin, senior professor and head of department of hepatology, director, Institute of Liver and Biliary Science (ILBS), Delhi; Dr Zarir F. Udwadia, consultant chest physician, Hinduja Hospital, Breach Candy Hospital and Parsee General Hospital, Mumbai; Secretary, MoHFW; and the Cabinet Secretary to the Union Government (also the convenor) as members of the task force.

Even after almost a month of the Union government taking steps to augment the supply of medical oxygen, twenty-six patients being treated for COVID-19 at the Goa Medical College and Hospital died on 11 May. While pushing for a probe by the high court into the early morning deaths at the state-run hospital, Goa Health Minister Vishwajit Rane said, 'I think there needs to be an inquiry into this (deaths) … it would also be fine if the high court enquires into this.' He was talking to reporters, hours after Chief Minister Pramod Sawant visited the hospital to assess the situation. High court approval was required for a probe by a judge, sitting or retired. Rane was quoted as saying in the media:

> We are facing a shortage of oxygen. Yesterday, we required 1,200 cylinders of oxygen but we got only 400. Because of interrupted oxygen supply, I think somewhere between the hours 2 a.m. to 6 a.m., there are a lot of deaths happening. Even today between 2 a.m. to 6 a.m., there were around 26 deaths.[19]

Two days later, on 13 May, another fifteen deaths were reported during the same hours. This, when the Bombay High Court had directed the state government to ensure there were no more deaths due to oxygen shortage.[20] On 30 July 2021, however, Rane in a written reply to a question in the Goa Assembly, said, 'No deaths due to lack of oxygen supplies have been reported in any government hospitals (sic) in the state till date.'[21]

Assuming that the production of oxygen had been resolved, supply chain problems continued. This, in fact, turned out to be tougher and remained unresolved, with the Union government blaming the states for it. Solicitor General Mehta had argued in the Supreme Court in April that there was no dearth of oxygen supply in the country and steps were being taken continuously to augment the supply of oxygen. Though he admitted that there had been a shortage of supply to certain states, he attributed this shortage to various factors, including the failure of state governments to lift the allocated quantity of oxygen from the supply point; transportation bottlenecks caused by interstate movement of tankers; and technical failure of certain plants leading to the reassessment of allocation on a real-time basis.[22]

Over a year after the pandemic struck the country, it would be hard to imagine that the non-availability of tankers would cost lives and choke the oxygen supply. Realizing that even import of oxygen would not be possible without the availability of tankers, the Union government started approving tanker imports as well. According to a government disposition in the Supreme Court in April, India had 1,224 oxygen tankers (16,732 tonne capacity) and efforts were made to increase this capacity to 2,000 tankers through conversion of nitrogen and argon tankers and import of 138 cryogenic tankers. When PIB issued a release on 10 May, it said the capacity of tankers was 12,480 tonne and their number was 1,040 in March 2020. This increased to 1,681 tankers with a total capacity of 23,056 tonne, which included 408 converted tankers and 101 imported tankers.[23] Considering that the capacity of tankers was 2.4 times the daily production of 9,446 tonne on 4 May, it can be said that for every tonne of production, 2.4 tonne of tanker capacity was available. This also meant that for a tonne of oxygen travelling to the demand side, another tonne and a little more tanker capacity could be assigned to run towards the production centre. The distance between the production and demand sites, however, added to the turnaround time. Under a plan to give Delhi 700 TPD, for instance, the turnaround time of four containers from Indian Oil Corporation and seven containers from DP World was four days.

As the crisis deteriorated, the Union government grappled with the problem of transportation. There was a mismatch between producing and consuming states, but equity among states was to be maintained, the Union government contended in a press release on 10 May.[24] One-third of the oxygen production was concentrated in east India, while 60 per cent of the demand was from north and south India, resulting in transportation challenges. 'Mapping of source and destination of oxygen has been completed to optimize transportation plan in consultation with States/UTs, manufacturers & other stakeholders,' it said. All modes of transport—air, sea, railway and road—had to be used to get the oxygen going.

Since oxygen had to travel long distances, the Madhya Pradesh and Maharashtra state governments in April 2021 approached the MoR to explore whether LMO tankers could be moved by train. To gauge its technical feasibility, a pilot was undertaken to transport tankers through roll-on-roll-off (RORO) service. This involves trucks rolling on or driving on to flat wagons and rolling or driving off once the journey is over. The right size of tankers had to be chosen due to restrictions of height, because of road overbridges (ROBs) and overhead equipment (OHE) at some places. The T1618 tanker, with a height of 3.32 m was found feasible. These tankers were to be placed on flat railway wagons used for moving army trucks. These wagons are called Defence Bogie Open Military or DBKM wagons, with a height of 1.29 m. One such wagon was placed at the Kalamboli goods shed in Mumbai on 15 April, where a tanker loaded with LMO belonging to INOX Air Products was loaded onto it.

INOX Air Products and the Indian Railways jointly took measurements. 'Based on these measurements, route clearances were taken and it was found that it would be possible to undertake movements as RORO as ODC (over dimensional consignment) with speed restrictions on some sections depending on overhead clearances. In order to enable commercial booking and freight payment for RO-RO movement of LMO in cryogenic tankers, the Ministry of Railways has brought out a circular on 16.04.2021 providing all the necessary details and guidance on the matter,' said a railway press release dated 18 April.[25] The previous day, a meeting was held between Railway Board officials, state transport commissioners and representatives of industry on transportation of LMO. It was decided that the transport commissioner of Maharashtra would arrange empty tankers, which would move from Kalamboli and Boisar railway stations near Mumbai. They were to head to Vishakhapatnam, Jamshedpur, Rourkela and Bokaro for loading of LMO. Zonal Railways were to receive the trailers and load them back. Ramps had to be built at Vishakhapatnam, Angul and Bhilai and the existing ramp at Kalamboli was strengthened. The Kalamboli ramp was to be readied in one day, and at other places, the ramps had to be ready by the time the tankers arrived.

A trial was organized at Boisar station in the Western Railway zone on 18 April, where a loaded tanker was placed on a flat wagon and all the required measurements were taken. While the railways placed DBKM wagons at Kalamboli, the Maharashtra government had to arrange ten empty tankers to dispatch the next day. Finally, however, seven empty tankers departed from the Kalamboli goods yard for Visakhapatnam steel plant in Andhra Pradesh at 8.05 p.m. on 19 April. This train crossed Vasai Road, Jalgaon, Nagpur, Raipur Junction and finally reached the Visakhapatnam steel plant siding in the East Coastal Railway zone.[26] A total of ten drivers accompanied these tankers. One tanker belonged to Taiyo Nippon Sanso, three to INOX Air Products, one to Air Liquide and two to Linde. But it took some time for the train to reach Vishakhapatnam, then get loaded and go back to Maharashtra. The return journey, with 126 tonne of oxygen, started on 22 April. Another Oxygen Express started its journey from Lucknow to Bokaro via Varanasi the same day.[27] For the movement of this train, a green corridor or a clear track with no stoppages was created between Lucknow and Varanasi. The distance of 270 km was covered by the train in four hours and twenty minutes, at an average speed of 62.35 kmph.

According to the Indian Railways, the Kalamboli-Vishakhapatnam route had to be mapped to assess various constraints, such as Ghat sections, road overbridges, tunnels, curves, platform canopies and overhead equipment. The Central Railway in its press statement said that because height was an important factor in this movement, the railways mapped the route via Vasai. The model of road tanker T1618, with a height of 3,320 mm, was found feasible to be placed on flat wagons. The longer route via Vasai was charted as over dimensional consignment (ODC) is not permitted to travel in the Western Ghat sections over the Mumbai division. Besides, since oxygen is a cryogenic and hazardous chemical, sudden acceleration and deceleration are avoided and pressure has to be monitored.

Trains were being used for long-distance movement since they were faster than road transport. They could run continuously, while truck drivers needed to take halts while moving by road. The distance between Kalamboli and Vishakhapatnam is more than 1,850 km, which was covered by the empty tanker rakes in about fifty hours. Seven tankers with more than 100 tonne of oxygen were loaded in ten hours and transported back to Nagpur in twenty-one hours. Three tankers were unloaded in Nagpur on 23 April and the remaining four tankers reached Nashik at 10.25 a.m. on 24 April.[28]

Once these two operations to Uttar Pradesh and Maharashtra were completed, requests from states such as Andhra Pradesh and Delhi also came in, and by 12 May, the Indian Railways had run 100 Oxygen Express trains with 6,260 tonne of oxygen in more than 396 tankers to various states across the country.[29]

This was the first time the Indian Railways was carrying oxygen. The other alternative, of airlifting oxygen over long distances, was not feasible because of the hazardous nature of the gas, so empty tankers were carried by air, and on the return journey, they travelled by road. One C-17 plane of the Indian Air Force, used for strategic airlift missions and transportation of troops and cargo, flew from Delhi to Durgapur in West Bengal with empty tankers while the other transported oxygen tankers between Hyderabad in Telangana and Angul in Odisha. Another C-17 of the Indian Air Force flew at

2 a.m. on 24 April 21 from Hindan Air Base near Delhi for Changi International Airport, Singapore.[30] The aircraft arrived at Singapore at 7.45 a.m. After loading four empty cryogenic oxygen containers, it went to Panagarh air base in West Bengal to offload the containers for filling at the Durgapur Steel Plant. Another C-17 of the Indian Air Force flew from Hindan Air Base at 8 a.m., headed to the Pune air base. The jet was loaded with two empty cryogenic oxygen container trucks, which were then flown to Jamnagar air base. The same C-17 aircraft took two more empty containers from Pune to Jamnagar. Another C-17 plane transported two empty containers from Jodhpur to Jamnagar on 24 April.

The Union government tried importing oxygen and, on 16 April, floated a global tender to import 50,000 tonne of oxygen. The effort, however, led to a firm commitment of only 500 tonne from a Gulf organization and about 3,000 tonne of supply commitment till 25 April. 'The worrying part is these imports will not come immediately and are priced very high. Some of the global suppliers are taking advantage of the shortage,' a senior government official was quoted as saying in a *Business Standard* article.[31] Later, in a 10 May press release, the Union government said quotations were obtained on 21 April, but these were just three quotations, received and approved for 3,500 tonne with delivery over three months. In addition, 2,285 tonne of LMO was imported from UAE, Bahrain, Kuwait and France.

The sea route was also used for importing oxygen. *INS Tarkash*, with two cryogenic containers filled with 20 tonne of LMO each and 230 oxygen cylinders, arrived at Mumbai on 12 May. The containers were facilitated by the French Mission as part of 'Oxygen Solidarity Bridge'. Some cylinders were gifted by the Indian diaspora in Qatar.[32] Earlier, on 5 May, Indian Naval Ship *Talwar* entered the port of New Mangalore in Karnataka ferrying two 27-tonne liquid oxygen tanks from Bahrain. The same day, *INS Kolkata*, deployed in Persian

Gulf, also departed Kuwait, loaded with two 27-ton oxygen tanks, 400 oxygen cylinders and forty-seven concentrators. The Indian Navy, under its Samudra Setu II operation, commissioned nine ships from all three Naval Commands in Mumbai, Visakhapatnam and Kochi.[33] They were deployed to ship LMO and other medical equipment from 'friendly foreign countries in the Persian Gulf and South East Asia'. Four warships sailed with around nine 27-tonne oxygen tanks and more than 1,500 oxygen cylinders from Qatar and Kuwait.

The volume being transported was not huge, but these mammoth exercises, across all modes of long-distance transport, were an all-out wartime-like effort to meet the demand for oxygen. It was necessary because a large number of people were dying due to the lack of oxygen and proper medical care. These deaths, and the deployment of these massive resources, could have been avoided if after one year of the pandemic breaking out and after witnessing a spike in September 2020, onsite oxygen generation units had been put up across all major hospitals in the country. Oxygen scarcity was not a new challenge for a country that had witnessed a huge controversy in 2017, when many child deaths were reported in government-run BRD Medical College hospital in Gorakhpur in Uttar Pradesh: in August of that year, sixty-three children had died at the hospital after its piped oxygen supply ran out.

If lessons had been learnt and pressure swing adsorption (PSA) plants at hospitals had been commissioned by 2021, it would have enabled self-sufficiency. These units, installed on hospital premises, derive oxygen from atmospheric air, which is purified and supplied through pipes to patients. When the second wave of COVID-19 was sweeping the country in April, the MoHFW submitted to the Supreme Court that it was in the process of commissioning 162 PSA plants of 154-tonne capacity, each.[34] The number of plants installed till 30 April was a mere thirty-eight.

Orders for 500 PSA units were finally placed in the fourth week of April, but they were expected to come up not before July. All it took was Rs 75 lakh and some taxes to build one such unit.[35] Four hundred and fifty plants were being set up by Tata Advance Systems, and the remaining fifty were being put up by Trident Pneumatics. Faced with criticism for the delay in setting up these plants, the government, on 25 April, announced that the PM Cares Fund had given in-principle approval to the allocation of funds for 551 dedicated PSAs inside public health facilities in the country.[36] These were to be set up in identified government hospitals in district headquarters in various states and Union territories. A rather unapologetic government statement that did not acknowledge the tragic losses that had already occurred said:

> Liquid medical oxygen (LMO) would serve as a 'top up' to the captive oxygen generation. Such a system will go a long way in ensuring that government hospitals in the districts do not face sudden disruption of oxygen supplies and have access to adequate uninterrupted oxygen supply to manage the COVID-19 patients and other patients needing such support.

That lives were lost for a month in the country's capital, even as the Delhi government fought a legal battle in the Supreme Court to get a higher oxygen quota from the Union government, appeared even more surreal when the state, in less than ten days, offered 'extra' oxygen to other states on 13 May because the demand had fallen and it needed only 582 TPD.[37]

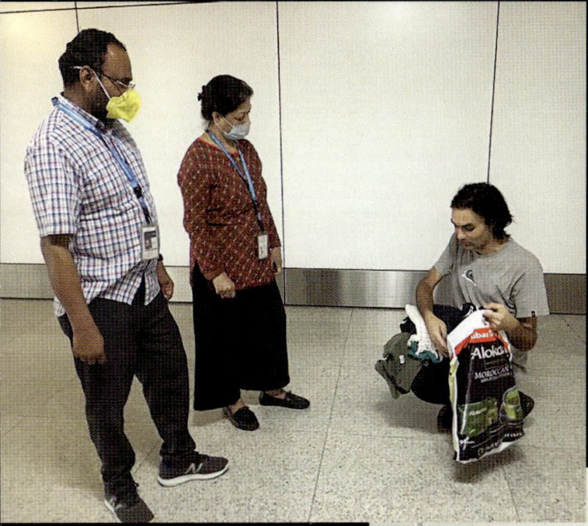

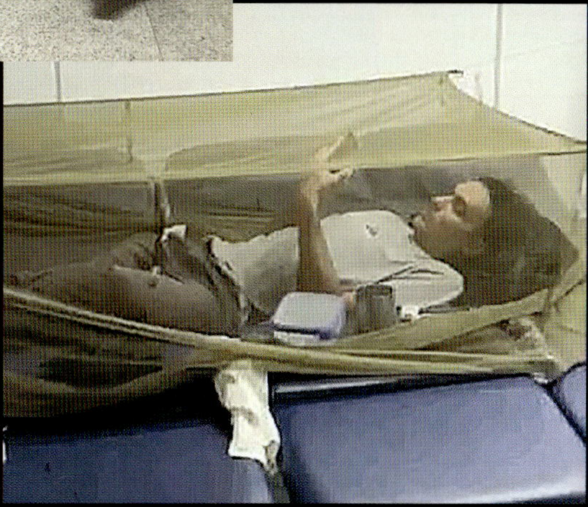

German national Edgard Ziebart, for whom Indira Gandhi International Airport became home or fifty-five days when international lights shut (Chapter 1). *Photo credit: Delhi International Airport Ltd*

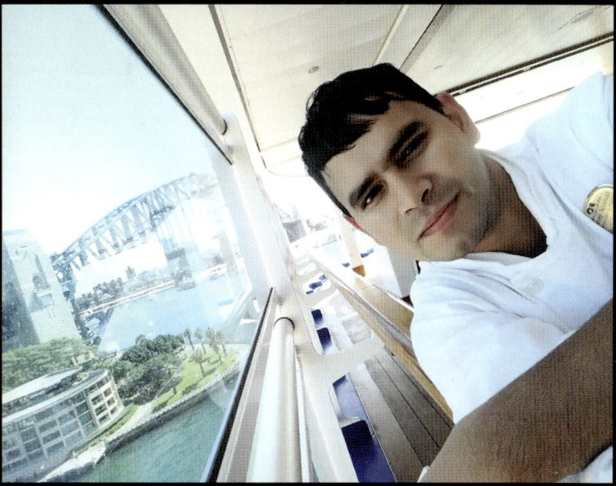

Binay Sarkar on board the *Diamond Princess* at Sydney Harbour in iappier times (Chapter 2). *Courtesy of Binay Sarkar*

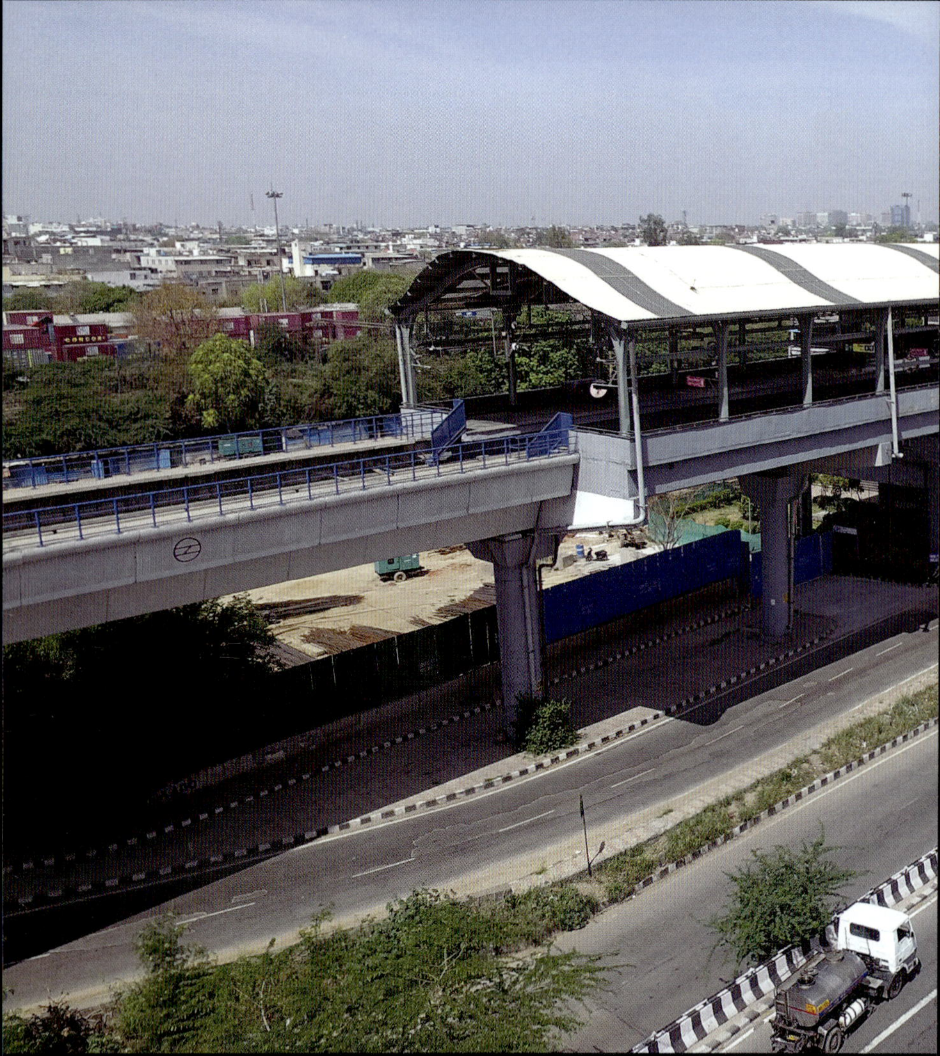

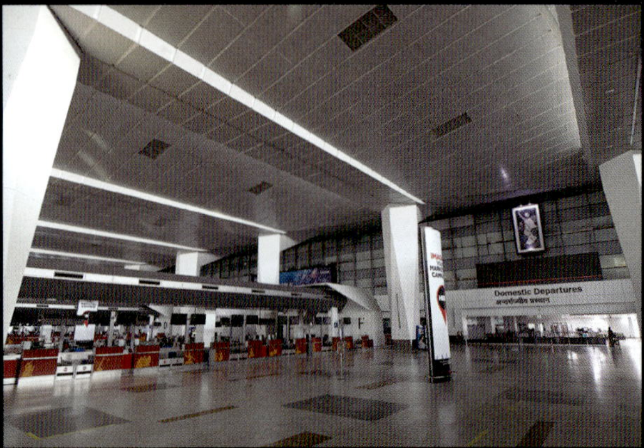

The domestic departure terminal at Indira Gandhi International Airport in Ne Delhi when flights were shu down (Chapter 4). *Photo credit: Delhi International Airport Ltd*

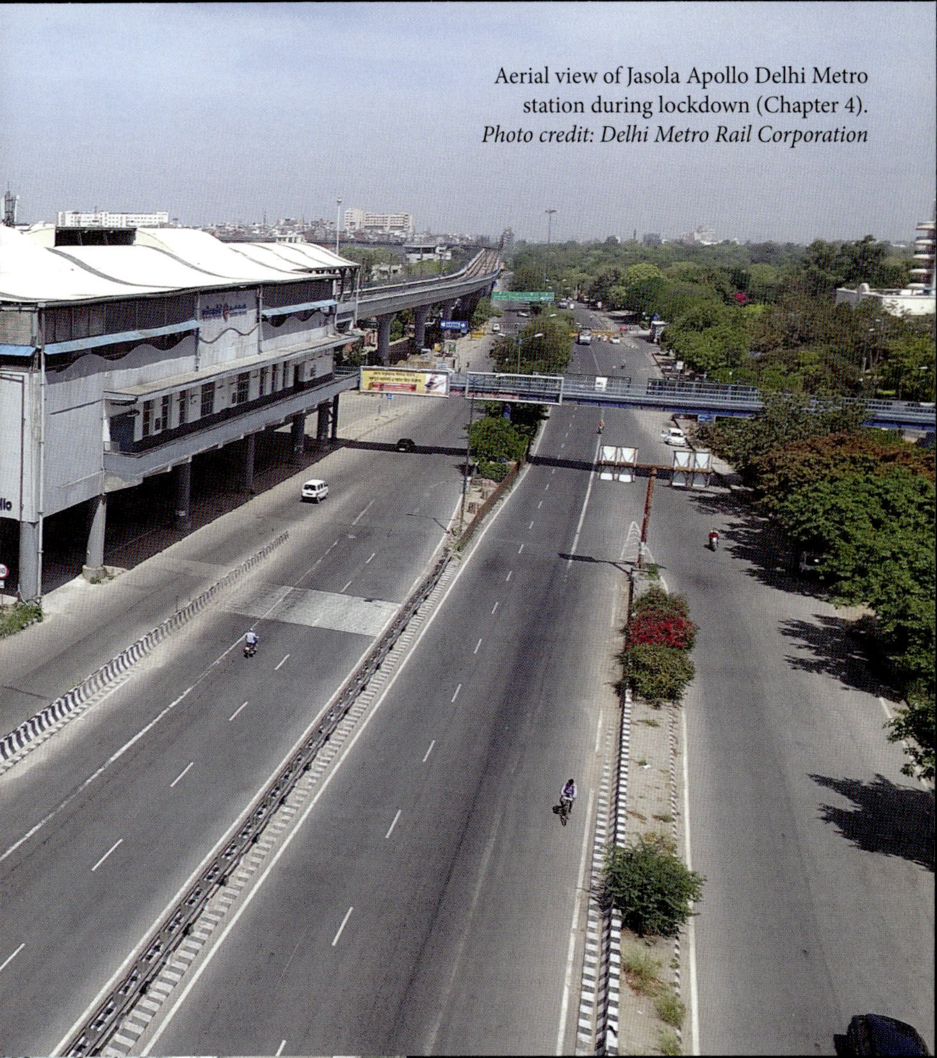

Aerial view of Jasola Apollo Delhi Metro station during lockdown (Chapter 4).
Photo credit: Delhi Metro Rail Corporation

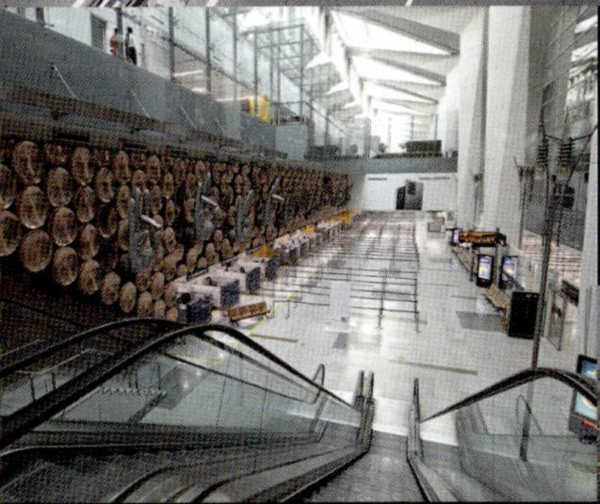

Vacant immigration counters at Indira Gandhi International Airport (Chapter 4).
Photo credit: Delhi International Airport Ltd

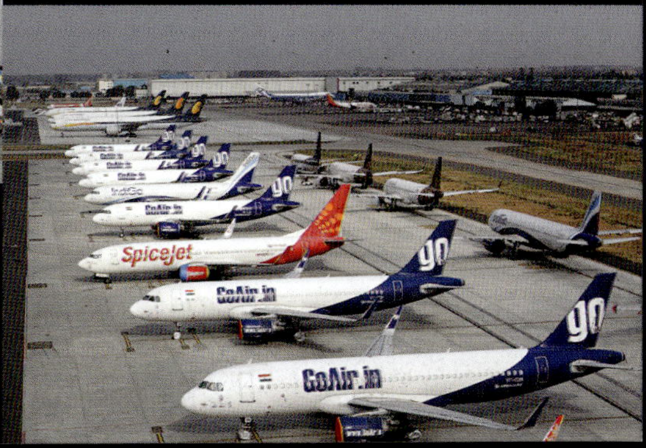

owhere to go: Aeroplanes parked at Indira Gandhi International Airport (Chapter 4).
hoto credit: Delhi International Airport Ltd

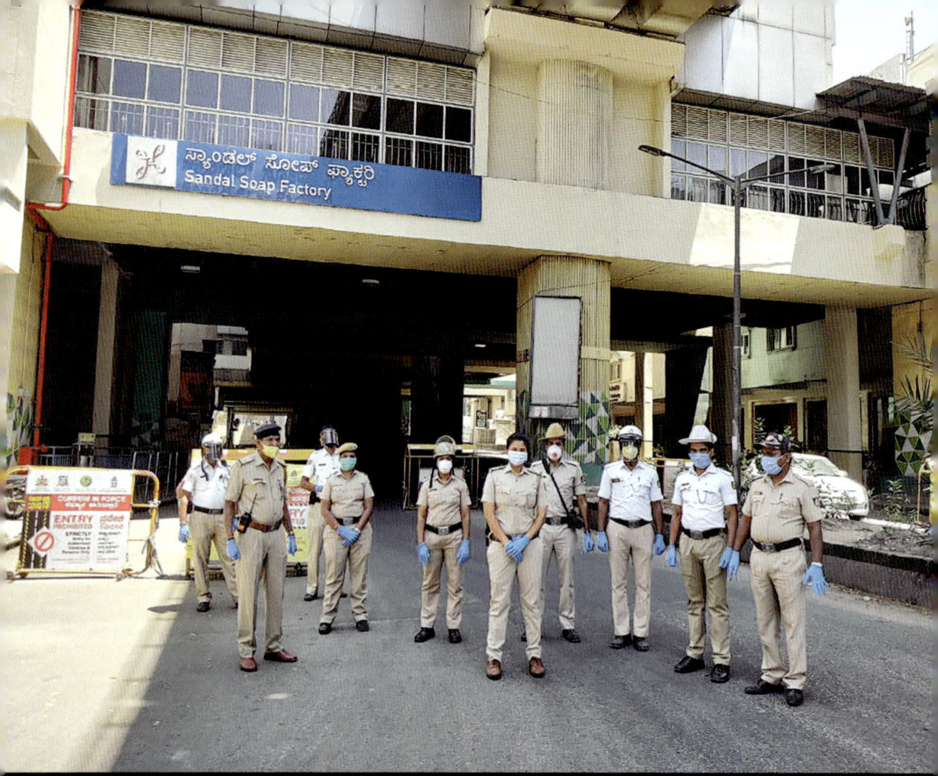

A Namma Metro station in Bengaluru during lockdown (Chapter 5). *Courtesy of the author*

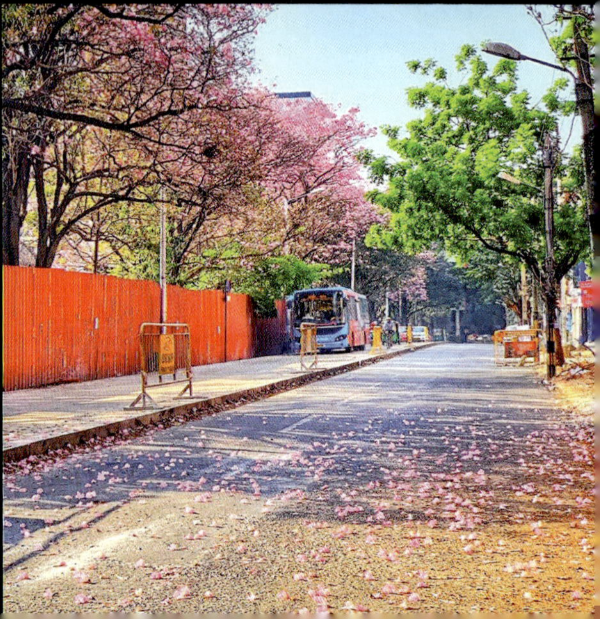

A locked-down street in Bengaluru (Chapter 5). *Courtesy of the author*

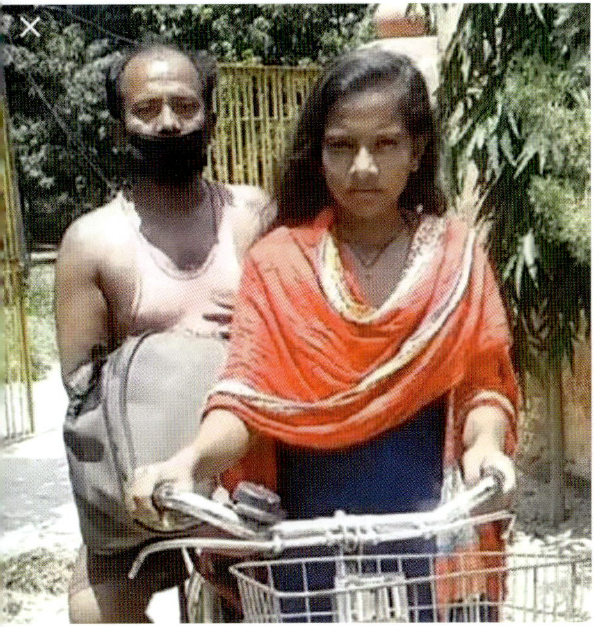

Jyoti Kumari with her father, Mohan Paswan, cycled from Gurugram to Bihar (Chapter 6). *Courtesy of Jyoti Kumari*

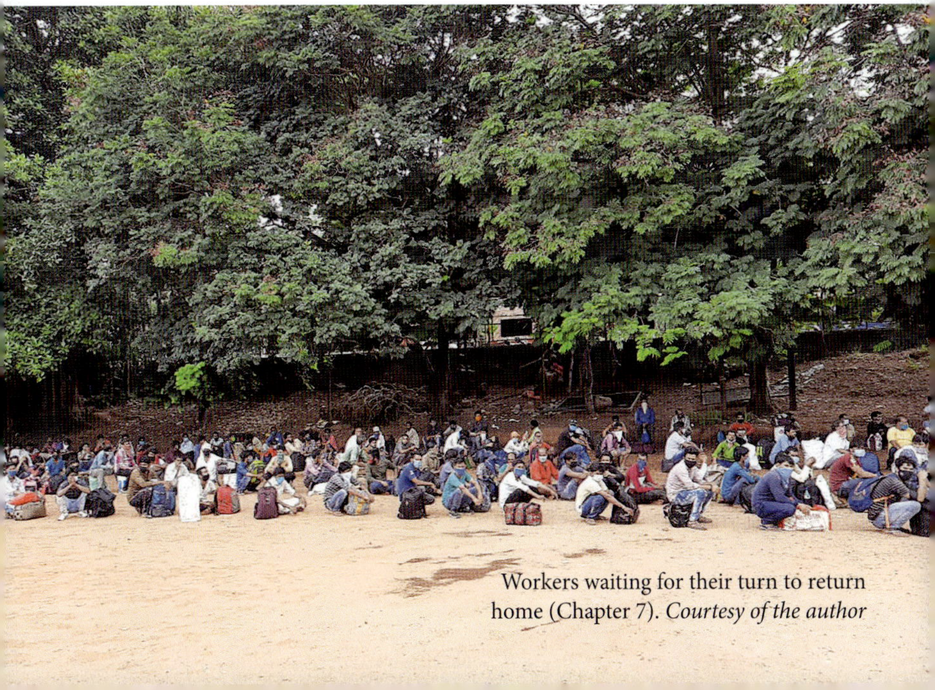

Workers waiting for their turn to return home (Chapter 7). *Courtesy of the author*

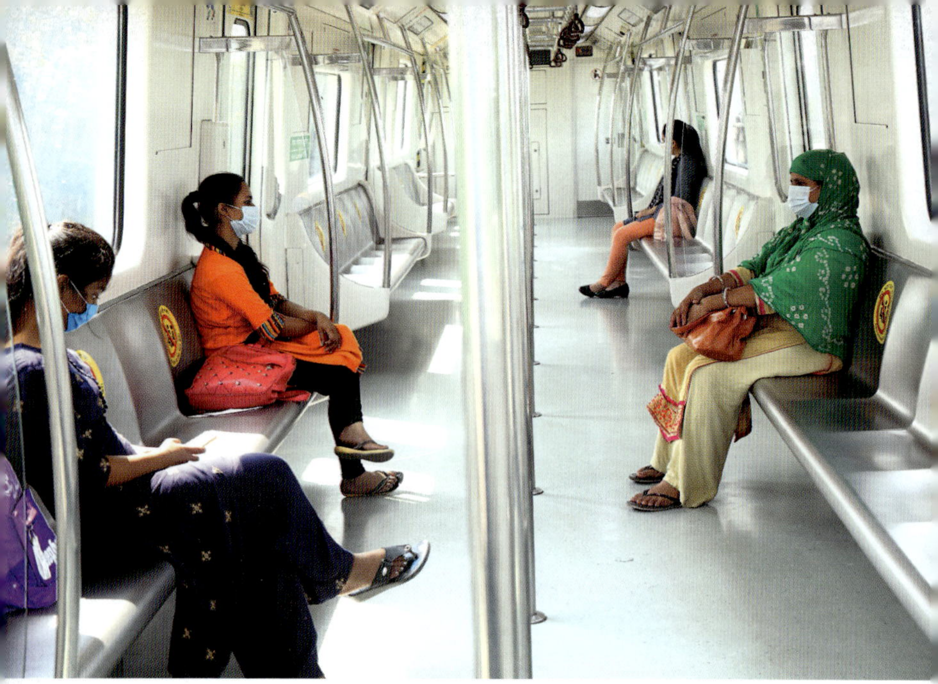

Limited seating in Delhi Metro coaches (Chapter 10).
Photo credit: Delhi Metro Rail Corporation

Social distancing at a security checkpoi
at a Delhi Metro station (Chapter 10
Photo credit: Delhi Metro Rail Corporatio

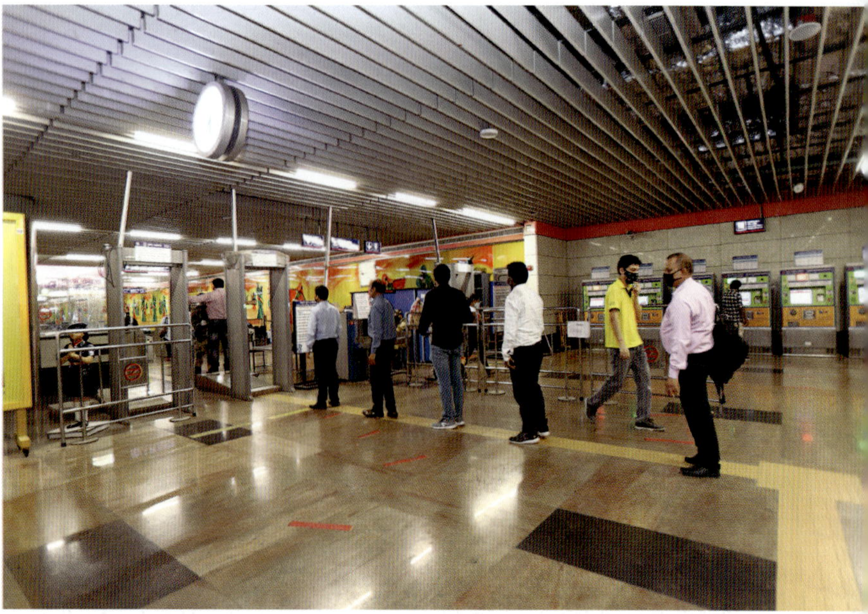

ixty-one-year-old Delphin Massey contracted COVID-19 and was one of the patients who died due to lack of oxygen (Chapter 13). *Photo credit: Erick Massey*

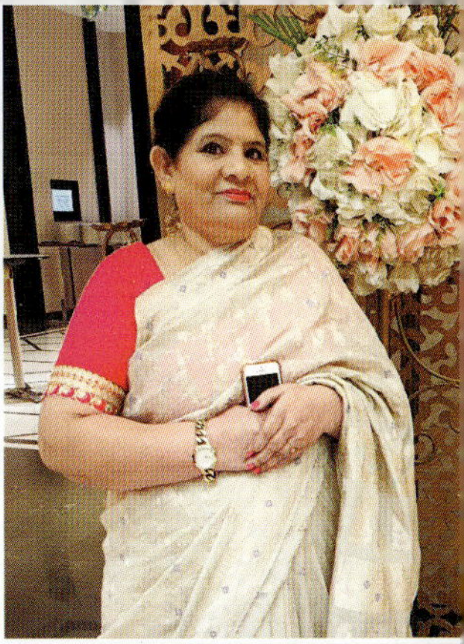

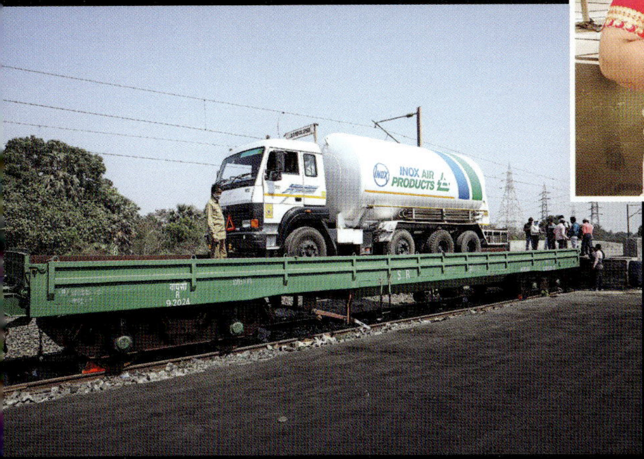

An Inox oxygen tanker being moved through railway (Chapter 13). *Photo credit: Inox*

COVID-19 detection dogs at Helsinki airport (Chapter 15). *Photo credit: Finavia Corp*

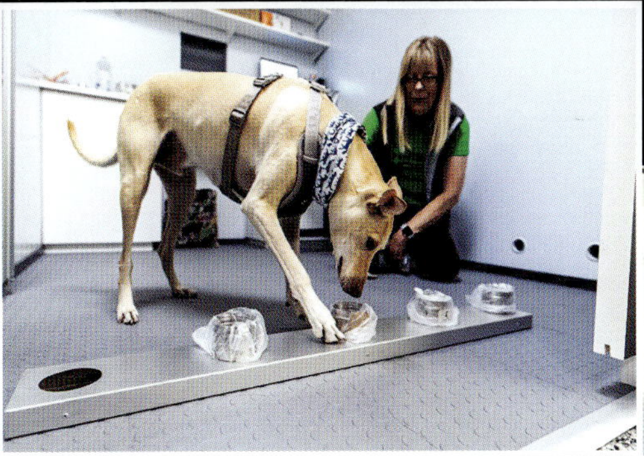

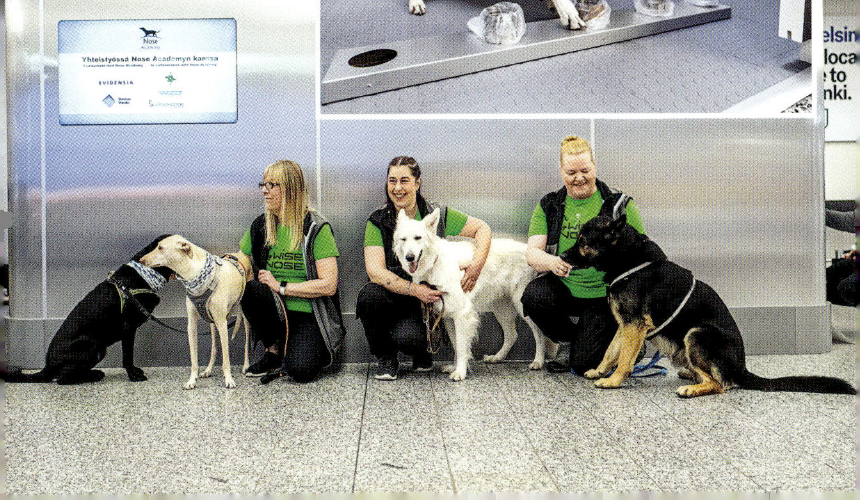

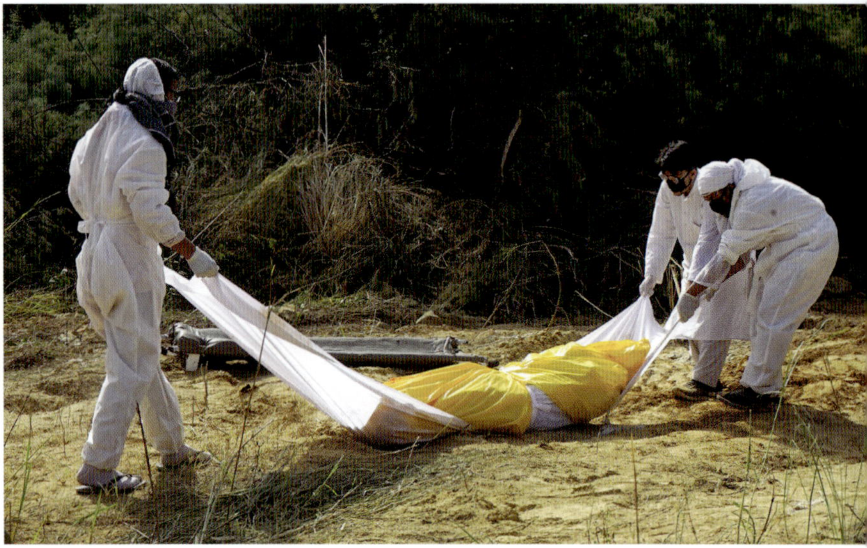

Burial of a COVID-19 victim at an Islamic burial ground in Delhi's ITO area. Family member were only allowed to view the burial from a distance with protective gear during the outbreak of COVID in 2020, otherwise called the first wave. *Photo credit: Shome Basu*

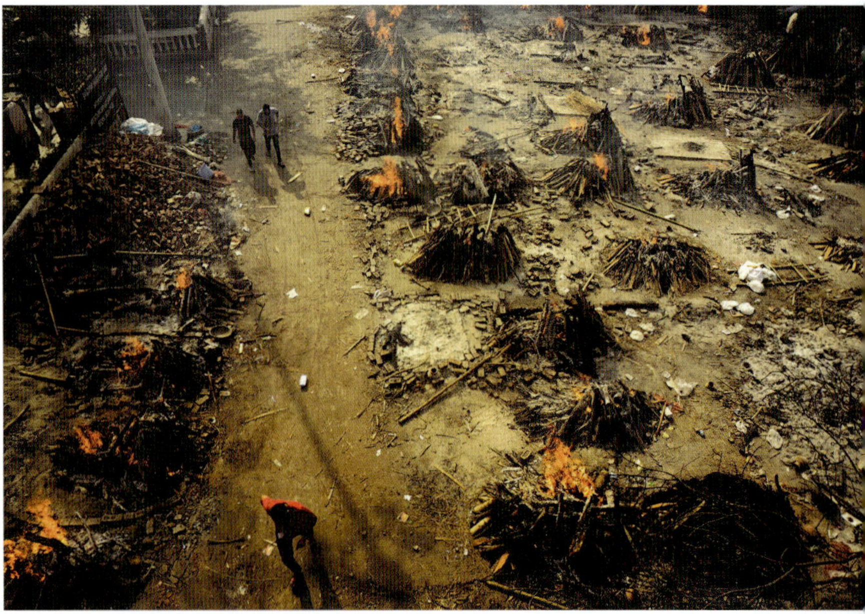

At a Hindu crematorium in East Delhi's Ghazipur where pyres were piled up. Clueless families wandered around to find their near ones who had died of COVID-19 during the second wave of the pandemic in 2021. *Photo credit: Shome Basu*

PART VI

THE ALTERNATIVES

14

WELL-TIMED ALTERNATIVES

BETWEEN THE SUMMER OF 2020 and that of 2021, the COVID-19 pandemic persisted in India. It resurrected, bringing death and trauma, from March 2021. In the interim, India had its own virus variants as well, though a needless controversy arose on whether the variants should be called 'Indian' or not. Then US President Donald Trump had called the coronavirus a 'China' virus in 2020, right at the onset of the pandemic, and the Narendra Modi government was upset that the variant in the second wave was being called Indian. The WHO also received communications from several countries and agencies to consider easy-to-pronounce and non-stigmatizing labels for variants of interest (VOI) and variants of concern (VOC).[1]

When the second wave had scarred the country, the Indian government thought one of the ways of fighting the global criticism of the deterioration of the COVID situation in the country was by issuing a clarification on the use of the term 'Indian variant' for a strain of the virus. On 12 May 2021, it said that media reports using the term were without any basis and unfounded. It said

WHO, while classifying B.1.617 as a variant of global concern, 'did not term it as an Indian Variant.'[2] WHO played it safe and started identifying them as 'variants first found in' a specific country. On 19 May 2021, it noted, 'There are four variants of concern that WHO is tracking around the world. The B.1.1.7, which was first identified in the United Kingdom, the B.1.351, which was first identified in South Africa, the P.1 variant which was first identified in Japan from travellers from Brazil. And now we've recently classified the B.1.617, which was first identified in India.'[3] But by 31 May, it had issued a new nomenclature. It said 'simple, easy-to-say and remember labels for key variants' of the virus using letters of the Greek alphabet were being assigned. It was simultaneously preventing the association of the coronavirus and its variants with countries.[4] So, it started using the Greek alphabets Alpha, Beta, Gamma and so on for virus variants, which it felt would be easier and more practical for discussion among non-scientific audiences.

Interestingly, after the variant Omicron, fifteenth in the Greek alphabet series, was first reported in South Africa on 24 November 2021, WHO skipped letters Nu and Xi.[5] A *New York Times* report said, 'Now the alphabet has created its own political headache. When it came time to name the potentially dangerous new variant that has emerged in southern Africa, the next letter in alphabetical order was Nu, which officials thought would be too easily confused with "new". The letter after that was even more complicated: Xi, a name that in its transliteration, though not its pronunciation, happens to belong to the leader of China, Xi Jinping. So they skipped both and named the new variant Omicron.' The report quoted Tarik Jasarevic, a spokesperson for WHO, saying '"Nu" is too easily confounded with "new," and "Xi" was not used because it is a common last name.[6]

B.1.617 or Delta, a deadlier strain of the coronavirus, had been circulating in India from February 2021. There were, in fact, four virus mutations found in the country. According to America's CDC, the first variant seen in India was in October 2020, followed by two in December 2020 and one in February 2021.[7]

Not only did infections and deaths spike in March, April and early May, the medical infrastructure turned out to be woefully deficient for the increase in cases. Established hospitals found they could not handle the load even when they had beds, because oxygen was in short supply. If this was the case with existing hospital facilities, the creation of additional COVID facilities was of no use to those who needed urgent medical support.

No one doubted in April 2021 that governments, states as well as Central, had let the past year go by without preparing to handle the second wave. The only people who perhaps did not think that way were decision-makers themselves, for whom the battle over COVID-19 had already been won, since in government analysis, the first wave had not caused much damage. In an April 2021 interview with *The Indian Express*, K. Vijay Raghavan, principal scientific advisor to the Government of India, said, 'The ferocity of the second wave took everyone by surprise. Prior to the first wave, the predictions were dire. The response to those predictions was electric and everyone came on board … The relatively lower severity in India during the first wave and the squelching of that wave have been discussed widely. Lockdowns, ensuring physical distancing, adoption of masks, and the extraordinary and rapid action from our health services all contributed, and had a strong impact. During and after the first wave, multiple measures were initiated by the Centre and states for revamping response infrastructure. This, and the flattening of the first wave, and the confidence from vaccine development all contributed to us not anticipating the size of this [second wave] surge.'[8] Clearly, he was crediting the government efforts for the 'low intensity' first wave, while citing this as the reason for not really estimating the severity of the second wave.

There are only two ways that strategies can be planned around a pandemic – one, by preventing it from spreading, which is what the Union government intended to do by imposing a lockdown in 2020; the other, by meeting the challenge through medical support when the infection has spread. Whether lessons were learnt from the first wave, and how far they were implemented, is not very clear because the government kept crediting itself with a successful lockdown. When the second wave broke out, however, it exposed another summer of government incompetence. At that point, any government or policy planner would think only of what could be done immediately, and in the short term, to prepare for another wave. The Union government took belated note of the second wave, leading to not only the loss of lives but also a situation where things went out of control. By the time systems were equipped to handle it, the crisis started receding in the second fortnight of May 2021, but this was only because the infection started decreasing, not because any government action contributed to it.

Between 2020 and 2021, there was a stark difference in what happened after the Union government tried to control the crisis unleashed by COVID-19. In 2020, COVID-19 was tackled through a national lockdown and the snapping of all transport links, leaving a huge section of the population in a disarray. This section was the most economically vulnerable. An uncertain employment situation made them walk through the streets of megacities to reach their villages on foot. Many came out to help this distressed lot but for some, it was simply an act of the 'uneducated' that could spell doom in the villages. They feared the contagion from cities would move to the hinterland. The government stepped in by first stopping these people from going back home from the cities, but eventually tried to remedy the situation by facilitating the travel of stranded people to their homes through special buses and trains. But in the interim, people suffered. A *Business Standard* article dated 30 March 2020 quoted Shanti Narain, former member (traffic), Railway Board, criticizing the government for not having any plan when it went into a national lockdown on 25 March 2020. He felt trains should have been allowed for about two to three days after the lockdown. 'Since railway ticketing is computerised, it is possible to know for which places there was a rush for tickets. For instance, if there were 5,000 people who needed to go to Uttar Pradesh from New Delhi, you could have ensured that people reach their destination,' he says.[9]

An RTI application filed with the Indian Railways, seeking reasons for the Shramik Special trains starting on 1 May 2020 and not earlier, was struck down by director TT (punctuality), Railway Board, Sudesh V.C., in his capacity as central public information officer, for being 'interrogatory' in nature. Since the information was denied, it put a question mark on whether the government had any reason at all not to start the trains earlier. Was 1 May just a symbolic date since it was International Workers' Day? When an appeal was filed, contesting the grounds that it was interrogatory, the appellate authority, executive director TT/Coaching, M.S. Bhatia, modified the reply with three attachments – the MHA's order to start of trains, the MoR's guidelines for these trains, and a list of nodal officers.

The desperation to travel, and hence, the crisis, would not have been so severe if special trains were provided for people with an urgent need to travel. This could have been accompanied by repeated advisories asking people to avoid coming out of their homes, especially for travel. The Indian Railways could have easily run special trains instead of imposing a complete shutdown since it handles the rush on particular routes by running special trains, especially during festivals, in normal times. For airlines, however, it would not have been as important to ensure operations, simply because the class of people who travel by air do not live at the edge of starvation, nor do they eke it out by earning a meagre wage for each day's work.

The reverse migration witnessed in 2020 also exposed the inability of governments when it came to maintaining a data bank on this population, and how to reach them for any kind of support. 'No one records that so many people have come from another state. No government agency records their movement, so there is a total mismatch. It is unorganized and that is the reason that this problem emerged. There are all kinds of workers who come [to one state from another], including seasonal workers,' says Seemant Kumar Singh, who was inspector general of police (administration) in Bengaluru during the migrant labourer crisis in 2020. He underscores the need to have a strong database. On whether there should have been such a harsh lockdown, he says:

> Decisions were taken at the government level and if so many people were allowed to rush back, it would have created chaos there [at the destination]. Bihar would have taken some 10 million from outside (the state). These people could have created problems in Bihar. It is not like Delhi and Mumbai, which can take a huge influx of people.

He, however, sees a silver lining in the fact that states were able to create a database after the crisis, since people needed to register before they could travel.

The other important requirement, according to Singh, is that employment opportunities be created in states where cheap labour is available. He says:

> Some people from Ranchi, for instance, work in Kerala and earn Rs 12,000. Why not keep them in Ranchi so that even if they earn Rs 6,000, they will be happy? Why cannot industry

> shift? The database can be of help in such things. We sent three trainloads of fishermen back to Ranchi from Mangalore. It was an eye-opener for me.

The Union government did try to remedy the situation in 2020 by opening up the transport network in a phased manner, but there was no national lockdown in 2021. States were left to decide for themselves how they wanted to deal with the situation. Most of them reacted with their own version of a lockdown, but long-distance travel continued and transport links remained unbroken. Even local transport services, like taxis and buses, were available. The Union government's silence and the abrogation of its responsibility were more pronounced in the initial phase of the second wave. It was also the time when political campaigning for assembly elections to four states and one Union territory was going on. Crowds at political rallies with no social distancing did not bother the Prime Minister and scores of Union ministers, including Home Minister Amit Shah. Modi was, in fact, criticized for boasting about a huge crowd at his election rally in Asansol in West Bengal. 'I have come here twice during Lok Sabha elections. Last time I came to seek votes for *Babulji* [Union Minister Babul Supriyo, who is the Asansol member of Parliament]. The first time I came for myself. But the crowd was only a quarter of this size' said Modi. '[B]ut today, in all directions I see huge crowds of people … have witnessed such a rally for the first time … Today, you have shown your power. The next step is more important—go and vote and take others also,' he added.[10]

While the decision to not impose a national lockdown in 2021 was perhaps dictated by political exigencies and the criticism it had invited in 2020, a more realistic approach would have been to impose restrictions simply on the congregation of people, whether in political rallies or at religious events such as the Mahakumbh. Strict

Central government monitoring of this, along with state government vigilance, could have helped keep the number of COVID-19 cases down. Another important step could have been to move to totally digital governance. In a city such as Delhi, which is the seat of both the Central and state governments, keeping government offices open just to send a signal that the government was working full-time was not exactly helping. The physical presence of government functionaries was adding to the number of COVID-19 cases in the city and, similarly, in other state capitals. This increased the burden on the health infrastructure, especially in apex government facilities. Besides, by the time the second wave arrived, COVID-19 was believed to be airborne, which meant that the disease could spread inside large housing complexes without the physical interaction of residents. In such a situation, locked-down streets and public spaces would not have made much difference.

When there is a medical emergency, the surest way of not losing the plot is not to lose time. If the disease was not coming under control, could treatment come on time? But between February 2020, when India became aware of the danger of COVID-19, and February 2021, the only lesson that the Union government seemed to have learnt was not to impose a lockdown. The very reason dished out to impose the lockdown in March 2020, however, was not visible when it was badly needed during the second wave. It was said India would use the period of lockdown to create more health infrastructure. This meant that while lockdown would keep the disease under control by forcefully imposing social distancing and keeping people inside their homes, the period would be used to create COVID-19 treatment facilities so that whenever the unlocking happened, the country would be better prepared. The MoHFW said in a statement on 21 May 2020:

> The period of the lockdown has been gainfully utilized to ramp up the health infrastructure in the country ... In collective efforts of central as well as state governments, as many as 3,027 dedicated Covid hospitals and Covid health centres along with 7013 Covid care centres have been identified. Additionally, more than 281,000 isolation beds, more than 31,250 ICU beds, and 109,888 oxygen supported beds have already been identified in dedicated Covid hospitals and Covid health centres. Also, [the] Government of India has supplied 6.5 million PPE coveralls and 10.107 million N95 masks to the states. Nearly 300,000 PPE coveralls and 300,000 N95 masks are now being manufactured per day by domestic producers, although they were not produced in the country earlier.[11]

An *India Today* analysis of government data of 2 May 2021, however, revealed that the number of oxygen-supported beds, ICU beds and ventilators saw a drastic decrease between September 2020 (when India saw the peak of the first COVID-19 wave) and end-January 2021 (just before the second wave started, around mid-February).[12] The analysis was done when the second wave was sweeping the country and was based on data collected from Parliament documents and official press releases. According to the analysis, India had 247,972 oxygen-supported beds, 66,638 ICU beds and 33,024 ventilators as of 22 September 2020. The numbers on 28 January 2021, however, fell to 157,344 oxygen beds, a 36.54 per cent fall; 36,008 ICU beds, a 46 per cent fall; and 23,618 ventilators, a 28 per cent fall. The primary reason for this cutting down of resources was that emergency facilities were pulled back after cases started declining. Governments were confident that COVID-19 would not return. The only way to remedy the situation was to again scale up the infrastructure. There were, however, two hindrances to that. The lack of enough oxygen supply was one. Besides, unlike the lockdown phase, when even healthy people were asked to stay at home and those with COVID-19 were taken away to quarantine facilities, people who were unwell came out scampering for medical support, putting others at risk.

Kerala and Mumbai, which had both seen high COVID-19 infections, however, were praised for their tackling of the health emergency. While hearing a petition regarding oxygen shortage in Delhi, the Supreme Court on 5 May 2021 observed:

> It has emerged before the court that efficient administrative modalities were placed into operation by the Municipal Corporation of Greater Mumbai during the second wave of the COVID-19 pandemic. In order to enable the GNCTD [government of national capital territory of Delhi] as well as the central government to have the benefit of these shared experiences, there has been a consensus before us that a team of officers comprised both of GNCTD as well as the Central Government will engage in the next three days with the officials and medical experts of the Municipal Corporation of Greater Mumbai as well as the team of expert private doctors set up by the government of Maharashtra and derive inputs from the modalities which were followed for augmenting the oxygen supply to Mumbai. Based on these experiences, steps can be taken in close collaboration between the Central Government and GNCTD for replicating the administrative arrangements which were arrived at in Mumbai to the extent they may be found to be feasible in their application to NCT of Delhi.[13]

Apart from ramping up the oxygen supply, there was also a conscious policy effort by the local administration in Mumbai. *Business Standard* reported that in 2020, municipal commissioner I.S. Chahal spearheaded the 'chase the virus' programme to track and test COVID-19 suspects. A 'chase the patient' programme for triaging and treatment of COVID-19 positive individuals was also done in 2021. What also helped was the creation of twenty-four-hour war rooms, manned by municipal teachers and doctors, in each of the twenty-four civic wards, to assist in assessing a COVID-19 patient's condition (asymptomatic, mild, severe) and making other arrangements such as allotting hospital beds.

Similar war rooms were created in Kerala so that patients could reach out for help. Such ground-level assistance at the level of the district administration could have helped in other states as well, but whether this outreach could be practically implemented in a short span in largely rural districts is doubtful. Nevertheless, it could have been established in the first year of the outbreak. Establishing such war or crisis management rooms is one part but delivering medical facilities is the crucial part. Through corporate sponsorships and adequate Centre–state planning, this part could have been fixed. Even if facilities created through such tie-ups would have been insufficient because of overwhelming cases, they would have still made a difference when the second wave surfaced.

Governments, whether state or Union, could remedy the hardships caused by the lockdown in 2020. Social welfare schemes and cash transfers did help bring relief to some, though it was not sufficient. The medical emergency of 2021, however, could not be remedied because death does not wait for policymakers and administrators to put in place systems that can halt its stride. If the pandemic was here to stay, only well-timed interventions and investment in health infrastructure could have prevented the colossal loss of lives in the summer of 2021.

15

TRAVEL WITH CAUTION

THE TWITTER HANDLE OF Medical Detection Dogs, a charity organization based out of Milton Keynes, England, introduces Cody, a black Labrador retriever, as one training to specialize in the subject 'open doors.' 'He's doing brilliantly in his training. Will soon be able to help open the door to normality,' says a 21 April 2021 tweet.[1] The dog was learning to detect the odour of COVID-19. The Twitter page, in fact, has many pictures and names of dogs who are training to detect diseases including life-threatening cancer and diabetes.

Asher, Kyp, Lexi, Marlow, Millie and Tala sniffed samples on a stand system that required a 'yes/no' decision by the dogs on each sample. 'When they found the odour of Covid-19, they made clear indications to their handlers such as a sit, nudge or stare. If they didn't detect the odour on what is known as a "blank run," with samples from non-Covid individuals, they walked past without indicating,' said Medical Detection Dogs in May 2021 after the completion of a study. Each time the dogs identified the sample correctly, they received a food reward or a game of ball, depending on their preference.[2]

Over 3,758 people across the UK, including the National Health Service staff, donated odour samples for the study. These were socks, face masks and shirts they had worn. These samples were processed by the research team, which chose 325 positive and 675 negative samples for testing and used them for training and testing the dogs. The training took a number of weeks.

The Helsinki airport in Finland was the first to use dogs to screen passengers for COVID-19. Unbelievable as it may sound, the dogs were deployed because of the deep faith in canine olfactory abilities. It is believed that they could detect the infection in a person even before symptoms appeared and even when laboratory tests failed. An eight-year-old greyhound mix called Kössi was among ten dogs that were deployed at the Helsinki Airport for the purpose. Kössi is no ordinary dog. It learnt the trick to identify the scent in just seven minutes.[3] It was the city of Vantaa, the location of the airport, which deployed the dogs as part of its effort to test new and efficient ways to reduce the spread of the pandemic.

The pilot project to use canine scent detection against COVID-19 at the airport started on 15 September 2020. A statement issued three days later, on 18 September, by Finavia, a Finnish airport company, quoted a research group at the Veterinary Faculty of the University of Helsinki as saying that dogs were able to smell the virus with almost 100 per cent success. 'Dogs are also able to identify COVID-19 from a much smaller sample than the PCR tests used by health care professionals. The difference is massive, as a dog only needs 10–100 molecules to identify the virus, whereas test equipment requires 18 million,' said the statement.[4]

The dogs deployed at the airport are trained by Wise Nose Academy, the research group's start-up company. 'In the future, customs dogs might replace the current operatives,' the airport said.

It assured passengers that taking a COVID-19 dog test would not include direct contact with the dog. Instead, the dog performed its work in a separate booth. Those taking the test would swipe their skin with a test wipe and drop it into a cup, which is then given to the dog. This protected the dog's handler from any exposure to infection. If the test result was positive, the passenger was to be directed to a health information point maintained by the city of Vantaa. Four dogs work at the airport during each shift. In total, nine dogs were used for testing volunteering passengers during the seven-month pilot at the airport.

'The sniffer dogs indicated 48 positive cases during this project. In total, just over 10,000 people were screened by sniffer dogs,' Wise Nose Academy said in emailed responses to questions. The dogs used were Labrador Retrievers, White Shepherds, German Shepherds and a mixed breed called Galgo. The dogs were owned by private persons, who were also the handlers, though they were trained by the Wise Nose Society. Four dogs were validated at the end of the study and overall, the sensitivity and accuracy of their work was around 90 per cent. Depending on the background, the training of an adult dog takes about two to three months.

The trained dogs were also used at construction companies. After the Helsinki airport pilot, the next part included training another two to four dogs to validate the findings of the pilot projects. 'The validation method will be a little different than at the airport, as the dogs that are next tested will work on samples taken at construction sites. But validation is, of course, performed and documented with equal precision and done as a triple-blind study,' says the spokesperson from the society. Soile Turunen, project planner and daily operative manager at the sniffer dog project at the airport, says it was a pilot project to study and develop the utilization of sniffer dogs to screen people with COVID-19.[5] 'The Covid-19 testing with RT-PCR began obligatory at the airport at the beginning of

2021. The regulations have been very tight for travellers, so the number of passengers participating in the scent test (done by a sniffer dog) went down. The scent test was unofficial for voluntary participants,' says Turunen. From the pilot project point of view, there were several observations and lessons learnt on how to operate and arrange this kind of sniffer dog testing. These included how long a dog can work, how many dogs and dog handlers are needed, development of the testing system etc., says Turunen.

Though the dogs were deployed at the Helsinki airport till April 2021, COVID-19 testing with trained dogs was not officially recognized and needed legislative amendment. Customs and police use service dogs for tasks such as sniffing drugs. For service dogs, the legislation would have needed to give permission for disease detection too. 'The legislation did not change because there was no scientific proof that dogs could detect COVID-19. Instead, the private sector is allowed to train COVID-19 detection dogs and their service is unofficial. Companies that use sniffer dogs in COVID-19 testing are still using RT-PCR tests if a dog indicates positive persons,' says Turunen.

Whether other countries would be using this low-cost, quick method of spot testing to screen passengers would depend on how reliable the dogs' training is and whether health experts consider the findings scientific enough. Wise Nose Society collaborates internationally with corona dog units and researchers in different countries.

Medical Detection Dogs, which has been working on disease testing by dogs for over twelve years, says its peer-reviewed research supports the theory that diseases have their own unique odours and that its experience says dogs can detect COVID-19. The organization says on its website:

> A dog's incredible sense of smell is thanks to the complex structure of its nose, which contains over 300 million scent receptors, compared to 5 million in a human. This means they have an incredible ability to detect odours, and are the best biosensors known to man which combined with their ability to learn makes them perfect for detection dog. They are already commonly used to detect odours associated with drugs, explosives, and food, which most of us will have encountered at airports, and our research has shown they can detect the odour of disease with high levels of accuracy.[6]

Their project is backed by the UK government and by public donations, and collaborators include the London School of Hygiene and Tropical Medicine and Durham University.

A California-based non-profit open-access publisher in science and medicine, *PLOS*, published a research paper in December 2020 that described a study on detection dogs: a total of 232 trials using thirty-three positive samples in France (Alfort and Ajaccio), and 136 trials for sixty-eight positive samples in Lebanon (Beirut).[7] The study says its objective was 'a proof-of-concept' one that did not aim to provide evidence that a whole population of trained dogs were able to detect COVID-19 positive samples, but 'rather to provide evidence that a well-trained dog' is able to detect COVID-19 positive samples. 'Such evidence is provided if one observes from one dog a higher proportion of successes than the one expected by chance alone. Therefore, the target population is not a population of dogs, but the whole population of trials (consisting of infinitive number of trials) for one dog, each dog being considered as a "diagnostic tool".' The study, however, did have its own challenges, since three search and rescue dogs had to be withdrawn for not being able to adapt to an 'olfactive' search on a line of samples and eight of the same category could not be included in the results since they were sent for retraining. Eighteen dogs were initially selected, but the final results were based on eight dogs who followed the whole process. 'The results of this first proof of concept study demonstrate that Covid-19 positive people produce an axillary (excessive) sweat that has a different odour, for the detection dog, than Covid-19 negative persons,' the study said.[8]

During the study, two negative samples were identified as positive by two dogs. This information was shared with the hospital from where the sample came through the anonymous sample codes, and tests were redone on the patients giving positive results. The study says the dogs sniff for specific molecules produced by the SARS-CoV-2 virus presence. It was ensured that there was no disturbance around the dogs during their work. The study defined success as a situation in which a dog identified the one box containing the COVID-19+ sweat sample, while a failure was when the dog alerted its handler to any of the other boxes. If the dog marked a negative sample first, the trial was considered as failed, even if the dog marked the sample as positive afterwards. A total of 198 armpit sweat samples were obtained from different hospitals. Eight dogs of the initial group that were included in the study were explosives detection dogs and colon cancer detection dogs. They performed a total of 368 trials. The percentages of the dogs' success in finding the positive sample in a line containing several other negative samples or mocks (two to six) were 100 per 100 for four dogs, and eighty-three, eighty-four, ninety and ninety-four per 100 for the others. 'All significantly different from the percentage of success that would be obtained by chance alone. We conclude that there is a very high evidence that the armpits sweat odour of COVID-19+ persons is different, and that dogs can detect a person infected by the SARS-CoV-2 [COVID] virus,' says the study.

Another technique for quick COVID-19 detection was developed by Breathonix, a spin-off company of the National

University of Singapore (NUS). This technique uses a breathalyser. Volatile organic compounds (VOC) in a person's exhaled breath, which are produced by biochemical reactions in human cells, are detected. 'VOC signatures in the breath of healthy people vary from that of people with illnesses, meaning that changes in VOCs can be measured as markers for diseases like Covid-19,' NUS and Breathonix said in a joint statement on 24 May.[9] The trials were conducted at the National Centre for Infectious Diseases (NCID) and at Changi Airport in Singapore, as well as in Dubai in collaboration with the Dubai Health Authority and the Mohammed Bin Rashid University of Medicine and Health Sciences. After Singapore's Health Sciences gave provisional authorization, the joint statement said Breathonix would work with the Singapore Ministry of Health to run a 'deployment trial of their technology' at one of the land checkpoints, where incoming travellers would undergo screening with the 'BreFence Go Covid-19 breath test' system.

From using dogs as a detection tool, which many countries and even travellers might not find reliable enough for adoption, to the use of laboratory tests at airports and other travel points, managers of transport services might use myriad screening methods to separate suspected infected persons from others before a journey begins or even after it ends.

The dependence on laboratory tests has been crucial for preventing the contagion due to travel. The insistence on getting a negative report seventy-eight hours before travel by various states in India, particularly for those flying in from high infection states, however, added to the stress on the testing system during the second wave of COVID-19. Both Maharashtra and Delhi, for instance, wanted people flying in from either of the states to get tested before they flew, and if that was not possible, to be tested at the destination airport once they landed. But getting tests done became a challenge in April 2021, since governments informally asked laboratories to cap the number of tests in order to grossly under-report the number of COVID-19 cases. At the same time, patients would not even get beds in hospitals without a positive report of infection. The MoHFW had to come out with a directive on 8 May saying '[The] requirement of a positive test for COVID-19 virus is not mandatory for admission to a Covid health facility.'[10] Hospitals, however, were running full, so admission was a challenge in itself. Doctors kept advising patients to start medicines for the disease right at the onset of symptoms. But with home collection of samples discontinued or delayed, a healthy person visiting a testing centre just because they wanted to travel meant increasing their chances of contracting the infection. At the same time, their report may turn out to be negative, infection picked up at the testing centre would not show in that report and surface only later, leading to infection being passed on during the journey. The shambolic nature of the whole process put a question mark on the testing infrastructure during the second wave, a marked change from the first one, when states were able to bring the pandemic under control through testing and tracing.

Even if the process of getting a test done had eased in India and governments did not reduce the number of tests to show lower infections, two challenges to using laboratory test results as a pass to travel would still remain, especially because of the sheer volume of the travelling population. These are false negatives and fake reports. According to a 1 May 2021 column in *The Indian Express,* up to 20 per cent of symptomatic COVID-19 patients were testing negative.[11] This apparent trend of false negative results might have led to hospital admission and critical care refusing to admit serious patients, while asymptomatic ones could move around and spread the virus, said the column. 'The trend has prompted experts, including AIIMS director Dr Randeep Guleria, to recommend Covid-19 treatment for everyone showing classic symptoms irrespective of RT-PCR results,' it said. The Indian Council of Medical Research (ICMR), which lays down medical protocol, says the reliability of an RT-PCR test is 95 per cent, leaving a scope of just 5 per cent for false negatives. Listing the various reasons for false negatives, the column said that one could be the quality of testing laboratories. The number of COVID test labs in India increased from fourteen in February 2020 to more than 2,400 in April 2021.

> Such a rapid expansion required approving hundreds of labs for RT-PCR testing and training thousands of technicians in a hurry. As a safeguard, ICMR in July 2020 listed 30 Quality Control labs to check on all the Covid labs it approved. Another 8 QC labs have been added since. However, sources in multiple labs across three states said 'only a few inspections of facilities and instruments' took place.

Other reasons cited by the column were the low viral load and a rapid fall in the prices of testing kits, which leads to a compromised testing system. If the RT-PCR test, considered the most reliable for diagnosis of COVID-19, was producing false negatives to the extent of 20 per cent, as claimed by media reports, then the big question for transport and public health managers was whether these test results could be used for allowing travel. It can, however, still be argued that there is no foolproof mechanism for testing other than the RT-PCR test, especially for asymptomatic carriers of the virus.

Nonetheless, while a false negative may not be intentional, a racket around testing evolved, offering negative reports to whoever wanted to travel. A *Business Standard* report of 27 April 2021 said the MoCA wrote to the MoHFW saying that only those RT-PCR certificates that had a QR code linking them to their original test report would be allowed as authentic for the purpose of travel by airlines and airports. 'Till now, airlines have been allowing test reports from the 634 labs approved by ICMR but the majority of them do not provide certificates embedded with a QR code. This makes it difficult for airlines to verify their authenticity,' says the report.[12] The airlines wanted to play safe, since the Delhi government had threatened to file criminal cases against IndiGo, Vistara, SpiceJet and AirAsia India for allegedly not checking the RT-PCR negative reports of passengers flying from Maharashtra into Delhi.[13]

The situation for overseas travel got even more complicated. Some forty-nine passengers on a Vistara flight from New Delhi to Hong Kong tested positive for COVID-19 just when Hong Kong decided to ban all flights from India because of the second wave. The passengers who tested positive flew into Hong Kong on 4 April. This number was higher than those being detected by Hong Kong domestically. A two-week ban on all flights from India, Pakistan and the Philippines was imposed on 19 April 2021 after it categorized them as 'extremely high risk.'

Indian states, on their part, were making testing and quarantine mandatory for travellers from areas with high caseloads, but these requirements were limited to airline passengers. States such as Maharashtra, Uttarakhand and Odisha, however, wrote to the Union government, asking for COVID-19 testing for inbound rail commuters when the second wave hit the country. These states wanted RT-PCR reports of passengers before the start of the journey. The Indian Railways, however, felt that it could not handle this load and decided to offer its help if the states would test passengers on arrival. Maharashtra issued orders in early May 2021 that passengers on trains from West Bengal and Uttarakhand, apart from those from Delhi, Gujarat, Rajasthan, Goa and Kerala (which were already on the list), would also be screened. This was despite an ICMR advisory on 4 May 2021 against requiring test reports of individuals travelling within the country. 'The need for RTPCR test in healthy individuals undertaking interstate domestic travel may be completely removed to reduce the load on laboratories. Non-essential travel and interstate travel of symptomatic individuals (COVID-19 or flu like symptoms) should be essentially avoided to reduce the risk of infection,' it said in recommended measures for optimizing RT-PCR testing during the second wave of COVID-19 in India.[14] Amid criticism of lower testing across all states, ICMR stated that the total number of molecular testing laboratories, including RT-PCR, TrueNat, CBNAAT and other platforms, was 2,506, and the total daily national testing capacity was close to 1.5 million tests, considering a three-shift operationalization of the existing laboratory network. 'At present, the laboratories are facing challenges to meet the expected testing target due to extraordinary case load and staff getting infected with Covid-19. In view of this situation, it is imperative to optimize the RT-PCR testing and simultaneously increase the access and availability of testing to all citizens of the country,' it said.

About five months before that, WHO, in its 16 December 2020 interim guidance, had categorically stated that 'international travellers should not be categorized as suspected COVID-19 cases.' It did not recommend healthy travellers as a priority group for COVID-19 testing, particularly when resources were limited, to avoid diverting resources from settings and patients where testing could have a higher public-health impact and drive action. 'In principle, high-risk settings and high-risk groups should be prioritized for testing, including people at risk of developing severe disease and vulnerable populations and health workers, in line with WHO's guidance,' it said.[15]

Despite this realistic observation, the world was dealing with the necessity to open up travel, both within and between countries, and the strategy for at least foreign travel hinged on testing and temporary bans on travel from certain countries whenever cases increased there. No one wanted to import infection and newer strains of the virus. India's strategy was the same, though it did not have a set criterion for taking decisions on banning travel from certain countries. In contrast, the US CDC evolved a mechanism in conjunction with the US Department of State Travel Advisory for grading risk from travel to other countries. Travel Health Notices (THNs) alerted travellers to health threats. Countries were categorized accordingly. At Level 4 were the countries with very high case numbers, where travellers were told to avoid all travel. At Level 3 were destinations with high numbers of COVID-19, where travellers were asked to avoid all non-essential travel. Level 2 were places with moderate levels of COVID-19, where travellers who were at increased risk of severe illness were asked to avoid all non-essential travel. And at Level 1 were countries with low numbers of COVID-19 infections, where travellers could go but with a mask, maintaining six feet distance from people who were not from the same travel group, avoiding crowds, washing hands, using sanitizers and watching their health for signs of illness. The CDC used COVID-19 data reported by WHO and other official sources to determine THN levels. 'If a destination does not provide data, their THN level is designated as "unknown" and travellers are advised to follow THN Level 4 recommendations,' said the CDC.[16]

For a Level 4 classification, the primary criterion for destinations with a population of over 200,000 was more than 100 incidence rate or cumulative new cases over the previous twenty-eight days per 100,000 population. For Level 3, it was an incidence rate of 51–100, 5–50 for Level 2 and less than 5 for Level 1. The primary criterion for destinations with a population of 200,000 or less was an incidence rate that was the same at Levels 4 and 3, but was 10–50 for Level 2 and less than 10 for Level 1. This implied that for more populated countries, the criterion was stricter. The CDC did not count identified imported cases (travellers who were exposed in another country) against a destination's total. The secondary criterion for determining THN levels was an assessment of testing capacity using two secondary metrics: population testing rate and test-to-case ratio. The population testing rate was the number of tests conducted per 100,000 people over twenty-eight days. The test-to-case ratio was the number of tests conducted for each case reported during the same twenty-eight-day period.

The WHO, however, presented a different risk-based approach to international travel in its 16 December 2020 interim guidance. It acknowledged that 'comprehensive public health measures adapted to the local epidemiologic context and capacities can mitigate the risk substantially but cannot achieve zero risk.'[17] Though this guidance was valid for only two years or till further modifications, it gave a broad overview on the dependence on testing before travel, quarantine and immunity after infection for determining whether a person be considered for international travel. Vaccination had already started in the UK on 8 December 2020 and in the US on 14 December 2020 but this guidance did not take these developments into account. It provided a step-by-step approach to decision-making for calibrating risk mitigation measures and establishing policies for international travel. There were three main sections: risk assessment, risk mitigation and risk communication, applicable to international travel via air, sea or land between countries, territories or sub-national areas. It also came out with an algorithm-based tool that countries could use to assess risk.

The WHO specified overarching questions to guide national and sub-national decision-making processes for implementing travel-related risk mitigation measures. For inbound travel, the questions were: will the number of cases to be imported from the country of departure likely have a significant impact on the current transmission level in the country of destination? What is the probability of individuals from the country of departure being infected? What is the travel volume across all routes (air, land and sea)? Are the current response capacities in the country of destination sufficient to cope with the potential rise of imported cases from the country of departure, including risk communication capacities to inform incoming travellers, in appropriate languages, about mechanisms for seeking care and public health and social-distancing measures in place? Can the current public health and social measures implemented in the country of destination support the introduction of international travellers? For advising individuals on outbound travel, the questions were: how likely are travellers to be infected in the country of destination compared to their likelihood of getting infected in the country of departure? Does the country of destination have sufficient response capacity to treat travellers who may need medical care while travelling? Does the country of departure have sufficient capacity to enforce mandatory public health and social measures on the return of travellers, if necessary?

During these global discussions on the ways of having people travel and yet prevent exposing the destination to fresh infections, the concept of 'immunity certificates' also came up, especially in the context of international travel. WHO, however, was against such certification, stating that it was:

> not currently supported by scientific evidence and is, therefore, not recommended by WHO … Beyond the scientific uncertainties around immunity passports, there are ethical, legal and human rights aspects related to privacy of personal data and medical confidentiality; the potential for falsification or engagement in risky behaviour based on a false sense of security; stigma; and discrimination.[18]

India, despite its failures of screening and testing, started linking passports with vaccination status from June 2021.[19] In fact, the government allowed priority vaccination of students and for those travelling abroad for work from 1 June. The National Health Mission revised the list of preferential groups for vaccination by adding four more groups: students going to foreign countries to pursue studies, those who wanted to travel outside the country for employment, workers of milk co-operative societies, and cable operators.

These moves were necessary, since countries were insisting on full vaccination for allowing entry to people from other countries. A vaccine passport or a certificate that allows those who are fully vaccinated to travel without giving proof of a test will increasingly gain credence. In India, for instance, the cities of Thane and Mumbai made vaccination compulsory for boarding city buses from November 2021. A strict adherence to the vaccination to allow travel within the country, however, is not the right thing to do since it is against the basic right to free movement. Assuming sporadic cases of infection remain in the country with no widespread 'wave', such a condition could build barriers within the country. Besides, vaccine penetration in a big country such as India would be low. Moreover, if vaccination were to be required annually for some time, then it would be near impossible to have a vast moving population, or migrant workers, adjust to such a rule.

In the US, however, vaccination has given people a free pass to travel without the need for a lab test or quarantine. In a Twitter post on 2 April 2021, the CDC said that those who were fully vaccinated could travel domestically without a pre- or post-travel test and without quarantining after travel. Such people could also travel internationally without a pre-travel test depending on the rules of the destination country.[20] Quarantining requirements of such international travellers were also waived. The CDC considered people fully vaccinated two weeks after their second dose in a two-dose series, such as those of Pfizer or Moderna vaccines, or two weeks after a single-dose vaccine, such as that of Johnson & Johnson's Janssen vaccine.

Thailand, which earned 10.4 per cent of its GDP, or $9,170 billion, from tourism pre-pandemic in 2019, set multi-layered requirements for tourists from 1 April 2021, which largely banked on a combination of vaccination and quarantine. According to data put out by World Travel & Tourism, Thailand saw tourism's contribution to its GDP fall to 5.5 per cent. At $4,671 billion in 2020, it was almost half of the share in 2019 when it contributed 10.4 per cent to GDP.[21] It, therefore, implemented a relaxation of COVID-19 measures from 1 April for entry into the kingdom. All travellers, Thais and non-Thais, did not require fit-to-fly certificates. Travellers from countries without COVID-19 variants, with the certificate of COVID-19 vaccine approved by the Food and Drug Administration (FDA) of Thailand, or approved by WHO, or authorized by the country's public health ministry, were to quarantine upon arrival in Thailand for at least seven days. There were seven such vaccines that were notified. Travellers from countries without COVID-19 variants, and without the vaccine certificate, had to quarantine for three more days. Travellers from countries with COVID-19 variants were asked to quarantine for at least fourteen days. The list of countries with COVID-19 variants included eleven African countries, but not India, though according to America's CDC, the first variant of the coronavirus was seen in India in October 2020, followed by two in December 2020 and one in February 2021.[22]

By 27 May, Thailand decided to open up tourism for all without any quarantine requirement in Phuket. In an announcement titled 'Phuket Sandbox starts on July 1, 2021,' the government announced this. Upon arrival, however, visitors were required to test negative.[23]

Countries such as the UK and the US, initially did not accept vaccines being administered in India for travel to their country without COVID-19 related quarantine requirements. It was only after eleven months of Covaxin, India's indigenously developed vaccine, being administered in the country that WHO approval came on 3 November 2021.[24] Union External Affairs Minister S. Jaishankar on 6 December said that India had worked out arrangements with over 100 countries to mutually recognize vaccine certifications in order to speed up international travel and restore livelihoods.[25]

Though WHO has been behind the curve in terms of adequate warnings and policy statements all through the pandemic, it made its views on a vaccine passport clear almost a month after the world's first vaccine against COVID-19 infection was given to a ninety-year-old woman in Coventry, UK. In its 5 February 2021 interim position paper on considerations regarding proof of COVID-19 vaccination for international travellers, WHO said:

> At the present time, it is WHO's position that national authorities and conveyance operators should not introduce requirements of proof of Covid-19 vaccination for international travel as a condition for departure or entry, given that there are still critical unknowns regarding the efficacy of vaccination in reducing transmission. In addition, considering that there is limited availability of vaccines, preferential vaccination of travellers could result in inadequate supplies of vaccines for priority populations considered at high risk of severe Covid-19 disease. WHO also recommends that people who are vaccinated

should not be exempt from complying with other travel risk-reduction measures.[26]

The February paper also noted the limited access to COVID-19 vaccines worldwide, particularly in low-income and lower-middle-income countries. It said 94 per cent of countries that had started vaccinating their population at that time were in the high- or high-middle-income category. WHO expressed concern that 'the inequitable distribution of Covid-19 vaccines could deepen already existing inequalities and introduce new ones.' Also, introducing the requirement of vaccination as a condition to travel could potentially hinder equitable global access to a limited vaccine supply and would be unlikely to maximize the benefits of vaccination for individual societies and overall global health, it said. 'While individual, economic and social benefits could potentially be promoted through such a policy, these benefits also have to be balanced against the risk to public health based on current scientific knowledge, including critical unknowns about the risks mitigated by vaccination.'

Another ethical consideration was equity in the general distribution of benefits and burdens. In the context of unequal vaccine distribution, individuals who did not have access to an authorized COVID-19 vaccine would be unfairly impeded in their freedom of movement if proof of vaccination status became a condition for entry to or exit from a country, said WHO in its paper. National authorities should choose public health interventions that least infringed on individual freedom of movement.

WHO's views on immunity certificates and vaccination passport notwithstanding, the European Union went ahead and forwarded a proposal to the European Parliament on 17 March 2021 for a Digital Green Certificate covering vaccination, testing and recovery.[27] The commission adopted the proposal to establish a common framework for an EU-level approach to issuing, verifying and accepting such certificates. The aim was 'to help holders to exercise their right to free movement within the European Union, as well as making it easier to wind down Covid-19 restrictions put in place in compliance with EU law.' A certificate would allow all European Union citizens and their family members to receive secure and interoperable validation, which could be used as proof, wherever relevant, to waive free movement restrictions—such as quarantine or testing requirements. 'It is important to stress that people without such a certificate must still be able to travel and that being in possession of a certificate is not a prerequisite of exercising the right to free movement or other fundamental rights. It is important to have trust in the certificates to allow for their acceptance,' said a European Commission communication.

Nevertheless, if and when countries adopted the vaccine passport concept, they would need to ensure that there was no fraud in the issuance of this pass to travel. To a large extent, this could be done by barcoding the physical vaccine certificate. Alongside that, a software application could show an individual's vaccine status and the history of their vaccination. India's vaccination drive is riding on CoWIN, a two-way technology platform that gives vaccination appointments to individuals and also aggregates data from vaccination centres. This is linked to Aarogya Setu, the contact-tracing application of the Union government, where a person's vaccine status would be shown through a single blue tick in case of one dose and double ticks in case of both doses. Individuals could also link their vaccine status to their passports through CoWIN.

Besides privacy concerns surrounding CoWIN, the vaccination drive itself had a slow start because of initial hesitation among the elderly population aged sixty and over. Later, non-availability of the vaccine, caused by a lack of planning and reluctance on the part of producers to ramp up production and instead bargain for a higher price, stalled speedy vaccination coverage. If not for this slow start, perhaps many serious cases and deaths could have been avoided, since a vaccinated person is said to be more resistant to a serious bout of the disease.

In the middle of the second wave on 20 April 2021, for instance, approximately 1.1 billion Indians had received the first dose of one of two coronavirus vaccines approved for use in the country. This translates to a mere 8.09 per cent of the country's 13.6 billion population. By that date, only 17.5 million people had received their second dose of vaccine, which was just 1.29 per cent of the total population. At this rate, according to a calculation by *Business Today*, at least one year and four months would be required to administer the first shot of the vaccine to 70 per cent of the population, and eight years and nine months for the second dose. To administer the first shot to the entire population would take one year and eleven months. Administering both doses to the entire population would require twelve years and six months.[28]

Among all the precautions that could be adopted for safe travel, particularly among nations, it is this concept of a vaccine passport that is likely to stay forever, with safety protocols, such as masking and sanitization, continuing in the short term. Allowing only vaccinated people to move from one country to another might be a restrictive measure in itself and its certification could risk privacy, but it would be similar to getting a yellow fever vaccine before travel to certain identified countries, such as Angola, Benin, Burkina Faso, Burundi, Cameroon and Chad. It is implementable, even if it takes a longer time, because there is no other way except through vaccination that the coronavirus can be fought. With or without a passport, only vaccines can keep the pace of travel going as and when countries open up their borders completely.

ACKNOWLEDGEMENTS

IT WAS PERHAPS JUST a question of a third desk at home. As a full-time writer for newspapers, I always wrote in the office. At home, it was the good old dining table or the sofa for pending office work to be done on the weekend. The world of office-goers, however, changed with lockdowns. There was the risk of a wrong posture but more than that, a pending book idea that needed its space. 'Get me a desk and I will give you a book,' I told my husband, Akshaya, sometime in October 2020. I had a thinking corner to myself soon. So Akshaya and our daughter, Jahnavi, studied, researched and wrote in their corners while I did in mine.

Akshaya, as a co-traveller in this journey of print journalism and writing, always encouraged me to continue, not to give up, despite the innumerable times I had this desire to move to the hills and even earlier, when the stress of being a young mother would take away my better judgement. He has been the bulwark against such thoughts, encouraging me to continue to do what I love most: just write.

The fourth member of our family never needed a desk of her own but if pets could be writers, my Bella would have been a co-author, just sitting next to my table in her own corner, getting up when I did, and of course, pulling my hands off the laptop and crying, like a human baby, when it was time to stretch muscles and just walk or get a quick snack.

Lockdowns also threw up the challenge of doing all the housework yourself, somehow an anathema for most Indians due to the sheer enormity of the task with dusty houses, big families, three elaborate meals and a preference for fresh food over frozen. We managed somehow, but my excellent house help Anjana Biswas's return to the household in early June 2020, and her taking over the kitchen and cleaning, gave us some more time to go to our desks.

My sister, Neeti Sharma, an excellent cook and manager of everything that seems impossible to handle, ensured that I finished my book by sending meals during the second COVID-19 wave. In April 2021, Anjana was on a trip to her village in West Bengal after a gap of three years. She wanted to cast her vote in the assembly elections. 'Don't come back yet. Neither is it safe to undertake the journey, nor will staying in Gurugram guarantee you medical help in case you get COVID-19. Let the deadly wave ease' was my advice to her. A one-month leave turned into a two-month forced stay at the village for her.

Neeti's affection has always kept me going, ever since we lost our mother, Krishna Sharma, aeons ago. Amma, I wish I could present my book or even my first newspaper byline of 1994 to you, since you chided me a couple of times for reading newspapers too keenly while school books waited.

Sanjay Kala, my late uncle who passed away in September 2020 during the peak of the first COVID-19 wave, always appreciated my writings and encouraged me in my journalistic pursuits. His wife, Vinita Kala, told me, 'Mama [maternal uncle] had a special place in his heart for you and would have been so proud' each time we discussed the upcoming book. This helped me to keep going despite the morbidity of the second wave.

My father, Prakash, from whom I inherited the fear-no-one-and-nothing spirit, has always been a pillar in our lives. Like a typical parent of the earlier times, he is never exuberant about his children's achievements, but will always softly say, 'Always do well.' He never asked me why I came late during my early news desk days in The Asian Age and The Financial Express in the early nineties, even when we were under the stress of bringing up a young Jahnavi. 'Put the child in a hostel,' he would say, much to our discomfort, when he found us often struggling to look for a caretaker. He spent days and nights teaching my daughter how to eat by herself and looked after her when she fell ill, since young children often fall ill.

The little Jahnavi is an adult now and is the first reader of some of the extracts of my new work. Her valuable inputs helped me gauge whether the book would appeal to students with an interest in history and public policy. An old friend, Amiti Sen, also read some extracts despite being weak and recovering from COVID-19. It is said that a photograph is worth a thousand words. Aadit Kumar Sharma, Anurav Singh, Anuj Dayal, Nayanima Basu, Shome Basu, Subhendu Ray and Gurinder Osan made inclusion of the crucial visual stories possible.

My colleague in Business Standard, Shine Jacob, wanted me to take my writings beyond pure play journalism. He added the subtle nudge that was needed beyond what Akshaya always told me.

A book manuscript could just end up being a mere personal journal on the desk if it fails to find a publisher but Krishan Chopra graciously went through my proposal, agreed to publish it and encouraged me to work on it by simply saying, 'It will be a good book.' My editor Shreya Lall took on the baton from him and was prompt in responding to my queries and coordinated the publishing of this work.

Arindam Majumdar, Aneesh Phadnis, Sachin P. Mampatta, Kalpana Pathak and Somit Sen responded to my messages promptly when I felt I could not find some information and sought their help. Aditi Divekar and Shreya Jai's exuberant 'wow' on knowing I was doing a book added the positivity that was missing on a grave subject like the pandemic.

I am particularly grateful to Anisha Datta of Hindustan Times, with whom I have hardly spoken beyond the occasional WhatsApp text messages, for doing wonderful reporting on the Indian Railways despite the government pressures of not doing 'negative reporting'.

Young overseas travellers Aishwarya Airy and Mihir Tak, Finavia Corporation, Nose Academy and Princess Cruises graciously replied to all my email queries, while senior police officials Seemant Singh and Usha Kundu agreed to give first-hand accounts of the challenges faced on the ground by government officers. This was essential for the narrative because it was equally important to know the other side of the story of the migrant crisis.

The experience of airline staff and how the pandemic made their jobs risky but crucial could not have been narrated without Megha. Government officials Ashish Kundra, Sanjay Chadha and Manu Srivastava were a big help in providing some important data on migrants who were wanting to leave Delhi, and also explaining complicated government terminology, like which level of officers could be made 'incident commanders', or what was a BOXN wagon. Retired railway officials Shakeel Ahmed and Shanti Narain gave their insights into railway functioning.

An old friend and an official in the West Bengal government, Sonam Wangdi, Press Trust of India photographer Atul Yadav, Gaon Connection's Mithilesh Dhar, Megha Manchanda and Shruti Srivastava helped me find the contact details of some of those caught in the middle of nowhere due to the lockdown. Without them, the narration of human sufferings would not have been possible. Anto T. Joseph, a former colleague, was particularly helpful in explaining how the triple lockdown during the second wave in Kerala was stricter than the 2020 one.

I am also grateful to the Delhi International Airport Ltd management for agreeing to brief me despite the lack of time and stressful business circumstances they were facing. Subhendu Ray was particularly helpful in facilitating the briefing.

COVID-19, lockdowns and the anxiety that came with job losses, salary cuts and the change in work culture have altered the lives of professionals and even of households. There is a struggle for an office space within a personal space, especially for those with young children. I was never personally in favour of working from home, especially for women who have a higher pressure of managing a household and thus get caught both in office as well as domestic work when at home. The book, nonetheless, would not have been possible without work from home.

NOTES

INTRODUCTION

1. Reverse migration is a term used for labourers going back from their place of work to place of their origin.
2. 'Bengal man's family says he died of police beating, police say he had heart ailment,' Kolkata: *India Today*, 26 March 2020.
3. ANI, 'Two Cops Suspended for Killing Vegetable Vendor in UP's Unnao,' Lucknow: *Hindustan Times*, 22 May 2021.
4. Case No. 2020AP765-OA, Wisconsin Legislature, versus Secretary-Designee Andrea Palm, Julie Willems Van Dijk and Lisa Olson, Executives of Wisconsin Department of Health Services. Original action opinion filed: 13 May 2020, Submitted on briefs: oral argument: 5 May 2020. https://www.wicourts.gov/sc/opinion/DisplayDocument.pdf?content=pdf&seqNo=260868
5. Case No. 20-C-760, Amended Decision and Order Granting Defendants' Motion to Dismiss, United States District Court Eastern District of Wisconsin, 18 July 2020. https://www.wpr.org/sites/default/files/easterndistlocalcoviddismiss.pdf

6. 'Federal Judge Dismisses Lawsuit Challenging Local Stay-At-Home Orders In Wisconsin,' Wisconsin Public Radio, 21 July 2020.
7. Amitabh Sinha, 'In Second Wave, Covid Hits Rural India: Cases and Deaths Quadruple,' Pune: The Indian Express, 8 May 2021.
8. *Collected Works of Mahatma Gandhi*, Volume 16: 1 September 1917–23 April 1918.
9. *India in the Years 1917–1918*, p. 182.
10. John M. Barry, *The Great Influenza*, Penguin Random House, New York, p. 364.
11. *India in 1919*, p. 72, Railway Diagram II, 'The numbers of passengers carried and the earnings therefrom on all Indian Railways.'
12. Narendra Modi (@narendramodi), 'Tomorrow, will be chairing high-level meetings to review the prevailing COVID-19 situation. Due to that, I would not be going to West Bengal.' Twitter, 22 April 2021, https://twitter.com/narendramodi/status/1385200406775672835?s=20
13. 'Coronavirus Disease (COVID-19): How Is It Transmitted?', World Health Organization, 30 April 2021 update. https://www.who.int/news-room/questions-and-answers/item/coronavirus-disease-covid-19-how-is-it-transmitted (accessed on 30 April 2021).
14. 'Modes of Transmission of Virus Causing COVID-19: Implications for IPC Precaution Recommendations,' World Health Organization scientific brief, 29 March 2020. https://www.who.int/news-room/commentaries/detail/modes-of-transmission-of-virus-causing-covid-19-implications-for-ipc-precaution-recommendations (accessed on 10 June 2021).

1: FROM CLOSING TO BEING SHUTTERED OUT

1. WHO, 'WHO Advice for International Travel and Trade in Relation to the Outbreak of Pneumonia Caused by a New Coronavirus in China', 10 January 2020. https://www.who.int/news-room/articles-detail/who-advice-for-international-travel-and-trade-in-relation-to-the-outbreak-of-pneumonia-caused-by-a-new-coronavirus-in-china (Accessed on 19 September 2020).

2. WHO MERS advice. https://www.who.int/news-room/articles-detail/who-advice-for-international-travel-and-trade-in-relation-to-the-outbreak-of-pneumonia-caused-by-a-new-coronavirus-in-china (Accessed on 16 December 2020).
3. WHO, International Health Regulation, 1 January 2016. https://www.who.int/publications/i/item/9789241580496 (Accessed on 16 December 2020).
4. Press Information Bureau, 17 January 2020, Release ID: 1599665, 'Health Ministry Reviews Preparedness for Novel Corona Virus (nCoV).' https://pib.gov.in/PressReleasePage.aspx?PRID=1599665 (Accessed on 16 December 2020).
5. Press Information Bureau, 17 January 2020, Release ID: 1599666, 'Novel Coronavirus Outbreak in China: Travel Advisory to Travelers Visiting China.' https://pib.gov.in/PressReleasePage.aspx?PRID=1599666
6. Press Information Bureau, 30 January 2020, Release ID: 1601095, 'Update on Novel Coronavirus: One Positive Case Reported in Kerala.'
https://pib.gov.in/PressReleasePage.aspx?PRID=1601095
7. Press Information Bureau, 21 January 2020, Release ID: 1600015, 'Thermal Screening of Passengers Arriving from China Including Hong Kong Expanded to Seven Airports Now.'
https://pib.gov.in/PressReleasePage.aspx?PRID=1600015
8. ndtv.com, Press Trust of India, 4 March 2020, 'Passengers of All International Flights To Be Screened For Virus: Centre.'
https://www.ndtv.com/india-news/union-health-minister-harsh-vardhan-all-international-flights-to-be-screened-for-coronavirus-2189659 (accessed on 4 June 2021).
9. WHO, 24 January 2020, 'Updated WHO Advice for International Traffic in Relation to the Outbreak of the Novel Coronavirus 2019-nCoV.'
https://www.who.int/news-room/articles-detail/updated-who-advice-for-international-traffic-in-relation-to-the-outbreak-of-the-novel-coronavirus-2019-ncov-24-jan/ (Accessed on 16 December 2020).

10. WHO, 14 April 2020, 'COVID19 Strategy Update.' https://www.who.int/publications/i/item/covid-19-strategy-update---14-april-2020, WHO The Strategy Preparedness and Response Plan (SPRP) Update (14 April 2020).
11. WHO, 21 May 2021, 'Evidence Review – Public Health Measures in the Aviation Sector in the Context of COVID-19: Quarantine and Isolation.' https://www.who.int/publications/i/item/evidence-review-public-health-measures-in-the-aviation-sector-in-the-context-of-covid-19-quarantine-and-isolation---21-may-2021 (Accessed on 4 June 2021).
12. WHO, 20 January 2020, 'Novel Coronavirus (2019-nCoV) Situation Report – 1, 21 January 2020. https://www.who.int/docs/default-source/coronaviruse/situation-reports/20200121-sitrep-1-2019-ncov.pdf?sfvrsn=20a99c10_4 (Accessed on 16 December 2020).
13. Footnote 9.
14. Ministry of Health and Family Welfare, 5 February 2020, Travel Advisory. https://www.mohfw.gov.in/pdf/Traveladvisory05022020.pdf (Accessed on 16 December 2020).
15. PricewaterhouseCoopers, Corporate Travel: Collaboration Is Essential for Successful COVID Recovery. https://www.pwc.com/us/en/industries/consumer-markets/library/corporate-travel-collaboration-essential-for-covid-19-recovery.html (Accessed on 4 June 2021).
16. Debasis Mohapatra and Neha Alawadhi, 'Coronavirus Outbreak: IT Services Companies Widen Travel Restrictions,' *Business Standard*, 2 March 2020. https://www.business-standard.com/article/economy-policy/coronavirus-outbreak-it-services-companies-widen-travel-restrictions-120030200051_1.html (Accessed on 17 December 2020).
17. Director General of Civil Aviation, 3 February 2020, Circular no. 4/1/2020-IR. https://dgca.gov.in/digigov-portal/jsp/dgca/homePage/

viewPDF.jsp?page=topHeader/COVID/Circular%20(Covid-19).pdf (Accessed on 17 December 2020).

18. 'WHO Director-General's Opening Remarks at the Media Briefing on COVID-19,' 11 March 2020 https://www.who.int/director-general/speeches/detail/who-director-general-s-opening-remarks-at-the-media-briefing-on-covid-19---11-march-2020. Accessed on 17 December 2020.
19. International Civil Aviation Organization, 18 March 2020. https://www.icao.int/safety/COVID-19OPS/Documents/046e.pdf (Accessed on 17 December 2020).
20. Director General of Civil Aviation, 12 March 2020, Circular no. 4/1/2020-IR. https://dgca.gov.in/digigov-portal/jsp/dgca/homePage/viewPDF.jsp?page=topHeader/COVID/Circular%20(Covid-19).pdf
21. Email interview with Mihir Tak.
22. Ministry of Health and Family Welfare, 10 March 2020, Additional Travel Advisory (I) for COVID-19 on Home Isolation. https://www.mohfw.gov.in/pdf/AdditionalTravelAdvisory1homeisolation.pdf (Accessed on 31 December 2020).
23. Interview with Videh Kumar Jaipuriar, CEO, Delhi International Airport Ltd.
24. Email interview with Aishwarya Airy.
25. Ibid.
26. Anvit Srivastava, 'Why German Stuck at Delhi's IGI Airport Turned Down Offer to Go Home,' *Hindustan Times*, 12 May 2020. https://www.hindustantimes.com/delhi-news/german-stuck-at-delhi-s-igi-airport-refused-to-go-home/story-YGHdm1PoqhYT8TVmo0DIMO.html (Accessed on 29 June 2021).
27. Office of the Director General of Civil Aviation, Circular no. 4/1/2020-IR, 19 March 2020. https://dgca.gov.in/digigov-portal/?dynamicPage=dynamicPdf/130618190&mainpublicNotices/0/0/viewAllService (Accessed on 16 December 2020).
28. Office of the Director General of Civil Aviation, 26 March 2020. https://dgca.gov.in/digigov-portal/jsp/dgca/homePage/viewPDF.jsp?page=topHeader/COVID/Circular%2026.3.2020.pdf (Accessed on 16 December 2020).

29. Office of Director General of Civil Aviation, 14 April 2020. https://dgca.gov.in/digigov-portal/jsp/dgca/homePage/viewPDF.jsp?page=topHeader/COVID/Circular%20Int.%20Ops-%2014.4.2020.pdf (Accessed on 16 December 2020).
30. Office of Director General of Civil Aviation, 2 May 2020. https://dgca.gov.in/digigov-portal/jsp/dgca/homePage/viewPDF.jsp?page=topHeader/COVID/Circular%202.5.2020.pdf (Accessed on 16 December 2020).
31. Office of Director General of Civil Aviation, 17 May 2020. https://dgca.gov.in/digigov-portal/jsp/dgca/homePage/viewPDF.jsp?page=topHeader/COVID/Circular%2017-05-2020-.pdf. Accessed on 16 December 2020).
32. Office of Director General of Civil Aviation, 30 May 2020. https://dgca.gov.in/digigov-portal/jsp/dgca/homePage/viewPDF.jsp?page=topHeader/COVID/Circular%2030-05-2020.pdf (Accessed on 16 December 2020).
33. Office of Director General of Civil Aviation, 26 June 2020. https://dgca.gov.in/digigov-portal/jsp/dgca/homePage/viewPDF.jsp?page=topHeader/COVID/Circular(26June2020).pdf (Accessed on 16 December 2020).
34. Office of Director General of Civil Aviation, 27 October 2020. https://dgca.gov.in/digigov-portal/jsp/dgca/homePage/viewPDF.jsp?page=topHeader/COVID/circular(27Oct2020).pdf (Accessed on 18 December 2020).
35. Office of Director General of Civil Aviation, 26 November 2020. https://dgca.gov.in/digigov-portal/jsp/dgca/homePage/viewPDF.jsp?page=topHeader/COVID/circular(26Nov2020).pdf (Accessed on 18 December 2020.
36. Office of Director General of Civil Aviation, 28 May 2021. https://www.dgca.gov.in/digigov-portal/Upload?flag=iframeAttachView&attachId=150428362 (Accessed on 24 June 2021).
37. Office of Director General of Civil Aviation, 7 October 2020. https://dgca.gov.in/digigov-portal/jsp/dgca/homePage/viewPDF.

jsp?page=topHeader/COVID/Circular(7Oct2020).pdf (Accessed on 5 January 2021).

38. APP, 23 January 2020, 'Pakistan Starts Screening at Four Major Airports for China Virus.' https://tribune.com.pk/story/2143063/1-pakistan-starts-screening-four-major-airports-china-virus-outbreak (Accessed on 5 January 2021).
39. Asif Shahzad and Syed Raza Hassan, 'Pakistan Limits Flights, Shuts Borders and Schools over Coronavirus,' *Reuters*, 13 March 2020. https://www.reuters.com/article/us-health-coronavirus-pakistan-idUSKBN21027M (Accessed on 18 December 2020).
40. Ikram Junaidi, 'Pakistan Suspends International Flights for Two Weeks,' *Dawn*, 22 March 2020. https://www.dawn.com/news/1542812 (Accessed on 16 December 2020).
41. Leslie Josephs, 'Coronavirus Forces Airlines to Consider a Once Unthinkable Possibility—Halting US Flights,' cnbc.com, 16 March 2020. https://www.cnbc.com/2020/03/16/coronavirus-makes-airlines-consider-chances-for-a-halt-to-us-flights.html (Accessed on 18 December 2020).
42. Donald J. Trump, 'Proclamation on Suspension of Entry as Immigrants and Nonimmigrants of Persons Who Pose a Risk of Transmitting 2019 Novel Coronavirus,' 31 January 2020. https://trumpwhitehouse.archives.gov/presidential-actions/proclamation-suspension-entry-immigrants-nonimmigrants-persons-pose-risk-transmitting-2019-novel-coronavirus/ / (Accessed on 7 October 2021).
43. American Airlines Newsroom, 2 February 2020, 'Government-Imposed Travel Restrictions Due to the 2019 Novel Coronavirus.' http://s21.q4cdn.com/616071541/files/doc_news/Government-Imposed-Travel-Restrictions-Due-to-the-2019-Novel-Coronavirus-OPS-DIS-02-2020.pdf (Accessed on 18 December 2020).
44. American Airlines Newsroom, 29 January 2020, 'Update on American Airlines Flights to China.'

http://news.aa.com/news/news-details/2020/Update-on-American-Airlines-Flights-to-China-OPS-DIS-01/default.aspx (Accessed on 18 December 2020).

45. American Airlines Newsroom, 30 April 2020, 'Additional Schedule Changes to Match Reduced Customer Demand Related to COVID-19.' http://news.aa.com/news/news-details/2020/Additional-Schedule-Changes-to-Match-Reduced-Customer-Demand-Related-to-COVID-19-OPS-DIS-04/default.aspx (Accessed on 18 December 2020).
46. A Proclamation on the Suspension of Entry as Nonimmigrants of Certain Additional Persons Who Pose a Risk of Transmitting Coronavirus Disease 2019, 30 April 2021. https://www.whitehouse.gov/briefing-room/presidential-actions/2021/04/30/a-proclamation-on-the-suspension-of-entry-as-nonimmigrants-of-certain-additional-persons-who-pose-a-risk-of-transmitting-coronavirus-disease-2019/ (Accessed on 18 December 2020).
47. US Mission India, 28 April 2021, 'Health Alert.' https://in.usembassy.gov/health-alert/ (Accessed on 5 June 2021).
48. COVID-19 – Global Travel Advisory for India Updated on 4 June 2021.' https://travel.gc.ca/destinations/india (Accessed on 5 June 2021).
49. Department of Transport, 19 April 2021, 'Guidance, Red, Amber and Green List Rules for Entering England. https://www.gov.uk/government/news/india-added-to-red-list-as-cases-of-new-variant-rise (Accessed on 5 June 2021).
50. HT Correspondent, 'India Raises Return of Students with Australia,' *Hindustan Times*, 11 September 2021. https://www.hindustantimes.com/india-news/india-raises-return-of-students-with-australia-101631377027579.html (Accessed on 10 October 2021).

2: AT SEA WITH THE PANDEMIC

1. Promotional Multimedia on Princess Cruises website. https://www.princess.com/cruise-tips-vacation-ideas/video/cruise-ships/diamond.html#:~:text=Diamond%20Princess%20Cruise%20Ship%20%2D%20Princess%20Cruises (Accessed on 3 January 2020).
2. Binay Kumar Sarkar Facebook post. https://www.facebook.com/binaykumar.sarkar (Accessed on 3 January 2021).
3. Nakazawa, E., Ino, H., and Akabayashi, A. (2020). Chronology of COVID-19 Cases on the Diamond Princess Cruise Ship and Ethical Considerations: A Report from Japan. *Disaster Medicine and Public Health Preparedness, 14*(4), 506-513. doi:10.1017/dmp.2020.50. https://www.cambridge.org/core/journals/disaster-medicine-and-public-health-preparedness/article/chronology-of-covid19-cases-on-the-diamond-princess-cruise-ship-and-ethical-considerations-a-report-from-japan/6D4183045C3AB3CDB3100EE1DE7AE9E1# (Accessed on 20 December 2020).
4. The Government of Hong Kong Special Administration Region, Press Release of 1 February 2020. https://www.info.gov.hk/gia/general/202002/01/P2020020100795.htm (Accessed on 20 December 2020).
5. Diamond Princess updates, 27 February 2020. https://www.princess.com/news/notices_and_advisories/notices/diamond-princess-update.html (Accessed on 20 December 2020).
6. Footnote 3.
7. Unstarred Rajya Sabha question number 2930 answered on 19 March 2020.
8. Princess Cruises announcement 12 March 2020. https://www.princess.com/news/news_releases/2020/03/princess-cruises-announces-a-voluntary-and-temporary-pause.html (Accessed on 20 December 2020).
9. Updated statement of 6 February 2020 regarding Westerdam. https://www.hollandamerica.com/blog/ships/ms-westerdam/statement-regarding-westerdam-in-japan/ (Accessed on 20 December 2020).
10. Footnote 3.

11. Footnote 8.
12. Bangkok Post, 11 February 2020, 'Thailand Denies Westerdam Cruise Ship Entry.' https://www.bangkokpost.com/thailand/general/1855034/thailand-denies-westerdam-cruise-ship-entry-china-virus-toll-passes-1-000 (Accessed on 20 December 2020).
13. bbc.com, 13 February 2020, 'Coronavirus: "Pariah" Cruise Ship Rejected by Five Ports Docks at Last.' https://www.bbc.com/news/world-asia-51484625 (Accessed on 20 December 2020).
14. Tedros Adhanom Ghebreyesus, Director General of World Health Organisation, 13 February 2020. https://twitter.com/DrTedros/status/1227963448048394241?s=20 (Accessed on 20 December 2020).
15. Footnote 8.
16. WHO, 'A Small Country with a Big Heart – Welcoming the Westerdam,' 25 June 2020. https://www.who.int/cambodia/news/feature-stories/detail/a-small-country-with-a-big-heart-welcoming-the-westerdam (Accessed on 20 December 2020).
17. Princess Cruises press release, 3 December 2020. https://www.princess.com/news/news_releases/2020/12/princess-cruises-global-fleet-to-feature-medallionclass-experience-in-2021.html (Accessed on 20 December 2020).
18. Ship itinerary of Holland America Line. https://www.hollandamerica.com/en_US/find-a-cruise. (Accessed on 15 May 2021).
19. Avinash Nair, *The Indian Express*, 2 January 2021 https://indianexpress.com/article/cities/ahmedabad/hit-by-covid-luxury-cruise-liners-queue-up-at-alang-7130194/ (Accessed on 15 May 2021).
20. Directorate General of Shipping (DGS), 'MS Notice No. 02 of 2020,' 28 January 2020. https://dgshipping.gov.in/writereaddata/ShippingNotices/202001290408252368177Ms_Notice_02of2020.pdf (Accessed on 20 December 2020).
21. Directorate General of Shipping, 'Order No. 2 of 2020,' 16 March 2020. https://dgshipping.gov.in/writereaddata/

News/202003160633573492901DGSORDER02OF2020.PDF (Accessed on 20 December 2020).

22. Aditi Divekar, *Business Standard*, Jawaharlal Nehru Port Trust Quarantined Ship from Iran Amid Coronavirus,' 17 March 2020. https://www.business-standard.com/article/current-affairs/jawaharlal-nehru-port-trust-quarantined-ship-from-iran-amid-coronavirus-120031701894_1.html (Accessed on 20 December 2020).
23. Department of Transport, UK Government, 'Joint Statement of the International Maritime Virtual Summit on Crew Changes, 9 July 2020. https://www.gov.uk/government/news/joint-statement-of-the-international-maritime-virtual-summit-on-crew-changes (Accessed on 20 December 2020).
24. TNN, *Times of India*, 'Sub-zero Temps, No Doctors: Indian Sailors Stranded in Chinese Waters Get Desperate in "Captivity."' 30 December 2020. https://timesofindia.indiatimes.com/india/sub-zero-temps-no-doctors-unless-someone-is-dying-a-suicide-attempt-indian-sailors-stranded-in-chinese-waters-get-desperate-in-captivity/articleshowprint/80023270.cms (Accessed 3 January 2021).
25. Mediterranean Shipping Company, 'MSC Ends Anastasia Cargo Ship Ordeal with Crew Change in Japan,' 9 February 2021. https://www.msc.com/ind/news/2021-february/msc-ends-anastasia-cargo-ship-ordeal-crew-change (Accessed 3 May 2021).
26. 'Lok Sabha Unstarred Question No. 349,' 3 February 2021. https://mea.gov.in/lok-sabha.htm?dtl/33449/QUESTION+NO349+INDIANS+STUCK+ON+CARGO+SHIPS (Accessed 3 May 2021).
27. Directorate General of Shipping, 'Clarification Regarding DGS Orders Numbered 4 and 5 of 2020.' https://www.dgshipping.gov.in/writereaddata/ShippingNotices/202003240659110012255202003240618285842704Clarification_regarding_DGSorderNo04and05of2020.pdf (Accessed 3 January 2021).
28. Directorate General of Shipping 'Order 35 of 2020,' 17 December 2020. https://dgshipping.gov.in/writereaddata/ShippingNotices/202012170427081387004DGS_Order_35of2020_17122020.PDF (Accessed 3 January 2021).

29. Interview with Binay Kumar Sarkar.

3: ONE NATION, MANY BOUNDARIES

1. Minutes of the meeting, Directorate General of Health Services, Public Health Wing IV, Government of National Capital Territory of Delhi, 4 March 2020. http://health.delhigovt.nic.in/wps/wcm/connect/cb3a77004d7297e6b220f7982ee7a5c7/MoMH.pdf?MOD=AJPERES&lmod=-1363861991&CACHEID=cb3a77004d7297e6b220f7982ee7a5c7 (Accessed on 8 January 2021).
2. Minutes of the meeting, Directorate General of Health Services, Public Health Wing IV, 9 March 2020. http://health.delhigovt.nic.in/wps/wcm/connect/59af3b004d81bb388ad8ff982ee7a5c7/MOM+STF+8-3-2020.pdf?MOD=AJPERES&lmod=-937627149&CACHEID=59af3b004d81bb388ad8ff982ee7a5c7 (Accessed on 8 January 2021).
3. Advisory, Health and Family Welfare Department, Government of National Capital Territory of Delhi, 19 March 2020. http://health.delhigovt.nic.in/wps/wcm/connect/97c8be004d9d5511ba1cff982ee7a5c7/advisory20.pdf?MOD=AJPERES&lmod=-160863242&CACHEID=97c8be004d9d5511ba1cff982ee7a5c7 (Accessed on 8 January 2021).
4. Government of Delhi, Health and Family Welfare Department Order, 22 March 2020. http://health.delhigovt.nic.in/wps/wcm/connect/deaf86804da4c3bb8687f7982ee7a5c7/lock.pdf?MOD=AJPERES&lmod=48689189&CACHEID=deaf86804da4c3bb8687f7982ee7a5c7 (Accessed on 8 January 2021).
5. DGCA tweet at 10.12 p.m. on 22 March 2020. https://twitter.com/DGCAIndia/status/1241767151398031360?s=20 (Accessed on 8 January 2021).
6. Press Information Bureau, Press Release ID:200619, 23 March 2020. https://pib.gov.in/PressReleasePage.aspx?PRID=1607740 (Accessed on 8 January 2021).
7. Haryana Health and Family Welfare Department Order (Endst No. 81-90/COVID/2020).

8. Government of Maharashtra Notification No: DMU/2020/CR. 92/ DisM-1 Dated 23 March 2020).
9. Interview with Sanjay Kumar Sharma.
10. COVID-19 Regulatory Package, Reserve Bank of India, 27 March 2020. https://www.rbi.org.in/Scripts/NotificationUser.aspx?Id=11835 (Accessed on 30 September 2021).
11. District Administration Gurugram, Order dated 30 May 2021 https://cdn.s3waas.gov.in/s325b2822c2f5a3230abfadd476e8b04c9/uploads/2021/05/2021053141.pdf (Accessed on 30 September 2021).
12. Health and Family Welfare Department, Government of Karnataka, Addendum dated 20 February 2021. https://covid19.karnataka.gov.in/storage/pdf-files/cir-hws/Circular-Special%20Surveillance%20Measures%20for%20arrivals%20from%20Kerala%20(into%20Karnataka%20including%20Bangalore)%20with%20immidiate%20effect.pdf (Accessed on 7 June 2021).
13. Government of Karnataka, Circular-Regarding Compulsory RT-PCR Report for Drivers and Assistants of Freight Transport Vehicles from Kerala and Maharashtra dated 3 March 2021. https://covid19.karnataka.gov.in/storage/pdf-files/cir-hws/Circular-Regarding%20having%20compulsory%20RT-PCR%20Examination%20Report%20for%20Drivers%20and%20Assistants%20of%20Freight%20Transport%20Vehicles%20from%20Kerala%20and%20Maharashtra%20States.pdf (Accessed on 7 June 2021).
14. Government of Karnataka circular on special surveillance measures for arrivals from Kerala, Maharashtra, Punjab and Chandigarh dated 22 March 2021. https://covid19.karnataka.gov.in/storage/pdf-files/cir-hws/Circular-Special%20Surveillance%20Measure%20for%20arrivals%20from%20Kerala,%20Maharashtra,%20Punjab%20and%20Chandigarh.pdf (Accessed on 7 June 2021).
15. Hannah Ritchie, Edouard Mathieu, Lucas Rodés-Guirao, Cameron Appel, Charlie Giattino, Esteban Ortiz-Ospina, Joe Hasell, Bobbie Macdonald, Diana Beltekian and Max Roser, 2020, 'Coronavirus Pandemic (COVID-19).' Published online at OurWorldInData.org.

https://ourworldindata.org/coronavirus (Accessed on 14 November 2021).

16. COVID-19 Community Mobility Report of Google 10 January 2021. https://www.gstatic.com/covid19/mobility/2021-01-10_IN_Mobility_Report_en-GB.pdf (Accessed on 7 June 2021).
17. covid19india.org data based on state press bulletins, government twitter handles, Press Information Bureau, Press Trust of India, ANI reports. https://www.covid19india.org/ (Accessed on 7 June 2021).
18. Footnote 15.
19. Vinod Kumar, *The Times of India*, 19 March 2020, 'Corona Outbreak: Punjab to Suspend Public Transport from Friday Midnight.' https://timesofindia.indiatimes.com/india/corona-outbreak-punjab-to-suspend-public-transport-from-friday-midnight/articleshow/74710266.cms (Accessed on 10 January 2021).
20. Romita Datta, *India Today*, 6 March 2020, 'West Bengal Screens over 1.4 Lakh People.' https://www.indiatoday.in/india/story/west-bengal-coronavirus-cases-positive-patients-screening-border-1653233-2020-03-06 (Accessed on 10 January 2021).
21. Anulekha Ray, *Mint*, 7 July 2020, 'West Bengal Bans Flights from Mumbai, Delhi and 4 Other Cities to Kolkata Airport Till Month-End.' https://www.livemint.com/news/india/covid-19-west-bengal-govt-bans-flights-from-mumbai-delhi-and-4-other-cities-till-month-end-11594996544222.html (Accessed on 10 January 2021).
22. Ministry of Home Affairs Order No. 40-3/2020-DM-I(A).
23. Abhishek Behl, *Hindustan Times*, 21 May 2020, 'Industrial Activity in Udyog Vihar As Workers Unable to Cross Border. https://www.hindustantimes.com/gurugram/industrial-activity-in-udyog-vihar-hit-as-workers-unable-to-cross-border/story-wQ2ve8kcrHq4o40GtcUf3L.html (Accessed on 10 January 2021).
24. Mohammad Ghazali, ndtv.com, 29 May 2020, 'Haryana to 'Completely Seal' Delhi Border, Essential Services Allowed. https://www.ndtv.com/india-news/coronavirus-haryana-minister-tweets-orders-issued-to-completely-seal-border-with-delhi-over-Covid-19-crisis-2236834 (Accessed on 10 January 2021).

25. The High Court of Delhi Judgement in *OP Gupta versus Union of India*, 14 May 2020. https://www.livelaw.in/pdf_upload/pdf_upload-374803.pdf (Accessed on 14 January 2021).
26. Annexure to the Ministry of Home Affairs Order No. 40-3/2020 dated 24 March 2020. https://www.mha.gov.in/sites/default/files/Guidelines_0.pdf (Accessed on 14 January 2021).
27. Government of Maharashtra Addendum No. DMU/2020/CR. 92/DisM-1, 15 April 2020.
28. Haryana Health and Family Welfare Department Order (Endst No. 81-90/COVID/2020).
29. The Government of West Bengal Memo No. 93-CS/2020 dated 27 April 2020. https://wb.gov.in/COVID-19/OC14.pdf (Accessed on 14 January 2021).
30. The Ministry of Home Affairs, Government of India order dated 25 March 2020. https://www.mha.gov.in/sites/default/files/MHA%20order%20with%20addendum%20to%20Guidelines%20Dated%2024.3.2020_0.pdf (Accessed on 14 January 2021).
31. Saket Sundria, *Bloomberg*, 8 April 2020, '90% of Trucks in India Are Now Off Roads Amid Coronavirus Lockdown.' https://www.business-standard.com/article/economy-policy/90-of-trucks-in-india-are-now-off-roads-amid-coronavirus-lockdown-120040800048_1.html (Accessed on 14 January 2021).
32. The Ministry of Home Affairs, Government of India, order dated 27 March 2020. https://www.mha.gov.in/sites/default/files/PR_SecondAddendum_27032020_0.pdf (Accessed on 14 January 2021).
33. 'Indian Railways' Initiatives,' 17 July 2020 presentation by Railway Board chairman.
34. Shine Jacob and Shreya Jai, *Business Standard*, 7 June 2020, 'Rail Freight Traffic Drops 28% in April–May Amid COVID-19 Lockdown.' https://www.business-standard.com/article/economy-policy/rail-freight-traffic-drops-28-in-april-may-amid-covid-19-lockdown-120060701026_1.html (Accessed on 14 January 2021).
35. Shine Jacob, *Business Standard*, 23 April 2020, How the Railways Readjusted Freight Operations to Cope with Lockdown.' https://www.business-standard.com/article/companies/how-

the-railways-readjusted-its-freight-operations-to-cope-with-lockdown-120042301698_1.html (Accessed on 14 January 2021).

36. 'Indian Railways Key Initiatives,' 18 December presentation by Railway Board chairman.
37. 'Important Policy Measures for Freight Customers,' The Indian Railways. https://www.fois.indianrail.gov.in/FOISWebPortal/resources/pdf/FreightPolicyMeasuresOnline.pdf (Accessed on 14 January 2021).
38. PIB Release ID: 1709006 dated 1 April 2021. https://pib.gov.in/PressReleasePage.aspx?PRID=1709006 (Accessed on 14 January 2021).
39. PIB Release ID: 1704371 dated 12 March 2021. https://pib.gov.in/PressReleasePage.aspx?PRID=1704371 (Accessed on 14 January 2021).
40. 'Major Ports Statistics,' Indian Ports Association. http://www.ipa.nic.in/ (Accessed on 14 January 2021).
41. The Ministry of Shipping, Government of India, 'Cargo Traffic Handled at Major Ports during and up to March 2021. https://shipmin.gov.in/sites/default/files/1%20Major%20March%2C%202021.pdf (Accessed on 14 November 2021).
42. Aditi Divekar, Arindam Majumder, Aneesh Phadnis and Shine Jacob, *Business Standard*, 10 April 2020, 'Shortage of Workers in Clearing Cargo Clogs Airports, Ports, Railways.
https://www.business-standard.com/article/current-affairs/shortage-of-workers-in-clearing-cargo-clogs-airports-ports-railways-120041001450_1.html (Accessed on 14 January 2021).
43. Directorate General of Shipping Order No. 07 of 2020 dated 29 March 2020. https://dgshipping.gov.in/writereaddata/News/202003290137384948107Advisoryonnon-chargingofcontainerdetentionchargesonimportandexportshipments.pdf (Accessed on 14 January 2021).
44. Aditi Divekar, Arindam Majumder, Aneesh Phadnis and Shine Jacob, *Business Standard*, 11 April 2020, 'Shortage of Workers in

Clearing Cargo Clogs Airports, Ports, Railways.' https://www.business-standard.com/article/current-affairs/shortage-of-workers-in-clearing-cargo-clogs-airports-ports-railways-120041001450_1.html (Accessed on 14 January 2021).

45. AAC 2 of 2020 R1 – Special Permission to Conduct Cargo Operations Using Passenger Category Aircraft during the COVID-19 Lockdown Period Dated 11 April 2020. https://dgca.gov.in/digigov-portal/jsp/dgca/homePage/viewPDF.jsp?page=topHeader/COVID/AAC02_2020R1.pdf (Accessed on 14 January 2021.).
46. Press Trust of India, The Economic Times, 14 November 2020, SpiceJet handles 10,000 cargo flights since lockdown in March. https://economictimes.indiatimes.com/industry/transportation/airlines-/-aviation/spicejet-handles-10000-cargo-flights-since-lockdown-in-march/articleshow/79224050.cms?from=mdr (Accessed on 14 January 2021).
47. Rhik Kundu, *Mint*, 4 November 2020, 'How a Cargo Craze Took Wing in Aviation.' https://www.livemint.com/news/india/how-a-cargo-craze-took-wing-in-aviation-11604412747478.html (Accessed on 14 January 2021).

4: A THREE-DAY COUNTDOWN TO LOCKDOWN

1. Press Information Bureau, Press Release ID: 1607248, 19 March 2020. https://pib.gov.in/PressReleaseIframePage.aspx?PRID=1607248 (Accessed on 3 March 2021).
2. Press Trust of India, *Business Standard*, 27 March 2020, 'Lockdown Address on Mar 24 Modi's Best in Terms of TV Ratings.' https://www.business-standard.com/article/pti-stories/lockdown-address-on-mar-24-modi-s-best-in-terms-of-tv-ratings-120032700821_1.html (Accessed on 3 March 2021).
3. Christian, W., *The Copenhagen Post*, 'Denmark Making Noise in Times of Fear and Isolation,' 20 March 2020. https://cphpost.dk/?p=111945 (Accessed on 3 March 2021).

4. Connor Perrett, *Business Insider US*, 'People Quarantined in Spain Leaning out of Windows to Applaud Frontline Medical Workers,' 18 March 2020.
https://www.businessinsider.co.za/spanish-lean-out-of-windows-thank-medical-workers-covid-19-2020-3 (Accessed on 3 March 2021).
5. Gartner Press Release, 'Gartner HR Survey Reveals 88% of Organizations Have Encouraged or Required Employees to Work From Home Due to Coronavirus,' 19 March 2020. https://www.gartner.com/en/newsroom/press-releases/2020-03-19-gartner-hr-survey-reveals-88--of-organizations-have-e (Accessed on 3 March 2021).
6. Haryana Health and Family Welfare Department Order (Endst No. 81-90/COVID/2020).
7. Delhi Metro Rail Corporation Tweet, 20 March 2020. https://twitter.com/OfficialDMRC/status/1240939400898301954?s=20 (Accessed on 3 March 2021).
8. Press Information Bureau, Press Release ID: 1607535, 21 March 2020. https://pib.gov.in/PressReleasePage.aspx?PRID=1607535 (Accessed on 4 March 2021).
9. Press Information Bureau, Press Release ID: 1606964, 18 March 2020. https://pib.gov.in/PressReleasePage.aspx?PRID=1606964 (Accessed on 4 March 2021).
10. Press Information Bureau, Press Release Release ID: 1607216, 19 March 2020. https://pib.gov.in/PressReleasePage.aspx?PRID=1607216 (Accessed on 4 March 2021).
11. Press Information Bureau, Press Release Release ID: 1606871, 11 March 2020. https://pib.gov.in/PressReleasePage.aspx?PRID=1606871 (Accessed on 8 March 2021).
12. Press Information Bureau, Press Release ID: 1607398, 20 March 2021. https://pib.gov.in/PressReleasePage.aspx?PRID=1607398 (Accessed on 8 March 2021).
13. Press Information Bureau, Press Release Release ID: 1607605, 22 March 2020. https://pib.gov.in/PressReleasePage.aspx?PRID=1607605 (Accessed on 8 March 2021).

14. *New York Times*, 'Strike of Indian Rail Workers Begins,' 8 May 1974.
15. https://www.nytimes.com/1974/05/08/archives/strike-of-indian-rail-workers-begins-tension-high-with-food.html (Accessed on 8 March 2021).
15. Interview with S. Dhasarathy.
16. Railway Budget Speech for 1974-75 presented on 27 February 1974.
17. Press Trust of India, *India Today*, 'L.N. Mishra Murder Case: 40 Years Later, 4 Get Life Term,' 18 December 2014. https://www.indiatoday.in/india/north/story/ln-mishra-murder-case-life-term-samastipur-railway-station-231798-2014-12-18 (Accessed on 18 February 2021).
18. Speech of Kamalapati Tripathi Introducing the Railway Budget for 1975-76, 20 February 1975. https://indianrailways.gov.in/railwayboard/uploads/directorate/finance_budget/Previous%20Budget%20Speeches/1975-76.pdf (Accessed on 18 February 2021).
19. Ibid.
20. Railway Board Chairman Media Presentation dated 3 June 2021; Monthly Evaluation Report of February 2021.
21. Press Information Bureau, Press Release ID: 1607535, 21 March 2020. https://pib.gov.in/PressReleasePage.aspx?PRID=1607535 (Accessed on 8 March 2021).
22. Press Information Bureau, Press Release ID: 1607740, 23 March 2020 https://pib.gov.in/PressReleasePage.aspx?PRID=1607740 (Accessed on 8 March 2021).
23. Press Trust of India, *Times of India*, 'Govt Responsible for Coronavirus Crisis as It Delayed Action: Kamal Nath,' 12 April 2020. http://timesofindia.indiatimes.com/articleshow/75106301.cms?utm_source=contentofinterest&utm_medium=text&utm_campaign=cppst (Accessed on 8 March 2021).
24. Jyoti Mukul, *Business Standard*, 'Railways' Move to Suspend Services Contradicts Social Distancing Message,' 31 March 2020. https://www.business-standard.com/article/current-affairs/railways-move-to-suspend-services-contradicts-social-distancing-message-120033101841_1.html (Accessed on 8 March 2021).
25. Ibid.

26. Ibid.
27. Prince Mathews Thomas, moneycontrol.com, 'Coronavirus Pandemic: Airlines Race against Time to Move Crew, Aircraft before March 24 Midnight Deadline,' 24 March 2020. https://www.moneycontrol.com/news/business/companies/coronavirus-pandemic-airlines-race-against-time-to-move-crew-aircraft-before-march-24-midnight-deadline-5065311.html (Accessed on 8 March 2021).
28. Manju V., *Times of India*, 'Air India Crew Being Ostracized by Neighbours, Housing Societies for Operating Flights to COVID-19 Countries,' 22 March 2020. http://timesofindia.indiatimes.com/articleshow/74761456.cms?utm_source=contentofinterest&utm_medium=text&utm_campaign=cppst (Accessed on 20 February 2021).
29. Press Information Bureau, Press Release ID: 1607531, 21 March 2020. https://pib.gov.in/PressReleasePage.aspx?PRID=1607531 (Accessed on 8 March 2021).
30. Press Information Bureau, Press Release ID: 1608804, 28 March 2020. https://pib.gov.in/PressReleasePage.aspx?PRID=1608804 (Accessed on 8 March 2021).
31. Press Trust of India, *The Hindu*, Railways Earned Rs 9000 Crore from Ticket Cancellation Charges, Non-cancellation of Wait-Listed Tickets, 25 February 2020. https://www.thehindu.com/news/national/railways-earned-9000-crore-from-ticket-cancellation-charges-non-cancellation-of-wait-listed-tickets/article30912651.ece (Accessed on 8 March 2021).
32. P. Manoj, *Business Line*, Railway Ticket Refund Excludes IRCTC's Convenience Fee, 20 April 2020. https://www.thehindubusinessline.com/news/railway-ticket-refund-excludes-irctcs-convenience-fee/article31390390.ece (Accessed on 22 February 2021).
33. Press Information Bureau, Press Release ID: 1614272, 14 April 2020. https://pib.gov.in/PressReleasePage.aspx?PRID=1614272 (Accessed on 22 March 2021).
34. Ministry of Civil Aviation, DT Section, Office Memorandum, 16 April 2020. https://dgca.gov.in/digigov-portal/jsp/dgca/homePage/

viewPDF.jsp?page=topHeader/COVID/Circular%2016.4.2020.pdf (Accessed on 22 February 2021).

35. Shine Jacob and Arindam Majumder, *Business Standard*, 'Covid-19 Lockdown Indecision: To Sell or Not to Sell Air and Train Tickets?, 13 April 2020. https://www.business-standard.com/article/current-affairs/covid-19-lockdown-indecision-to-sell-or-not-to-sell-air-and-train-tickets-120041300028_1.html (Accessed on 22 February 2021).
36. Director General of Civil Aviation, Government of India, Circular No. 4/1/2020 dated 19 April 2020. https://dgca.gov.in/digigov-portal/jsp/dgca/homePage/viewPDF.jsp?page=topHeader/COVID/Circular%2019.4.2020-final.pdf (Accessed on 22 February 2021).
37. Supreme Court of India Judgement in Pravasi Legal Cell and Others versus Union of India and Others, 1 October 2020. https://main.sci.gov.in/supremecourt/2020/10966/10966_2020_35_1501_24201_Judgement_01-Oct-2020.pdf (Accessed on 22 February 2021).
38. Footnote 36.
39. Bombay Stock Exchange filing, Financial Results Summary. https://www.bseindia.com/stock-share-price/interglobe-aviation-ltd/indigo/539448/financials-results/ (Accessed on 8 March 2021).
40. Directorate General of Civil Aviation, Monthly Traffic and Operating Statistics (Scheduled Domestic Service) for 2019 and 2020 https://www.dgca.gov.in/digigov-portal/?page=jsp/dgca/InventoryList/dataReports/aviationDataStatistics/airTransport/domestic/monthly/indigo20.PDF&main259/4184/servicename (Accessed on 8 March 2021).
41. Jyoti Mukul, *Business Standard*, 'IRCTC Struggles to Stay on Track as Travel Worst Impacted Due to Covid-19,' 28 December 2020. https://www.business-standard.com/article/indian-railways/irctc-struggles-to-stay-on-track-as-travel-worst-impacted-due-to-covid-19-120122700711_1.html (Accessed on 8 March 2021).
42. Ministry of Civil Aviation, Rajya Sabha Unstarred Question No. 980, 10 February 2021. https://pqars.nic.in/annex/253/AU980.pdf (Accessed on 9 March 2021).

43. Note from Ronojoy Dutta, CEO, IndiGo, 20 July 2020. https://www.goindigo.in/content/dam/goindigo/investor-relations/press-releases/2020-21/200720-Important-update-from-indigo.pdf (Accessed on 9 March 2021).
44. Press Trust of India, *Mint*, 'Air Deccan Ceases Operations, All Employees Put on Sabbatical Without Pay,' 5 April 2020. https://www.livemint.com/companies/news/air-deccan-ceases-operations-all-employees-put-on-sabbatical-without-pay-11586077400459.html (Accessed on 9 March 2021).
45. Ministry of Civil Aviation, Rajya Sabha, Unstarred Question No. 186, 3 February 2021. https://pqars.nic.in/annex/253/A186.pdf (Accessed on 9 March 2021).
46. Saurabh Sinha, *The Times of India*, 'Top Flight Caterer Shuts Shop at Delhi and Mumbai Airports,' 19 February 2021. https://timesofindia.indiatimes.com/city/delhi/top-flight-caterer-shuts-shop-at-delhi-mumbai-airports/articleshow/81098004.cms (Accessed on 9 March 2021).

5: A NATION LOCKED DOWN

1. WHO, 25 March 2020, Situation Report 65. https://www.who.int/docs/default-source/coronaviruse/situation-reports/20200325-sitrep-65-covid-19.pdf?sfvrsn=ce13061b_2 (Accessed on 28 March 2021).
2. Press Information Bureau, 24 March 2020, Text of PM's address to the nation on vital aspects relating to the menace of COVID-19. https://pib.gov.in/PressReleseDetail.aspx?PRID=1607995 (Accessed on 28 March 2021).
3. Ibid.
4. WHO, 25 March 2020, Director-General's opening remarks at the media briefing on COVID-19. https://www.who.int/director-general/speeches/detail/who-director-general-s-opening-remarks-at-the-media-briefing-on-covid-19---25-march-2020 (Accessed on 28 March 2021).

5. Central Government Status Report filed in the Supreme Court, *Alakh Alok Srivastava versus Union of India* case, 31 March 2020. https://www.mha.gov.in/sites/default/files/Status%20Report%20 COVID19.pdf (Accessed on 28 March 2021).
6. ourworldindata.org, 'COVID-19: Stay at Home Restrictions.' https://ourworldindata.org/covid-stay-home-restrictions (Accessed on 28 March 2021).
7. BBC, 7 April 2020, 'Coronavirus: The World in Lockdown in Maps and Charts.' https://www.bbc.com/news/world-52103747 (Accessed on 28 March 2021).
8. WHO, 23 January 2020, *Situation Report 3.* https://www.who.int/docs/default-source/coronaviruse/situation-reports/20200123-sitrep-3-2019-ncov.pdf?sfvrsn=d6d23643_8 (Accessed on 28 March 2021).
9. Nectar Gan, *CNN*, 8 April 2020, 'China Lifts 76-Day Lockdown on Wuhan As City Reemerges from Coronavirus Crisis.' https://edition.cnn.com/2020/04/07/asia/coronavirus-wuhan-lockdown-lifted-intl-hnk/index.html (Accessed on 28 March 2021).
10. Press Information Bureau, Press Release ID: 1610559, 3 April 2020. https://pib.gov.in/PressReleseDetail.aspx?PRID=1610559 (Accessed on 28 March 2021).
11. Power System Operation Corporation Ltd, May 2020, Report on Pan India Lights Off Event on 5 April 2020 Impact on Indian Power System. https://posoco.in/wp-content/uploads/2020/05/Report-on-Pan-India-Lights-Off-Event-9-PM-9-Minutes-on-5th-April-2020.pdf (Accessed on 28 March 2021).
12. Footnote 1.
13. Hale, Thomas, Sam Webster, Anna Petherick, Toby Phillips, and Beatriz Kira (2020). 'Oxford Covid-19 Government Response Tracker, Blavatnik School of Government.' https://ourworldindata.org/grapher/covid-stringency-index?stackMode=absolute&time=2020-03-25&region=World (Accessed on 2 April 2021).
14. Press Information Bureau, Press Release ID: 1608009, 24 March 2020. https://pib.gov.in/PressReleseDetail.aspx?PRID=1608009 (Accessed on 2 April 2021).

15. Ministry of Home Affairs, Order Number 40-3/2020-DM-I(A), 29 March 2020. https://www.mha.gov.in/sites/default/files/MHA%20Order%20restricting%20movement%20of%20migrants%20and%20strict%20enforement%20of%20lockdown%20measures%20-%2029.03.2020.pdf (Accessed on 2 April 2021).
16. Press Information Bureau, 29 March 2020, 'Initiation of Disciplinary Proceedings Against Four Officers of Government of National Capital Territory of Delhi for Dereliction of Duty Regarding Containment of Spread of COVID-19.' https://www.mha.gov.in/sites/default/files/PR_InitiationofDisciplinary_29032020.pdf (Accessed on 2 April 2021).
17. Government of National Capital Territory of Delhi, Health and Family Welfare Department Order, 13 March 2020. http://health.delhigovt.nic.in/wps/wcm/connect/bd9d8c804d883e3a976ff7982ee7a5c7/BAN+IPL.pdf?MOD=AJPERES&lmod=-754254481&CACHEID=bd9d8c804d883e3a976ff7982ee7a5c7 (Accessed on 3 April 2021).
18. TNN. *Times of India*, 1 April 2020, 'Delhi's Nizamuddin Congregation: FIR Registered Against Maulana, Others of Tablighi Jamaat. https://timesofindia.indiatimes.com/city/delhi/fir-registered-against-maulana-others/articleshow/74920881.cms (Accessed on 3 April 2021).
19. 'Tabligh Activities in India'. https://www.mha.gov.in/sites/default/files/PR_TablighactivitiesinIndia_31032020.pdf (Accessed 3 April 2021).
20. Abhinav Rajput, *Indian Express*, 29 March 2021, 'A Year on, Nizamuddin Markaz Reopens Its Doors.' https://indianexpress.com/article/cities/delhi/a-year-on-nizamuddin-markaz-reopens-its-doors-7249866/ (Accessed on 3 April 2021).
21. Home Secretary Ajay Bhalla's letter to state chief secretaries, 14 April 2020. https://www.mha.gov.in/sites/default/files/MHA DO letter dt.14.4.2020 to Chief Secretaries and Administrators for strict implementation of Lockdown Order during extended period.pdf (Accessed on 3 April 2021).

22. Ministry of Home Affairs, Government of India, Order dated 15 April 2020. https://www.mha.gov.in/sites/default/files/MHA%20order%20dt%2015.04.2020%2C%20with%20Revised%20Consolidated%20Guidelines_compressed%20%283%29.pdf (Accessed on 3 April 2021).
23. Ministry of Home Affairs, Government of India, Order dated 1 May 2020. https://www.mha.gov.in/sites/default/files/MHA%20Order%20Dt.%201.5.2020%20to%20extend%20Lockdown%20period%20for%202%20weeks%20w.e.f.%204.5.2020%20with%20new%20guidelines.pdf (Accessed on 3 April 2021).
24. Press Information Bureau, 12 May 2020, English rendering of Prime Minister Shri Narendra Modi's address to the nation on 12 May 2020. https://pib.gov.in/PressReleseDetail.aspx?PRID=1623418 (Accessed on 3 April 2021).
25. Home Secretary Ajay Bhalla's letter to state chief secretaries, 17 May 2020. https://www.mha.gov.in/sites/default/files/MHADOLrDt17052020.PDF (Accessed on 5 April 2021).
26. Asit Ranjan Mishra, livemint.com, 6 May 2020, 'India April Services PMI at Record Low of 5.4.' https://www.livemint.com/news/india/india-april-services-pmi-hits-record-low-of-5-4-11588742610136.html (Accessed on 5 April 2021).
27. Economic Survey 2020-21, Volume 1.
28. ourworldindata.org, COVID-19 Stringency Index. https://ourworldindata.org/covid-stay-home-restrictions (Accessed on 4 April 2021).

6: THE LONG ROAD HOME

1. Interview with Keerat Kori.
2. Interview with Mohan Paswan.
3. Swati Sharma, ndtv.com, 1 June 2021, 'Father of Bihar Girl, Who Cycled 1,200 km for Him during Lockdown, Dies.' https://www.ndtv.com/india-news/father-of-bihar-girl-jyoti-kumari-who-cycled-1-200-km-for-him-during-lockdown-dies-2453439 (Accessed on 25 November 2021).

4. Stranded Workers Action Network (SWAN), 16 June 2021, 'No Country for Workers: A Report.' http://strandedworkers.in/mdocuments-library/ (Accessed on 25 June 2021).
5. Ugo Gentilini, Mohamed Almenfi, and Pamela Dale, *World Bank*, 11 December 2020, 'Social Protection and Jobs Responses to COVID-19: A Real-Time Review of Country Measures.' https://documents1.worldbank.org/curated/en/467521607723220511/pdf/Social-Protection-and-Jobs-Responses-to-COVID-19-A-Real-Time-Review-of-Country-Measures-December-11-2020.pdf (Accessed on 25 June 2021).
6. Unstarred Lok Sabha question number 990, answered on 8 February 2021. http://loksabhaph.nic.in/Questions/QResult15.aspx?qref=19783&lsno=17 (Accessed on 8 April 2021).
7. Press Information Bureau, Press Release ID: 1608345, 26 March 2020. https://pib.gov.in/PressReleaseIframePage.aspx?PRID=1608345 (Accessed on 8 April 2021).
8. pmindia.gov.in, 30 June 2020, 'PM addresses nation and announces extension of Pradhan Mantri Garib Kalyan Anna Yojana.' https://www.pmindia.gov.in/en/news_updates/pm-addresses-nation-and-announces-extension-of-pradhan-mantri-garib-kalyan-anna-yojana/ (Accessed on 8 April 2021).
9. Interview with Seemant Singh.
10. Interview with Dharmendra Chauhan.
11. A report by the Stranded Workers Action Network; 5 June 2020. http://strandedworkers.in/mdocuments-library/ (Accessed on 8 April 2021)
12. India Today Webdesk, indiatoday.in, 14 April 2020, 'Photos, Videos Show Chaos at Mumbai Stations as Migrants Pack Their Bags to Leave Maharashtra.' https://www.indiatoday.in/india/story/mumbai-photos-videos-show-chaos-at-bandra-station-as-thousands-gather-to-go-home-1666937-2020-04-14 (Accessed on 9 April 2021).
13. Mohamed Thaver, indianexpress.com, 16 April 2020, 'TV Reporter Arrested for Bandra Migrant Gathering, Channel Calls It Outrageous.' https://indianexpress.com/article/coronavirus/mumbai-bandra-crowd-abp-tv-journalist-6364561/ (Accessed on 9 April 2021).

14. Ibid.
15. Sukanya Shantha, thewire.in, 8 August 2020, 'Mumbai Police Exonerates Journalist Arrested for "Fake News," Says FIR Based on "Mistaken Facts."' https://thewire.in/media/mumbai-police-exonerates-journalist-arrested-for-generating-fake-news (Accessed on 9 April 2021).
16. Union health and family welfare secretary Preeti Sudan's letter to chief secretaries of all states and union territories, 1 April 2020. https://www.mha.gov.in/sites/default/files/DO%20Lr.%20Dt.%2012.4.2020%20to%20Chief%20Secretaries%20and%20Administrators%20reg.%20welfare%20activities%20towards%20migrants.pdf (Accessed on 9 April 2021).
17. Ministry of Health and Family Welfare, 'Understanding the Issues of the Migrant Population-COVID-19.' https://www.mohfw.gov.in/pdf/RevisedPsychosocialissuesofmigrantsCOVID19.pdf (Accessed on 9 April 2021).
18. Ministry of Home Affairs' status report in the Supreme Court, 31 March 2020. https://www.mha.gov.in/sites/default/files/ Status%20Report%20COVID19.pdf (Accessed on 9 April 2021).
19. Hindustan Times, 8 May 2020, 'Tired Migrants Sat on Tracks for Rest, Fell Asleep. 16 Run Over by Train.' https://www.hindustantimes.com/india-news/14-migrant-workers-mowed-down-by-goods-train-in-maharashtra/story-Z6V8QkOY2CGvdKNHv2uPvI.html (Accessed on 9 April 2021).
20. Press Information Bureau, Press Release ID: 1622252, May 8, 2020.
21. Aman, Kanika Sharma, Krushna R. and Thejesh GN. (2020). India Non-virus Deaths During lockdown (Version 20200730) [Data set]. Zenodo. http://doi.org/10.5281/zenodo.4630198 (Accessed on 18 June 2021).
22. Unstarred Lok Sabha Question number 2044, answered on 22 September 2020.
23. Centre for Sustainable Employment, Azim Premji University, 2020, COVID-19 Livelihoods Survey https://cse.azimpremjiuniversity.edu.in/wp-content/uploads/2020/06/Compilation-of-findings-APU-

COVID-19-Livelihoods-Survey_Final.pdf (Accessed on 9 April 2021).

24. Freedom House, March 2021, Freedom in the World 2020 report. https://freedomhouse.org/country/india/freedom-world/2020 (Accessed on 10 April 2021).
25. Press Information Bureau, Press Release ID: 1702697, 5 March 2021. https://pib.gov.in/PressReleseDetail.aspx?PRID=1702697 (Accessed on 10 April 2021).
26. Footnote 8.
27. Lok Sabha unstarred question number 327, answered on 15 September 2020.
28. Harsh Mander, Speaking Tiger, 2021, *Locking Down the Poor: The Pandemic and India's Moral Centre*, p. 39.

7: THREE SETS OF TRAINS AND A BUS BACK HOME

1. Ministry of Home Affairs, Order Number 40-3/2020-DM-I (A), 29 March 2020. https://www.mha.gov.in/sites/default/files/MHA%20Order%20restricting%20movement%20of%20migrants%20and%20strict%20enforement%20of%20lockdown%20measures%20-%2029.03.2020.pdf (Accessed on 10 April 2021).
2. WHO, *Coronavirus Disease 2019 (COVID-19) Situation Report-69*, 29 March 2020. https://www.who.int/docs/default-source/coronaviruse/situation-reports/20200329-sitrep-69-covid-19.pdf?sfvrsn=8d6620fa_8 (Accessed on 10 April 2021).
3. Alok Pandey and Manish Kumar, ndtv.com, 18 April 2020, '"Injustice to Lockdown" Says Nitish Kumar on Buses for Students.' https://www.ndtv.com/india-news/injustice-nitish-kumar-on-up-sending-buses-to-evacuate-students-amid-lockdown-2213696 (Accessed on 10 April 2021).
4. Ibid.
5. Ministry of Home Affairs, Order Number 40-3/2020-DM-I (A), 29 April 2020. https://www.mha.gov.in/sites/default/files/MHAordernew_29042020.PDF (Accessed on 10 April 2021).

6. Sukhbir Siwach, *The Indian Express*, 30 April 2020, 'Rajasthan Starts Sending Stranded Migrant Labourers Back to Haryana in Buses.' https://indianexpress.com/article/india/rajasthan-starts-sending-stranded-migrant-labourers-back-to-haryana-in-buses-6387825/ (Accessed on 10 April 2021).
7. DGP Haryana Police (@DGHaryana) Tweet, 15 January 2021. https://twitter.com/DGPHaryana/status/1350018623633457161?s=20 (Accessed on 10 April 2021).
8. Interview with Usha Kundu.
9. Bagish Jha, *The Times of India*, 30 May 2020, 'Haryana: 3.5 Lakh Registered to Leave from Gurugram, 40,000 Took Trains, Buses.' https://timesofindia.indiatimes.com/city/gurgaon/3-5-lakh-registered-to-leave-from-gurgaon-40k-took-trains-buses/articleshow/76100328.cms (Accessed on 10 April 2021).
10. Ministry of Home Affairs, Order Number 40-3/2020-DM-I (A), 1 May 2020. https://www.mha.gov.in/sites/default/files/Orderdated01052020.pdf (Accessed on 10 April 2021).
11. news18.com, 30 April 2020, 'Seven States Oppose Govt Plan to Send Migrant Workers by Bus as Impractical, Say Process Could Take Months.' https://www.news18.com/news/india/states-seek-special-non-stop-trains-to-facilitate-return-of-migrant-workers-2599997.html (Accessed on 11 April 2021).
12. Press Information Bureau, Release ID: 202717, 1 May 2020. https://archive.pib.gov.in/newsite/PrintRelease.aspx?relid=202717 (Accessed on 11 April 2021).
13. HT Correspondent, *Hindustan Times*, 3 May 2020, '54 Passengers Per Coach, Non-stop Run: All You Need to Know About "Shramik Express" Trains.' https://www.hindustantimes.com/india-news/54-passengers-per-coach-non-stop-run-all-you-need-to-know-about-shramik-express-trains/story-WZqYPHBYXQCCFx4G753N3O.html (Accessed on 11 April 2021).
14. Ibid.
15. Interview with Seemant Singh.
16. Press Information Bureau, Press Release ID: 1620532, 2 May 2020. https://pib.gov.in/PressReleasePage.aspx?PRID=1620532 (Accessed on 11 April 2021).

17. Press Information Bureau, Press Release ID: 1622664, 10 May 2020. https://pib.gov.in/PressReleasePage.aspx?PRID=1622664 (Accessed on 11 April 2021).
18. Press Information Bureau, Press Release ID: 1622963, 11 May 2020. https://pib.gov.in/PressReleasePage.aspx?PRID=1622963 (Accessed on 11 April 2021).
19. Press Information Bureau, Press Release ID: 1626187, 22 May 2020. https://pib.gov.in/PressReleasePage.aspx?PRID=1626187 (Accessed on 11 April 2021).
20. Shine Jacob, *Business Standard*, 12 May 2020, 'IRCTC Site Starts with 2-hour Lag; Howrah-Delhi Tickets Gone in 10 Minutes.' https://www.business-standard.com/article/current-affairs/gone-in-just-10-min-irctc-site-starts-with-a-lag-but-not-tickets-sale-120051101374_1.html (Accessed on 11 April 2021).
21. Press Information Bureau, Press Release ID: 1625228, 19 May 2021. https://pib.gov.in/PressReleasePage.aspx?PRID=1625228 (Accessed on 11 April 2021).
22. Congress (@INCIndia) Tweet, 4 May 2020. https://twitter.com/INCIndia/status/1257140652913000448?s=20 (Accessed on 11 April 2021).
23. Shine Jacob, *Business Standard*, 4 May 2020, 'Railway Board in a Huddle as Congress Offers to Pay for Travel of Migrants.' https://www.business-standard.com/article/current-affairs/raliway-board-in-a-huddle-after-cong-offers-to-pay-for-travel-of-migrants-120050400354_1.html (Accessed on 11 April 2021).
24. Railway Board letter No. TC-11/2020/Spl Trains-Covid-19, dated 1.05.2020.
25. No. DTP/2020/05/17 Principal Executive Director (Coaching), Railway Board to General Managers of zonal railways, chief secretaries and administrators of states/union territories.
26. Express Webdesk, *The Indian Express*, 4 May 2020, 'Students Won't Have to Pay Train Fare; Migrants to Get Full Reimbursement: Bihar CM Nitish Kumar.' https://indianexpress.com/article/india/bihar-migrants-train-fare-students-lockdown-6393474/ (Accessed on 11 April 2021).

27. Interview with Ekdashi Kumar.
28. RTI Reply No. TC-II/MORLY/R/E/21/01183 dated 30 March 2021.
29. Press Information Bureau, Press Release ID: 1623773, 14 May 2020. https://pib.gov.in/PressReleasePage.aspx?PRID=1623773 (Accessed on 11 April 2021).
30. ANI Video, 15 May 2020, 'Several States Aren't Giving Permission for "Shramik" Trains Which Pains Me: Piyush Goyal.' https://fb.watch/9xZuV86SrG/ (Accessed on 12 April 2021).
31. Press Information Bureau, Press Release ID: 1624541, 16 May 2020. https://pib.gov.in/PressReleasePage.aspx?PRID=1624541 (Accessed on 12 April 2021).
32. Ministry of Home Affairs, Order Number 40-3/2020-DM-I (A), 19 May 2020. https://www.mha.gov.in/sites/default/files/MHA%20Order%20Dt.%2019.5.2020%20reg.%20revised%20SoPs%20on%20movement%20of%20stranded%20workers%20by%20trains.pdf (Accessed on 11 April 2021).
33. Express News Service, *The Indian Express*, 25 May 2020, 'Maharashtra: War of Words between Govt, Railways over Shramik Trains.' https://indianexpress.com/article/cities/mumbai/maharashtra-war-of-words-between-govt-railways-over-shramik-trains-6425651/ (Accessed on 11 April 2021).
34. Piyush Goyal (@PiyushGoyal) Tweet, 24 May 2020. https://twitter.com/PiyushGoyal/status/1264552758016761857?s=20 (Accessed on 11 April 2021).
35. Piyush Goyal (@PiyushGoyal) Tweet, 25 May 2020. https://twitter.com/PiyushGoyal/status/1264657825705259008?s=20 (Accessed on 11 April 2021).
36. Nitish Chandra, indiatvnews.com, 27 May 2020, 'Hearthbreaking Videos of Toddler Trying to Wake Dead Mother Brings out Hardships of Migrant Workers.' https://www.indiatvnews.com/news/india/heartbreaking-video-bihar-muzaffarpur-child-waking-dead-mother-migrant -workers-621002 (Accessed on 11 April 2021).

37. Press Information Bureau, Press Release ID: 16727561, 29 May 2020. https://pib.gov.in/PressReleasePage.aspx?PRID=1627561 (Accessed on 11 April 2021).
38. Anisha Dutta, *Hindustan Times*, 30 May 2020, 'Railway Protection Force Reports 80 Deaths on Shramik Trains.' https://www.hindustantimes.com/india-news/railway-protection-force-reports-80-deaths-on-shramik-trains/story-psJl3EenY4B0uUYMRvkChL.html (Accessed on 11 April 2021).
39. Press Trust of India, livemint.com, 24 May 2020, 'Shramik Special: "Horror Trip" Ends, Diverted Train Finally Reaches Gorakhpur.' https://www.livemint.com/news/india/shramik-special-horror-trip-ends-diverted-train-finally-reaches-gorakhpur-11590333359166.html (Accessed on 11 April 2021).
40. Press Information Bureau, Press Release ID: 1627722, 29 May 2020. https://pib.gov.in/PressReleseDetailm.aspx?PRID=1627722 (Accessed on 11 April 2021).
41. Press Information Bureau, Press Release ID: 1627493, 28 May 2020. https://pib.gov.in/PressReleasePage.aspx?PRID=1627493 (Accessed on 11 April 2021).
42. Shine Jacob, *Business Standard*, 30 May 2020, 'Rly Food Stalls Seek Force Majeure Extension Citing Rioting, Unviable Biz.' https://www.business-standard.com/article/current-affairs/rly-food-stalls-seek-force-majeure-extension-citing-rioting-unviable-biz-120053000467_1.html (Accessed on 22 June 2021).
43. Economic Survey 2021, Volume II, Chapter 01.
44. Indian Railways, 2021, Monthly Evaluation Report for February 2021. https://indianrailways.gov.in/railwayboard/uploads/directorate/stat_econ/2021/MER-Feb21.pdf (Accessed on 22 June 2021).
45. Press Information Bureau, Press Release ID: 1655124, 16 September 2020. https://pib.gov.in/PressReleasePage.aspx?PRID=1655124 (Accessed on 22 June 2021).
46. IRCTC press release dated 7 October 2020.
47. IRCTC press release dated 23 November 2020.
48. IRCTC press release dated 29 January 2021.

49. Bombay Stock Exchange filing, 26 April 2021, 'Temporary Suspension of Operation of Train No. 82901-02, ADI-MMCT-ADI Tejas Express Till 30th June, 2021.' https://www.bseindia.com/xml-data/corpfiling/AttachHis/5618318f-ded6-452d-815a-f730a85342aa.pdf (Accessed 22 June 2021).
50. Press Information Bureau, Press Release ID: 1700491, 24 February 2021. https://pib.gov.in/PressReleasePage.aspx?PRID=1700491 (Accessed on 22 June 2021).
51. Railway Board, 'COVID-19 Review of HSP Fare,' 12 November 2021. https://digitalscr.in/bzadiv/circulars/misc_circulars/uploads/Operation_train_services_shortly.pdf (Accessed on 28 November 2021).
52. Railway Board, Monthly Evaluation Reports of October 2021 and October 2019. https://indianrailways.gov.in/railwayboard/uploads/directorate/stat_econ/2021/MER-Oct-21.pdf https://indianrailways.gov.in/railwayboard/uploads/directorate/stat_econ/MTHSTAT/2019/MER_Oct_2019.pdf (Accessed on 28 November 2021).

8: TAKING OFF AGAIN WITH A BUBBLE AND MORE

1. Director General of Civil Aviation, Government of India, Circular number 4/1/2020-IR, 21 May 2020. https://www.dgca.gov.in/digigovportal/jsp/dgca/homePage/viewPDF.jsp?page=topHeader/COVID/Circular%2021.5.2020.pdf (Accessed on 18 April 2021).
2. Pranav Mukul & Anil Sasi, *The Indian Express*, 23 May 2020, 'Explained: Why the Govt Changed Its Mind in Just Three Days and Allowed Flights.' https://indianexpress.com/article/explained/why-the-govt-changed-its-mind-in-just-three-days-and-allowed-flights-6421673/ (Accessed on 18 April 2021).
3. Purva Chitnis, ndtv.com, 24 May 2020, 'No Passenger Flights For Now, Next 15 Days Crucial, Says Uddhav Thackeray.' https://www.ndtv.com/india-news/uddhav-thackeray-says-spoke-with-

aviation-minister-we-need-more-time-to-prepare-for-resuming-flights-2234285 (Accessed on 18 April 2021).

4. Ministry of Civil Aviation, Government of India, State-wise Quarantine Regulations. https://www.civilaviation.gov.in/sites/default/files/State_wise_quarantine_regulation-converted.pdf (Accessed on 18 April 2021).
5. Ministry of Civil Aviation, Government of India, Office Memorandum, 29 June 2020. https://www.civilaviation.gov.in/sites/default/files/MoCA_OM_dated_29_06_2020.pdf (Accessed on 18 April 2021).
6. Ministry of Civil Aviation, Government of India, Order dated 21 May 2020. https://www.civilaviation.gov.in/sites/default/files/Order_of_MoCA_dated_21st_May_2020.pdf (Accessed on 18 April 2021).
7. Ministry of Civil Aviation, Government of India, 21 May 2020, Guidelines for Air Passengers. https://www.civilaviation.gov.in/sites/default/files/Guidelines_for_Air_Passengers_21May.pdf (Accessed on 18 April 2021).
8. Ministry of Civil Aviation, Government of India, Order Number 01/2020, 21 May 2020. https://www.civilaviation.gov.in/sites/default/files/DOC052220-05222020133918.pdf (Accessed on 18 April 2021).
   https://www.dgca.gov.in/digigov-portal/jsp/dgca/homePage/viewPDF.jsp?page=topHeader/COVID/Circular%2021.05.2020.pdf
9. Ministry of Civil Aviation, Addendum, 25 May 2020. https://www.civilaviation.gov.in/sites/default/files/Addendum_to_Order_02_2020.pdf (Accessed on 18 April 2021).
10. Hardeep Singh Puri (@HardeepSPuri) Tweet, 23 August 2020. https://twitter.com/HardeepSPuri/status/1297433841833881600?s=20 (Accessed on 18 April 2021).
11. Ministry of Civil Aviation, Government of India, Order Number 11/2020 dated 3 December 2020. https://www.civilaviation.gov.in/sites/default/files/DOC120320-12032020182905.pdf (Accessed on 18 April 2021).

12. Anisha Dutta, *Hindustan Times*, 28 May 2021, 'Govt Cuts Seating Capacity in Domestic Flights to 50%, Fares Could Go Up.' https://www.hindustantimes.com/india-news/govt-cuts-seating-capacity-in-domestic-flights-to-50-fares-could-go-up-101622226192664.html (Accessed on 22 June 2021).
13. Ministry of Civil Aviation, Government of India, 14 June 2021, Detailed Monthly Information for the Month of May 2021. https://www.civilaviation.gov.in/sites/default/files/monthly%20 summary-06172021114841.pdf (Accessed on 22 June 2021).
14. Press Information Bureau, Press Release ID: 1701648, 1 March 2021. https://pib.gov.in/PressReleasePage.aspx?PRID=1701648 (Accessed on 22 June 2021).
15. Unstarred Lok Sabha question number 5012, answered on 25 March 2021. http://loksabhaph.nic.in/Questions/QResult15.aspx?qref=24059&lsno=17 (Accessed on 22 June 2021).
16. Unstarred Lok Sabha question number 5038, answered on 25 March 2021. http://loksabhaph.nic.in/Questions/QResult15.aspx?qref=24064&lsno=17 (Accessed on 22 June 2021).
17. Neha Tripathi, *Hindustan Times*, 13 October 2021, 'Domestic Flights to Operate at 100% Capacity from Oct 18.' https://www.hindustantimes.com/india-news/domestic-flights-to-operate-at-100-capacity-from-oct-18-101634076334390.html (Accessed on 30 November 2021).
18. Press Trust of India, *Business Standard*, 27 February 2020, 'Coronavirus: IAF Aircraft Brings 76 Indians, 36 Foreigners from Wuhan' https://www.business-standard.com/article/pti-stories/iaf-aircraft-brings-back-76-indians-36-foreigners-from-china-s-coronavirus-hit-wuhan-120022700156_1.html (Accessed on 19 April 2021).
19. ET Online and Agencies, economictimes.indiatimes.com, 7 May 2020, 'First Two Air India Flights of Vande Bharat Mission Land in Kerala.' https://economictimes.indiatimes.com/news/politics-and-nation/first-two-air-india-flights-of-vande-bharat-mission-land-in-kerala/

articleshow/75610241.cms?utm_source=contentofinterest&utm_medium=text&utm_campaign=cppst (Accessed on 19 April 2021).

20. Lok Sabha unstarred question number 1729, answered on 21 September 2020. http://164.100.24.220/loksabhaquestions/annex/174/AU1729.pdf (Accessed on 19 April 2021).
21. Fang Liu, Secretary General, International Civil Organization, 15 April 2020, Letter Reference: EC 6/3 – 20/55. https://www.icao.int/safety/Covid-19OPS/Documents/055e.pdf (Accessed on 19 April 2021).
22. Ministry of Home Affairs, Government of India, 5 May 2020, Order Number 40-3/2020-DM-I (A). https://www.mha.gov.in/sites/default/files/4MHA%20SOPs%20Dt.%205.5.2020%20reg%20movement%20of%20Indian%20nationals%20stranded%20outside%20the%20country%20and%20of%20specified%20perso-ns%20to%20travel%20abroad.pdf (Accessed on 19 April 2021).
23. Ministry of Health and Family Welfare, Government of India, 24 May 2020, Office Memorandum, FNo Z.28015/19/2020-EMR (Pt). https://www.mha.gov.in/sites/default/files/MHAOrderDt24052020forspecifiedpersonstotravelabroad.pdf (Accessed on 19 April 2021).
24. Ramesh Babu, Anisha Dutta, Anvit Srivastava and Neha LM Tripathi, *Hindustan Times*, 8 August 2020, '20 Dead in Kerala as Repatriation Flight Skids Off Runway, Breaks in Two.' https://www.hindustantimes.com/india-news/vande-flight-with-190-on-board-skids-off-runway-breaks-into-2/story-id2Sqz17JWy6bOHBOac0FL.html (Accessed on 19 April 2021).
25. Ramesh Babu, Anisha Dutta, Anvit Srivastava and Neha LM Tripathi, *Hindustan Times*, 8 August 2020, '20 Dead in Kerala as Repatriation Flight Skids Off Runway, Breaks in Two.' https://www.hindustantimes.com/india-news/vande-flight-with-190-on-board-skids-off-runway-breaks-into-2/story-id2Sqz17JWy6bOHBOac0FL.html (Accessed on 19 April 2021).
26. Ministry of Civil Aviation, Government of India, About Air Transport Bubbles. https://www.civilaviation.gov.in/en/about-air-transport-bubbles (Accessed on 19 April 2021).

27. Saurab Sinha, *Times of India*, 24 June 2020, 'UAE Says No Passengers on Vande Bharat Flights to Dubai, Its Airline Seeks Nods to Operate Charters from India.' https://timesofindia.indiatimes.com/business/india-business/uae-says-no-passengers-on-repatriation-flights-to-dubai-specific-nod-of-mission-needed-to-do-so-ai/articleshow/76548305.cms (Accessed on 19 April 2021).
28. Hardeep Singh Puri (@HardeepSPuri) Tweet, 17 July 2020. https://twitter.com/HardeepSPuri/status/1283832547508490240?s=20 (Accessed on 19 April 2021).
29. Saurab Sinha, *Times of India*, 24 June 2020, 'UAE Says No Passengers on Vande Bharat Flights to Dubai, Its Airline Seeks Nods to Operate Charters from India.' https://timesofindia.indiatimes.com/business/india-business/uae-says-no-passengers-on-repatriation-flights-to-dubai-specific-nod-of-mission-needed-to-do-so-ai/articleshow/76548305.cms (Accessed on 19 April 2021).
30. Jüri Ratas (@ratasjuri) Tweet, 6 May 2020. https://twitter.com/ratasjuri/status/1257960686489161733?s=20 (Accessed on 20 April 2021).
31. Lativian Public Broadcasting, 14 May 2020, 'What You Need to Know About the "Baltic Bubble" Travel Rules.' https://eng.lsm.lv/article/economy/transport/what-you-need-to-know-about-the-baltic-bubble-travel-rules.a359869/ (Accessed on 19 April 2021).
32. apnews.com, 11 September 2020, 'Latvia Bursts Baltic Travel Bubble as COVID19 Cases Surge.' https://apnews.com/article/estonia-denmark-latvia-travel-virus-outbreak-d1822eaeb66d3ff28514878b83f7f6a9 (Accessed on 19 April 2021).
33. The Government of Hong Kong Special Administrative Region, Press Releases, 11 November 2020, 'Designated Flights under HK-Singapore Air Travel Bubble to Launch November 22.' https://www.info.gov.hk/gia/general/202011/11/P2020111100217.htm (Accessed on 19 April 2021).
34. The Government of Hong Kong Special Administrative Region, Press Releases, 21 November 2020, 'Inaugural Flights under HK-Singapore Air Travel Bubble Deferred for Two Weeks.' https://www.info.gov.

hk/gia/general/202011/21/P2020112100656.htm (Accessed on 19 April 2021).

35. Denise Tsang and Phila Siu, *South China Morning Post*, 31 March 2021, 'Coronavirus: Hong Kong's Travel Bubble Hopes for Singapore, Australia and Beyond Depend on Pandemic Control, Vaccination Rate.' https://www.scmp.com/news/hong-kong/hong-kong-economy/article/3127677/coronavirus-hong-kongs-plans-restart-travel (Accessed on 19 April 2021)
36. Reuters Staff, *Reuters*, 6 April 2021, 'New Zealand-Australia Travel Bubble to Start on April 19.' https://www.reuters.com/article/us-health-coronavirus-newzealand-austral-idUSKBN2BT0B7?taid=606bf1dec8c94b0001857549&utm_campaign=trueanthem&utm_medium=trueanthem&utm_source=twitter (Accessed on 19 April 2021).
37. Press Trust of India, theprint.in, 8 April 2021, 'New Zealand Suspends Entry of Travelers from India as 17 Test Positive for Covid.' https://theprint.in/diplomacy/new-zealand-suspends-entry-of-travellers-from-india-as-17-test-positive-for-covid/636199/ (Accessed on 19 April 2021).
38. Ministry of external affairs; Rajya Sabha unstarred question number 564, answered on 17 September 2020.
39. Ministry of Civil Aviation, Government of India, 21 June 2021, Total number of Vande Bharat flights. https://www.civilaviation.gov.in/sites/default/files/flights_and_flawn-21-6-2021.pdf (Accessed on 22 June 2021).
40. Office of the Director General of Civil Aviation, 21 December 2020, Circular regarding temporary suspension of flights from United Kingdom to India. http://www.airindia.in/images/pdf/UK_circular_21-12-2020.pdf (Accessed on 22 June 2021).
41. Office of the Director General of Civil Aviation, Ministry of Civil Aviation, Government of India, 26 November 2021, Circular: Resumption of scheduled commercial international passenger services to/from India. https://www.dgca.gov.in/digigov-portal/Upload?flag=iframeAttachView&attachId=150798370 (Accessed on 1 December 2021).

42. WHO statement, 26 November 2021, Classification of Omicron (B.1.1.529): SARS-CoV-2 Variant of Concern. https://www.who.int/news/item/26-11-2021-classification-of-omicron-(b.1.1.529)-sars-cov-2-variant-of-concern (Accessed on 1 December 2021).
43. Special Correspondent, *The Hindu*, 27 November 2021, 'Omicron COVID-19 Variant—Review Plan to Start All International Flights: PM.' https://www.thehindu.com/news/national/omicron-covid-19-variant-review-plan-to-start-all-international-flights-narendra-modi/article37717858.ece (Accessed on 1 December 2021).
44. Office of the Director General of Civil Aviation, Ministry of Civil Aviation, Government of India, 1 December 2021 circular. https://www.dgca.gov.in/digigov-portal/Upload?flag=iframeAttachView&attachId=150807818 (Accessed on 1 December 2021).

9: THE WEB OF INTERSTATE TRAVEL

1. ourworldindata.org, COVID-19: Stay at Home Restrictions https://ourworldindata.org/grapher/covid-stringency-index?stackMode=absolute&time=2020-03-25&region=World (Accessed on 28 April 2021).
2. Press Information Bureau, Daily Bulletin on COVID-19, Press Release ID: 1628374, 1 June 2020. https://pib.gov.in/PressReleasePage.aspx?PRID=1628374 (Accessed on 28 April 2021).
3. WHO, 2 June 2020, Situation Report-134. https://www.who.int/docs/default-source/coronaviruse/situation-reports/20200602-covid-19-sitrep-134.pdf?sfvrsn=cc95e5d5_2 (Accessed on 28 April 2021).
4. Ministry of Home Affairs, Government of India, 30 May 2020, Order Number: 40-3/2020-DM-I (A). https://www.mha.gov.in/sites/default/files/MHAOrderDt_30052020.pdf (Accessed on 28 April 2021).
5. Ministry of Home Affairs, Government of India, 19 April 2020, Order Number: 40-10/2020-DM-I (A). https://www.mha.gov.in/sites/default/files/WestBengal_20042020.pdf (Accessed on 28 April 2021).

6. Press Information Bureau, 20 April 2020, 'Central Government Constitutes Six Inter-Ministerial Teams to Make Assessment of Situation and Augment State Efforts to Fight and Contain Spread of COVID-19 Effectively.' https://www.mha.gov.in/sites/default/files/press_20042020_0.pdf (Accessed on 28 April 2021).
7. Government of West Bengal, 30 May 2020, Memo Number 218-CS/2020. https://wb.gov.in/Covid-19/Lockdown_30may.pdf (Accessed on 28 April 2021).
8. Shiv Sahay Singh, *The Hindu*, 21 July 2020, 'West Bengal to Have Two-Day Lockdown Every Week.' https://www.thehindu.com/news/cities/kolkata/wb-to-have-two-day-lockdown-every-week/article32143818.ece (Accessed on 28 April 2021).
9. Government of Tamil Nadu, 31 May 2020, Revenue and Disaster Management (DM-II) Department GO.Ms.No.262. https://cms.tn.gov.in/sites/default/files/go/revenue_e_262_2020.pdf (Accessed on 28 April 2021).
10. Government of Tamil Nadu, 31 July 2020, Revenue and Disaster Management (DM-II) Department GO (Ms) No 396. https://cms.tn.gov.in/sites/default/files/go/revenue_e_396_2020.pdf (Accessed on 28 April 2021).
11. Government of Himachal Pradesh, March 2021, Executive Summary, Economic Survey 2020-21. https://himachalservices.nic.in/economics/pdf/Economic_Survey_eng2020-21.pdf (Accessed on 28 April 2021).
12. National Health Mission Himachal Pradesh, 1 June 2020, File No NHMHP-IDSP/1/2020. http://covidorders.hp.gov.in/frontend/web/writeData/Shimla/bcf4788c69e56aa5e5233801f5c37f563ee29651.pdf (Accessed on 28 April 2021).
13. Himachal Pradesh government, 2 July 2020, Revenue Department (Disaster Management Cell) (C) 20-2/2020-Covid-19. https://himachaltourism.gov.in/wp-content/uploads/2020/07/ORDER-Guidelines-of-Unlock-2-Revenue-Department-DM-Cell.pdf (Accessed on 29 April 2021).

14. Order issued by Ashish Kumar Srivastava, District Magistrate, Dehradun, 4 June 2020. https://health.uk.gov.in/files/1234.pdf (Accessed on 29 April 2021).
15. Health Bulletin of Uttarakhand State Control Room, 4 June 2020. https://health.uk.gov.in/files/2020.06.04_Health_Bulletin.pdf (Accessed on 29 April 2021).
16. Uttarakhand chief secretary Utpal Kumar Singh's letter, 8 June 2020, serial number 285/USDMA/792 (2020). https://health.uk.gov.in/files/CamScanner_06-08-2020_23.03.59.pdf (Accessed on 29 April 2021).
17. Uttarakhand chief secretary's Om Prakash letter, 19 September 2020, serial number 625/USDMA/792(2020). https://health.uk.gov.in/files/Rivised_order_covind-19_unlock-4_1.pdf (Accessed on 29 April 2021).
18. Uttarakhand chief secretary Om Prakash's letter, 1 October 2020, serial number 663/USDMA/792(2020). https://health.uk.gov.in/files/Adobe_Scan_01_Oct_2020_2.pdf (Accessed on 29 April 2021).
19. Union home secretary Ajay Bhalla's letter, 12 June 2020, DO No 40-10/2020-DM-I (A). https://www.mha.gov.in/sites/default/files/MHADOChiefSecretaries_12062020.pdf (Accessed on 29 April 2021).
20. Ministry of Home Affairs, Government of India, 29 June 2020, Order number 40-3/2020-DM-I (A). https://www.mha.gov.in/sites/default/files/MHAOrder_29062020.pdf (Accessed on 29 April 2021).
21. Ministry of Home Affairs, Government of India, 29 June 2020, DO number 40-3/2020-DM-I (A). https://www.mha.gov.in/sites/default/files/MHADOLr_29062020.pdf (Accessed on 29 April 2021).
22. Ministry of Home Affairs, Government of India, 29 July 2020, Order number 40-3-2020-DM-I (A). https://www.mha.gov.in/sites/default/files/Unlock3_29072020.pdf (Accessed on 29 April 2021).
23. Ministry of Home Affairs, Government of India, 29 August 2020, Oder number 40-3/2020-DM-I (A). https://www.mha.gov.in/sites/default/files/MHAOrder_Unlock4_29082020.pdf (Accessed on 29 April 2021).

24. Siddharth Tiwari, *Times of India*, 1 March 20201, 'No Buses, Girls in Nuh Forced to Pool Money for Auto, Hitchhike to school.' https://timesofindia.indiatimes.com/city/gurgaon/no-buses-girls-in-nuh-forced-to-pool-money-for-auto-hitchhike-to-school/articleshow/81263276.cms (Accessed on 29 April 2021).
25. Press Information Bureau, Press Release ID: 1684156, 28 December 2020. https://pib.gov.in/PressReleasePage.aspx?PRID=1684156 (Accessed on 29 April 2021).
26. Home secretary Ajay Bhalla's letter, 19 March 2021, DO number 40-34/2020-DM-I(A). https://www.mha.gov.in/sites/default/files/DOtoCSandAdministrators_19032021.pdf (Accessed on 29 April 2021).
27. Home secretary Ajay Bhalla's letter, 26 March 2021, Number 40-34/2020-DM-I (A). https://www.mha.gov.in/sites/default/files/DOAdministrators_26032021.pdf (Accessed on 29 April 2021).

10: LIFTING OF THE METRO GATES

1. DMRC Office Order Number PP/3026/2020.
2. Jyoti Mukul and Megha Manchanda, *Business Standard*, 17 August 2020, 'All Retail Outlets on Metro Premises Say They Can't Pay Us: Delhi Metro MD.' https://www.business-standard.com/article/current-affairs/all-retail-outlets-on-metro-premises-say-they-can-t-pay-us-delhi-metro-md-120081600543_1.html (Accessed on 30 April 2021).
3. Delhi Metro Rail Corporation Annual Report 2019-20. http://www.delhimetrorail.com/OtherDocuments/DMRC-English-Annual-Report-2019-20.pdf (Accessed on 30 June 2021).
4. DMRC reply to Right to Information application, 27 May 2021.
5. Megha Manchanda and Amritha Pillay, *Business Standard*, 21 August 2020, 'Pvt Metro Systems Suffer Revenue Loss, DMRC Cuts 'Non-essential' Costs.' https://www.business-standard.com/article/companies/pvt-metro-systems-suffer-revenue-loss-as-dmrc-cuts-non-essential-costs-120082000841_1.html (Accessed on 30 April 2021).

6. Special Correspondent, *The Hindu*, 14 September 2020, 'Kolkata Metro to Resume Services from Today.' https://www.thehindu.com/news/cities/kolkata/kolkata-metro-to-resume-services-from-today/article32595696.ece (Accessed on 30 April 2021).
7. Lok Sabha Unstarred Question Number 875, answered on 17 September 2020. http://164.100.24.220/loksabhaquestions/annex/174/AU875.pdf (Accessed on 30 April 2021).
8. Delhi Metro Rail Corporation press release, 6 September 2020, 'Delhi Metro Ready to Resume Its Service after 169 days.' http://www.delhimetrorail.com/PressReleaseDocuments/PRESS-RELEASE-06092020.pdf (Accessed on 30 April 2021).
9. Delhi Metro Rail Corporation Press Release, 10 September 2020, 'Metro Services on Last Major Line to Resume from Tomorrow; Operational Timings to Be Also Extended.' http://www.delhimetrorail.com/PressReleaseDocuments/PRESS-RELEASE-10092020.pdf (Accessed on 30 April 2021).
10. Megha Manchanda & Amritha Pillay, *Business Standard*, 16 September 2020, 'All Delhi Metro Lines Operational But Ridership Just a Fraction of Earlier.' https://www.business-standard.com/article/current-affairs/all-delhi-metro-lines-operational-but-ridership-just-a-fraction-of-earlier-120091500817_1.html (Accessed on 30 April 2021).
11. Express News Service, *The Indian Express*, 20 November 2021, 'DDMA Nod to 30 Standing Passengers per Coach in Delhi Metro.' https://indianexpress.com/article/cities/delhi/ddma-nod-to-30-standing-passengers-per-coach-in-delhi-metro-7633329/ (Accessed on 2 December 2021).
12. ANI, economictimes.indiatimes.com, 19 October 2020, 'Mumbai Metro Services Resume in Graded Manner.' https://economictimes.indiatimes.com/industry/transportation/railways/watch-mumbai-metro-services-resume-in-graded-manner/videoshow/78744874.cms (Accessed on 30 April 2021).
13. Manthan K Mehta, *The Times of India*, 21 March 2021, 'Mumbai: Metro to increase total number of services to 280 from Monday.'

https://timesofindia.indiatimes.com/city/mumbai/mumbai-metro-to-increase-total-number-of-service-to-280-from-monday/articleshow/81618418.cms?utm_source=twitter.com&utm_medium=social&utm_campaign=TOIMumbaiNews (Accessed on 30 April 2021).

14. Western Railway, 28 January 2021, Press Release Number 2021/01. https://wr.indianrailways.gov.in/view_detail.jsp?lang=0&id=0,4,268&dcd=5722&did=1611838678979697 83B97451BC2D650D5F620EC9626B7 (Accessed on 30 April 2021).
15. Piyush Goyal (@PiyushGoyal) Tweet, 20 October 2020. https://twitter.com/PiyushGoyal/status/1318514139136815104?s=20 (Accessed on 30 April 2021).
16. Piyush Goyal (@PiyushGoyal) Tweet, 12 February 2021. https://twitter.com/PiyushGoyal/status/1360148757841641474?s=20 (Accessed on 30 April 2021).
17. Press Trust of India, *Hindustan Times*, 8 November 2020, 'Railways to Run 696 Suburban Services in West Bengal from Nov 11.' https://www.hindustantimes.com/india-news/railways-to-run-696-suburban-services-in-west-bengal-from-nov-11/story-8IAZPaBFByOgUZWLXxDB5I.html#:~:text=The%20Railways%20will%20run%20696,due%20to%20the%20coronavirus%20outbreak. (Accessed on 30 April 2021).
18. MyGovIndia (mygovindia) Tweet, 19 April 2021. https://twitter.com/mygovindia/status/1384118415204372489?s=20 A (Accessed on 30 April 2021).
19. Delhi Metro Rail Corporation statement, 9 May 2021. http://www.delhimetrorail.com/press_reldetails.aspx?id=MrdFgJyXYRMlld (Accessed on 30 April 2021).

11: THIS TIME NO ONE WALKING

1. Department of Revenue and Forest, Disaster Management, Relief and Rehabilitation, Government of Maharashtra, 4 April 2021, Order number: DMU/2020/CR. 92/DisM-1. https://www.

maharashtra.gov.in/Site/Upload/Government%20Resolutions/Marathi/202104051005324619.pdf (Accessed on 7 May 2021).

2. Laxman Singh, Tabassum Barnagarwala and Jayprakash S. Naidu, *The Indian Express*, 5 April 2021, 'Mumbai: With New Curbs, Migrants Consider Going Home, Fear Stopping of Trains.' https://indianexpress.com/article/cities/mumbai/mumbai-with-new-curbs-migrants-consider-going-home-fear-stopping-of-trains-7258952/ (Accessed on 7 May 2021).
3. Ashok Kumar, Anuj Kumar and Shinjini Ghosh, *The Hindu*, 13 April 2021, 'Crowds Reappear at Transport Hubs, But Not Out of Lockdown Fear.' https://www.thehindu.com/news/cities/Delhi/crowds-reappear-at-transport-hubs-but-not-out-of-lockdown-fear/article34306324.ece (Accessed on 8 May 20221).
4. Delhi Disaster Management Authority, Government of NCT of Delhi, 15 April 2021, Order 373. http://ddma.delhigovt.nic.in/wps/wcm/connect/DOIT_DM/dm/home/covid-19/orders+of+ddma+on+covid+19/order+373 (Accessed on 8 May 20221).
5. Delhi Disaster Management Authority, Government of NCT of Delhi, 19 April 2021, Order 381. http://ddma.delhigovt.nic.in/wps/wcm/connect/DOIT_DM/dm/home/covid-19/orders+of+ddma+on+covid+19/order+381 (Accessed on 8 May 20221).
6. hindustantimes.com, 20 April 2021, 'Migrant Workers Start Leaving Delhi, Say Kejriwal Should've Given More Time Before Announcing Lockdown.' https://www.hindustantimes.com/cities/delhi-news/migrant-workers-say-kejriwal-should-ve-given-more-time-before-declaring-lockdown-101618884796305.html (Accessed on 8 May 2021).
7. Mahender Singh Manral, *The Indian Express*, 19 April 2021, 'Deal with Migrant Workers Tactfully to Prevent Exodus: Advisory to Officers.' https://indianexpress.com/article/cities/delhi/counsel-migrant-workers-and-send-them-back-home-or-to-shelters-if-they-start-moving-out-of-delhi-police-7278723/ (Accessed on 8 May 2021).

8. Government of Madhya Pradesh, 29 April 2021, Order Number 0141/administration/Transport Commissioner/21.
9. Ranjan, *Hindustan Times*, 4 May 2020, 'Thousands of Migrants Made to Wait in Madhya Pradesh as UP Shuts Border.' https://www.hindustantimes.com/india-news/thousands-of-migrants-made-to-wait-in-madhya-pradesh-as-up-shuts-border/story-QICTsKo7vjLA8XIT0onNJP.html (Accessed on 8 May 2021).
10. Interview with Jitendra Yadav.
11. Shally Seth Mohile, *Business Standard*, 30 April 2021, 'Auto Firms to Halt Production for up to 15 Days Amid Raging Second Wave.' https://www.business-standard.com/article/companies/auto-firms-to-halt-production-for-up-to-15-days-amid-raging-second-wave-121042901430_1.html (Accessed on 9 May 2021).
12. Leena Dhankhar and Abhishek Behl, *Hindustan Times*, 15 May 2021, Caught in Lockdown, Thousands of Workers in Gurugram Have Nowhere to Go.
https://www.hindustantimes.com/cities/gurugram-news/caught-in-lockdown-thousands-of-workers-in-gurugram-have-nowhere-to-go-101621078504052.html (Accessed on 20 June 2021).
13. Special report of Delhi Transport Department, on transport arrangements for migrants wanting to leave Delhi to go to their native places on commencement of lockdown from 19 April 2021 during the second surge of Covid-19; Government of NCT; May 2021.
14. Suo Motu Write Petition (Civil) No 6/2020 in RE: Problems and Miseries of Migrant Labourers, 13 May 2021, Record of Proceedings. https://main.sci.gov.in/supremecourt/2020/11706/11706_2020_36_1_28023_Order_13-May-2021.pdf (Accessed on 15 May 2021).
15. Footnote 13.
16. Delhi Disaster Management Authority, Government of NCT of Delhi, 6 May 2021, Order (HQ)/Misc Matters/COVID/411. http://ddma.delhigovt.nic.in/wps/wcm/connect/DOIT_DM/dm/home/covid-19/orders+of+ddma+on+covid+19/order+411 (Accessed on 15 May 2021).

17. lnoor Peermohamed, Apoorva Mittal and Ratna Bhushan, *The Economic Times*, 23 April 2021, 'Ecommerce Companies Step Up Hiring to Meet Staff Shortage.' https://economictimes.indiatimes.com/tech/technology/ecommerce-companies-step-up-hiring-to-meet-staff-shortage/articleshow/82202772.cms?from=mdr (Accessed on 15 May 2021).
18. Press Information Bureau, 28 January 2021, Prime Minister Narendra Modi's Speech at World Economic Forum Davos Dialogue. https://pib.gov.in/Pressreleaseshare.aspx?PRID=1693046 (Accessed on 15 May 2021).

12: NOT SO LOCKED DOWN

1. Election Commission of India, 26 February 2021, 'General Election to the Legislative Assemblies of Assam, Kerala, Tamil Nadu, West Bengal and Puducherry, 2021.' https://eci.gov.in/files/file/12919-general-election-to-the-legislative-assemblies-of-assam-kerala-tamil-nadu-west-bengal-and-puducherry-2021/ (Accessed on 16 May 2021).
2. HT Correspondent, *Hindustan Times*, 20 March 2021, 'Devotees Faith Will Overcome Fear of Covid-19 in Mahakumbh: CM Rawat.' https://www.hindustantimes.com/cities/others/devotees-faith-will-overcome-fear-of-covid-19-in-mahakumbh-cm-rawat-101616253395877.html (Accessed on 16 May 2021).
3. WHO, 21 April 2021, Situation Update Report-64. https://cdn.who.int/media/docs/default-source/wrindia/situation-report/india-situation-report-64.pdf?sfvrsn=7bf31dc6_4 (Accessed on 16 May 2021).
4. pmindia.gov.in, 20 April 2021, PM's Address to the Nation on the COVID-19 Situation. https://www.pmindia.gov.in/en/news_updates/pms-address-to-the-nation-on-the-covid-19-situation/?tag_term=pmspeech&comment=disable (Accessed on 16 May 2021).
5. Government of Maharashtra, 13 April 2021, Break the Chain, Order Number: DMU/2020/CR.92DisM-1.

6. Allahabad High Court order, 19 April 2021, Public Interest Litigation No 574. https://www.theleaflet.in/wp-content/uploads/2021/04/WPILA_574_2020-1.pdf (Accessed on 3 December 2021).
7. The Wire Staff, *The Wire*, 19 April 2021, 'UP: Allahabad HC Orders Lockdown in 5 Cities; Govt Says No to Complete Shutdown.' https://thewire.in/law/allahabad-high-court-uttar-pradesh-lockdown-prayagraj-lucknow-varanasi (Accessed on 20 May 2021).
8. Livelaw News Network, livelaw.in, 20 April 2021, 'Breaking: Supreme Court Stays Allahabad High Court Order Which Imposed Lockdown in 5 UP Cities.' https://www.livelaw.in/top-stories/supreme-court-stays-allahabad-high-court-judgment-which-imposed-lockdown-in-5-up-cities-172834?infinitescroll=1 (Accessed on 20 May 2021).
9. Awanish Kumar Awasthi, additional chief secretary, Uttar Pradesh administration, 3 May 2021, Letter number 786/2021. https://www.ciicovid19update.in/uploads/1/3/1/3/131362769/up-_4__5_may.pdf (Accessed on 20 May 2021).
10. Office of Awanish Kumar Awasthi, additional chief secretary, 30 April 2021, Order to police officers. https://www.ciicovid19update.in/uploads/1/3/1/3/131362769/notification_for_staff.pdf (Accessed on 20 May 2021).
11. Ishita Mishra, *The Times of India*, 9 May 2021, '9th Seer Dies of Covid after Kumbh, Over 250 Infected So Far' https://timesofindia.indiatimes.com/city/dehradun/9th-seer-dies-of-covid-after-kumbh-over-250-infected-so-far/articleshow/82485572.cms#:~:text=DEHRADUN%3A%20A%20mahamandaleshwar%20of%20the,concluded%20Maha%20Kumbh%20at%20Haridwar (Accessed on 20 May 2021).
12. Manoj Singh, *The Wire*, 18 May 2021, 'UP: Over 1600 Teachers Died of COVID-19 After Poll Duty for Panchayat Election.'. https://thewire.in/rights/uttar-pradesh-panchayat-elections-teachers-covid-19 (Accessed on 20 May 2021).
13. timesofindia.com, 26 February 2021, 'Election Commission to Announces Poll Dates for West Bengal, Assam, Kerala, Tamil Nadu,

Puducherry: Key Points.' https://timesofindia.indiatimes.com/india/election-commission-to-announce-poll-dates-for-four-states-one-ut-key-points/articleshow/81227165.cms (Accessed on 20 May 2021).

14. Arun Janardhanan, *The Indian Express*, 27 April 2021, 'Irresponsible … Must Perhaps Face Murder Charge: Madras HC on Election Commission.' https://indianexpress.com/article/india/eci-responsible-for-spreading-covid-19-says-madras-hc-7289824/ (Accessed on 21 May 2021).
15. Supreme Court of India, 6 May 2021, Civil Appeal No. 1767 of 2021. https://main.sci.gov.in/supremecourt/2021/11474/11474_2021_35_1502_27915_Judgement_06-May-2021.pdf (Accessed on 21 May 2021).
16. Ibid.
17. Narendra Modi (@narendramodi) Tweet, 22 April 2021. https://twitter.com/narendramodi/status/1385200406775672835?s=20 (Accessed on 21 May 2021).
18. Meghna Sen, livemint.com, 17 April 2021, 'PM Modi Says "Kumbh Mela Should Now Only Be Symbolic to Strengthen Covid-19 Fight."' https://www.livemint.com/news/india/pm-modi-says-kumbh-mela-should-now-only-be-symbolic-to-strengthen-covid-19-fight-11618630984604.html (Accessed on 21 May 2021).
19. Revenue and Disaster Management (DM-IV) Department, Government of Tamil Nadu, 8 April 2021, GO (Ms) No 342. https://cms.tn.gov.in/sites/default/files/go/revenue_e_342_2021.pdf (Accessed on 21 May 2021).
20. Revenue and Disaster Management (DM-IV) Department, Government of Tamil Nadu, 3 May 2021, GO (Ms) No 364. https://cms.tn.gov.in/sites/default/files/go/revenue_e_364_2021.pdf (Accessed on 21 May 2021).
21. Government of West Bengal order No 647-ISS/2M-22/2020 dated 15 May 2021.
22. Government of Kerala, 6 May 2021, GO (Ry) No 404/2021/DMD. https://kerala.gov.in/documents/10180/ec2395b2-9a5e-41fa-ac5e-ee91c3a0534a (Accessed on 21 May 2021).

13: THE LONG HAUL FOR OXYGEN

1. Interview with Erick Massey.
2. Supreme Court, 30 April 2021, Order, Suo Motu Writ Petition (Civil) No.3 of 2021. https://main.sci.gov.in/supremecourt/2021/11001/11001_2021_35_301_27825_Judgement_30-Apr-2021.pdf (Accessed on 9 May 2021).
3. Delhi High Court, 4 May 2021, Order, W.P. (C) No. 3031/2020 and all connected matters. https://www.livelaw.in/pdf_upload/16201557503482021-392893.pdf (Accessed on 9 May 2021).
4. Delhi High Special Leave Petition (Civil) Diary No (s).11622/2021, *Union of India Petitioner (s) versus Rakesh Malhotra & ANR*, 5 May 2021. https://www.livelaw.in/pdf_upload/supreme-court-oxygen-case-covid-delhi-392933.pdf (Accessed on 9 May 2021).
5. Kumar Kunal, Indiatoday.in, 24 April 2021, '25 Patients Die Due to Oxygen Shortage: Jaipur Golden Hospital to Delhi HC.' https://www.indiatoday.in/coronavirus-outbreak/story/20-covid-19-patients-die-due-to-oxygen-shortage-at-jaipur-golden-hospital-in-delhi-1794499-2021-04-24 (Accessed on 10 May 2021).
6. Astha Saxena, *The Indian Express*, 1 May 2021, 'Delhi's Batra Hospital Says 12 in ICU, Including Doctor, Dead during Oxygen Shortage.' https://indianexpress.com/article/cities/delhi/delhi-batra-hospital-oxygen-shortage-deaths-7297942/ (Accessed on 10 May 2021).
7. Express News Service, *The Indian Express*, 4 May 2021, '21 Patients Died of 'Respiratory Failure' and Not Due to Lack of Medical Oxygen, Delhi Govt Tells HC.'
https://indianexpress.com/article/cities/delhi/delhi-jaipur-golden-hospital-deaths-oxygen-govt-hc-7301714/ (Accessed on 10 May 2021).
8. Supreme Court, Special Leave Petition (Civil) against Union of India Diary Number 11694/2021, Order Dated 7 May 2021. https://main.sci.gov.in/supremecourt/2021/11694/11694_2021_35_1_28003_Order_07-May-2021.pdf (Accessed on 15 June 2021).

9. Darshan Devaiah BP, *The Indian Express*, 4 May 2021, 'Karnataka: 23 Die as Covid-19 Facility in Chamarajnagar Runs Out of Oxygen.' https://indianexpress.com/article/india/karnataka-23-dead-in-chamarajanagar-district-hospital-due-to-oxygen-shortage-7300205/ (Accessed on 15 June 2021).
10. Footnote 2.
11. Footnote 2.
12. Directorate General of Health Services, Central Drugs Standard Control Organisation (DCGI Secretariat), File Number DCGI/Msix/2020(96), 7 May 2020. https://cdsco.gov.in/opencms/opencms/system/modules/CDSCO.WEB/elements/download_file_division.jsp?num_id=NTgzNQ== (Accessed on 12 May 2021).
13. Ministry of Home Affairs, DO No 17/S(HFW)/MO/2021, 18 April 2021. https://www.mha.gov.in/sites/default/files/MHADOletterUT_18042021.pdf (Accessed on 12 May 2021).
14. Press Information Bureau, Press Release ID: 1716301, 5 May 202.1 https://pib.gov.in/PressReleasePage.aspx?PRID=1716301 (Accessed on 12 May 2021).
15. Press Trust of India, *Business Standard*, 24 April 2021, 'Long Queues Outside BHEL to Get Oxygen Cylinders Refilled in Madhya Pradesh.' https://www.business-standard.com/article/current-affairs/long-queues-outside-bhel-to-get-oxygen-cylinders-refilled-in-madhya-pradesh-121042400595_1.html (Accessed on 12 May 2021).
16. Press Information Bureau, Press Release ID:1717459, 10 May 2021. https://pib.gov.in/PressReleasePage.aspx?PRID=1717459
17. Supreme Court, Record of Proceedings Special Leave Petition (Civil) Diary No(s).11622/2021, 6 May 2021. https://main.sci.gov.in/supremecourt/2021/11622/11622_2021_35_35_27915_Order_06-May-2021.pdf (Accessed on 12 May 2021).
18. Ibid.
19. Gerald de Souza, *Hindustan Times*, 11 May 2021, '26 Deaths at Goa Medical College in 4 Hours. Health Minister Pushes for HC Probe' https://www.hindustantimes.com/india-news/26-deaths-at-goa-medical-college-in-4-hours-health-minister-pushes-for-hc-probe-101620752309311.html (Accessed on 12 May 2021).

20. Mayura Janwalkar, *The Indian Express*, 14 May 2021, 'Nightmare Runs on in Goa Hospital: 15 More Die as Oxygen Dips.' https://indianexpress.com/article/india/covid-second-wave-nightmare-runs-on-in-goa-hospital-15-more-die-as-oxygen-dips-7314298/ (Accessed on 12 May 2021).
21. Lisa Monteiro, *Times of India*, 31 July 2021, 'In U-turn, Goa Health Minister Says No Deaths Due to Oxygen Shortage in State.' https://timesofindia.indiatimes.com/india/in-u-turn-goa-health-minister-says-no-deaths-due-to-oxygen-shortage-in-state/articleshow/84907490.cms (Accessed on 10 December 2021).
22. Footnote 2.
23. Press Information Bureau, Press Release ID: 1717459, 10 May 2021. https://pib.gov.in/PressReleasePage.aspx?PRID=1717459 (Accessed on 12 May 2021).
24. Ibid.
25. Press Information Bureau, Press Release ID: 1712553, 18 April 2021. https://pib.gov.in/PressReleasePage.aspx?PRID=1712553 (Accessed on 12 May 2021).
26. Press Information Bureau, Press Release ID: 1712767, 19 April 2021. https://pib.gov.in/PressReleasePage.aspx?PRID=1712767 (Accessed on 12 May 2021).
27. Press Information Bureau, Press Release ID: 1713395, 22 April 2021. https://pib.gov.in/PressReleasePage.aspx?PRID=1713395 (Accessed on 12 May 2021).
28. Central Railway Press Release, 28 April 2021. https://cr.indianrailways.gov.in/view_detail.jsp?lang=0&dcd=6347&id=0,4,268 (Accessed on 12 May 2021).
29. Press Information Bureau, Press Release ID: 1717954, 12 May 2021. https://pib.gov.in/PressReleasePage.aspx?PRID=1717954 (Accessed on 12 May 2021).
30. Indian Air Force Press Release. https://indianairforce.nic.in/content/covid-19-relief-efforts-indian-air-force (Accessed on 14 May 2021).
31. Jyoti Mukul, *Business Standard*, 26 April 2021, 'Big Groups Plan O2 Storage, Transport; PM Cares Fund for 551 Plants.' https://

www.business-standard.com/article/companies/big-groups-plan-o2-storage-transport-pm-cares-fund-for-551-plants-121042600035_1.html (Accessed on 14 May 2021).

32. Indian Navy Operation Samudra Setu II - INS Tarkash Brings Medical Oxygen Consignment from Qatar. (Accessed on 14 June 2021).
33. Indian Navy, Press Release. https://indiannavy.nic.in/content/indian-navy-steps-covid-relief-operations-nine-warships-transporting-oxygen-medical (Accessed on 14 June 2021).
34. Footnote 2.
35. Jyoti Mukul, *Business Standard*, 30 April 2021, 'Tata Group Company to Set Up 450 Oxygen Units Worth Rs 75 Lakh Each.' https://www.business-standard.com/article/companies/tata-group-company-to-set-up-450-oxygen-units-worth-rs-75-lakh-each-121043001442_1.html (Accessed on 14 June 2021).
36. Press Information Bureau, Press Release ID: 1713904, 25 April 2021. https://pib.gov.in/PressReleasePage.aspx?PRID=1713904 (Accessed by 14 June 2021).
37. Express News Service, *The Indian Express*, 13 May 2021, 'Divert Surplus Oxygen from Delhi Quota to Other States, Says Manish Sisodia'
https://indianexpress.com/article/cities/delhi/divert-surplus-oxygen-from-delhi-quota-to-other-states-says-manish-sisodia-7313449/ (Accessed on 14 June 2021).

14: WELL-TIMED ALTERNATIVES

1. WHO, Tracking SARS-COV-2 variants. https://www.who.int/en/activities/tracking-SARS-CoV-2-variants/ (Accessed on 24 May 2021).
2. Press Information Bureau, Press Release ID: 1717876, 12 May 2021. https://pib.gov.in/PressReleasePage.aspx?PRID=1717876 (Accessed on 24 May 2021).
3. WHO, 19 May 2021, Science Conversation Episode #39-Update on Virus Variants. https://www.who.int/emergencies/diseases/

novel-coronavirus-2019/media-resources/science-in-5/episode-39---update-on-virus-variants (Accessed on 24 May 2021).

4. WHO, Departmental News, 31 May 2021, 'WHO Announces Simple, Easy-to-Say Labels for SARS-CoV-2 Variants of Interest and Concern.' https://www.who.int/news/item/31-05-2021-who-announces-simple-easy-to-say-labels-for-sars-cov-2-variants-of-interest-and-concern (Accessed on 24 May 2021).
5. WHO Statement, Classification of Omicron (B.1.1.529): SARS-CoV-2 Variant of Concern, 26 November 2021. https://www.who.int/news/item/26-11-2021-classification-of-omicron-(b.1.1.529)-sars-cov-2-variant-of-concern (Accessed on 1 December 2021).
6. Steven Lee Myers, *The New York Times*, 27 November 2021, 'The WHO skips forward two Greek letters, avoiding a Xi variant.' https://www.nytimes.com/2021/11/28/world/asia/omicron-variant-name-covid.html (Accessed on 1 December 2021).
7. Centers for Disease Control and Prevention, 1 December 2021, SARS-CoV-2 Variant Classifications and Definitions. https://www.cdc.gov/coronavirus/2019-ncov/cases-updates/variant-surveillance/variant-info.html (Accessed on 24 May 2021).
8. Amitabh Sinha, *The Indian Express*, 29 April 2021, 'None of the Scientists Forecast Second Wave of Such Vehemence.' https://indianexpress.com/article/india/none-of-the-scientists-forecast-second-wave-of-such-vehemence-7293093/ (Accessed on 24 May 2021).
9. Jyoti Mukul, *Business Standard*, 31 March 2021, 'Railways Move to Suspend Services Contradicts Social Distancing Message.' https://www.business-standard.com/article/current-affairs/railways-move-to-suspend-services-contradicts-social-distancing-message-120033101841_1.html (Accessed on 24 May 2021).
10. Monideepa Banerjie, Ndtv.com, 18 April 2021, '"Have Witnessed Such A Rally for the First Time...": PM Modi in Bengal.' https://www.ndtv.com/india-news/west-bengal-assembly-election-2021-prime-minister-narendra-modi-in-west-bengal-have-witnessed-such-a-rally-for-the-first-time-2416162

11. Press Information Bureau, Press Release ID: 162581, 21 May 2020. https://pib.gov.in/PressReleasePage.aspx?PRID=1625819 (Accessed on 24 May 2021).
12. Mukesh Rawat, indiatoday.in, 3 May 2021, 'Just Before 2nd Covid Wave Hit India, ICU Beds Decreased by 46%, Oxygen Ones by 36%.' https://www.indiatoday.in/coronavirus-outbreak/story/just-before-2nd-covid-wave-hit-india-icu-beds-decreased-by-46-oxygen-ones-by-36-1796830-2021-05-03 (Accessed on 24 May 2021).
13. Supreme Court of India, Special Leave Petition 11622/2021, Record of Proceedings dated 5 May 2021. https://main.sci.gov.in/supremecourt/2021/11622/11622_2021_35_1_27996_Order_05-May-2021.pdf (Accessed on 24 May 2021).

15: TRAVEL WITH CAUTION

1. Medical Detection Dogs (@MedDetectDogs) Tweet, 21 April 2021 https://twitter.com/MedDetectDogs/status/1384763839007399938?s=20 (Accessed on 25 June 2021).
2. Medical Detection Dogs, COVID-19-the Nose Knows Research Results. https://www.medicaldetectiondogs.org.uk/Covid-19-detection-dogs/ (Accessed on 25 June 2021).
3. Finavia, 18 September 2020, 'COVID-19 Dogs Arrive at the Airport—Able to Identify the Virus Earlier Than Laboratory Tests.' https://www.finavia.fi/en/newsroom/2020/Covid-19-dogs-arrive-airport-able-identify-virus-earlier-laboratory-tests (Accessed on 25 June 2021).
4. Ibid.
5. Interview with Soile Turunen.
6. Medical Detection Dogs. https://www.medicaldetectiondogs.org.uk/covid-19-dogs/ (Accessed on 2 May 2021).
7. D. Grandjean, R. Sarkis, C. Lecoq-Julien, A. Benard, V. Roger, E. Levesque, et al., 'Can the Detection Dog Alert on Covid-19 Positive Persons by Sniffing Axillary Sweat Samples? A Proof-of-Concept Study', PLoS ONE 15(12): e0243122. https://doi.org/10.1371/journal.pone.0243122, (Accessed on 2 May 2021).

8. Ibid.
9. Breathonix statement, 24 May 2021. https://breathonix.com/breathonix-covid-19-breath-test-gets-provisional-authorisation-in-singapore-to-undergo-trial-at-land-checkpoint/ (Accessed on 29 June 2021).
10. Press Information Bureau, Press Release ID: 1717009, 8 May 2021. https://pib.gov.in/PressReleasePage.aspx?PRID=1717009 (Accessed on 29 June 2021).
11. Jay Mazoomdaar, *The Indian Express*, 1 May 2021, 'Explained: Why Many People with Covid-19 Symptoms Have Been Testing Negative.' https://indianexpress.com/article/explained/covid-tests-rt-pcr-coronavirus-negative-result-7297329/ (Accessed on 29 June 2021).
12. Arindam Majumder, *Business Standard*, 27 April 2021, 'Airlines Stall Indians Travelling with Fake Covid-Negative Reports.' https://www.business-standard.com/article/companies/airlines-demanding-qr-coded-rt-pcr-tests-on-spike-in-fake-Covid-19-reports-121042500741_1.html (Accessed on 29 June 2021).
13. Saurabh Sinha, *Times of India*, 18 April 2021, 'Delhi Govt Orders FIR Against Four Airlines for Not Checking Negative RT-PCR Reports of Flyers from Maharashtra.' https://timesofindia.indiatimes.com/india/delhi-govt-orders-fir-against-four-airlines-for-not-checking-negative-rt-pcr-reports-of-flyers-from-maharashtra/articleshow/82129820.cms#:~:text=NEW%20DELHI%3A%20The%20Delhi%20government,from%20Maharashtra%20to%20the%20capital. (Accessed on 29 June 2021).
14. Indian Council of Medical Research, 4 May 2021, Advisory for COVID-19 Testing during the Second Wave of the Pandemic. https://www.icmr.gov.in/pdf/covid/strategy/Advisory_COVID_Testing_in_Second_Wave_04052021.pdf (Accessed on 20 June 2021).
15. WHO, 16 December 2020, Considerations for Implementing a Risk-Based Approach to International Travel in the Context of COVID-19: Travel, Points of Entry and Border Health. https://

www.who.int/publications/i/item/WHO-2019-nCoV-Risk-based-international-travel-2020.1 (Accessed on 29 June 2021).

16. Centers for Disease Control, How CDC Determines the Level for COVID-19 Travel Health Notices. https://www.cdc.gov/coronavirus/2019-ncov/travelers/how-level-is-determined.html (Accessed on 2 May 2021).
17. Footnote 15.
18. Footnote 15.
19. Aarogya Setu (@SetuAarogya) Tweet, 24 June 2021. https://twitter.com/SetuAarogya/status/1408007003868327941?s=20 (Accessed on 30 May 2021).
20. CDC (@CDCgov), 2 April 2021. https://twitter.com/CDCgov/status/1378028747681595396?s=20 (Accessed on 30 May 2021).
21. World Travel and Tourism Council. https://wttc.org/Research/Economic-Impact (Accessed on 10 December 2021).
22. Centers for Disease Control, SARS-CoV-2 Variant Classifications and Definitions. https://www.cdc.gov/coronavirus/2019-ncov/variants/variant-classifications.html?CDC_AA_refVal=https%3A%2F%2Fwww.cdc.gov%2Fcoronavirus%2F2019-ncov%2Fvariants%2Fvariant-info.html (Accessed on 10 December 2021).
23. The Phuket News, 28 May 2021. https://www.thephuketnews.com/phuket-sandbox-starts-on-july-1-tat-80136.php (Accessed on 10 June 2021).
24. WHO News, 3 November 2021, 'WHO Issues Emergency Use Listing for Eighth COVID-19 Vaccine.' https://www.who.int/news/item/03-11-2021-who-issues-emergency-use-listing-for-eighth-covid-19-vaccine (Accessed on 10 December 2021).
25. Elizabeth Roche, Mint, 'India Has Deals with 100+ Nations for Mutual Vax Certificate Recognition', 6 December 2021. https://www.livemint.com/news/india/india-has-pacts-with-100-nations-to-recognise-covid-jab-certificates-jaishankar-11638695463161.html (Accessed on 10 December 2021).

26. WHO, 5 February 2021, 'Interim Position Paper: Considerations Regarding Proof of COVID-19 Vaccination for International Travelers.' https://www.who.int/news-room/articles-detail/interim-position-paper-considerations-regarding-proof-of-Covid-19-vaccination-for-international-travellers (Accessed on 10 December 2021).
27. European Commission, 17 March 2021. https://eur-lex.europa.eu/legal-content/EN/TXT/PDF/?uri=CELEX:52021DC0129&from=EN (Accessed on 25 June 2021).
28. BusinessToday.in, 21 April 2021, 'COVID-19 Vaccination: India Needs 8 Yrs 9 Months to Achieve Herd Immunity.' https://www.businesstoday.in/latest/economy-politics/story/covid-19-vaccination-india-needs-8-yrs-9-months-to-achieve-herd-immunity-293987-2021-04-21 (Accessed on 25 June 2021).

INDEX

ABOUT THE AUTHOR

Jyoti Mukul is a policy analyst and a former journalist who has worked with *Business Standard*, the *Asian Age*, and the Indian Express, the Dainik Bhaskar and Deccan Chronicle groups. A commentator on the Indian economy, and transport and infrastructure sectors, she has travelled widely to rural heartlands and energy installations in India during the course of her reporting career. She lives in Gurugram with her husband, Akshaya; daughter, Jahnavi; and pet, Bella.